PHYSIOLOGY TEXTBOOK SERIES

These volumes may be purchased individually in a hard binding or paper covered.

PHYSIOLOGY and BIOPHYSICS of the CIRCULATION (2d Edition)

ALAN C. BURTON, PH.D., *Professor and former Head of the Department of Biophysics, Medical School, University of Western Ontario*

PHYSIOLOGY of RESPIRATION

JULIUS H. COMROE, JR., M.D., *Director, Cardiovascular Research Institute, and Professor of Physiology, University of California Medical Center, San Francisco*

PHYSIOLOGY of the DIGESTIVE TRACT (3d Edition)

HORACE W. DAVENPORT, PH.D., D.SC. (OXON.), *Professor and Chairman, Department of Physiology, The University of Michigan*

PHYSIOLOGY of the NERVOUS SYSTEM

CARLOS EYZAGUIRRE, M.D., *Professor and Chairman, Department of Physiology, University of Utah College of Medicine*

PHYSIOLOGY of the KIDNEY and BODY FLUIDS (2d Edition)

ROBERT F. PITTS, PH.D., M.D., *Professor of Physiology and Chairman of the Department of Physiology and Biophysics, Cornell University Medical College*

METABOLIC and ENDOCRINE PHYSIOLOGY (2d Edition)

JAY TEPPERMAN, M.D., *Professor of Experimental Medicine, Department of Pharmacology, State University of New York Upstate Medical Center, Syracuse*

PHYSIOLOGY
AND
BIOPHYSICS
OF THE
CIRCULATION

PHYSIOLOGY
and BIOPHYSICS

ALAN C. BURTON, Ph.D.

Professor and former Chairman of the Department of Biophysics, Medical School
University of Western Ontario, London, Ontario, Canada

of the CIRCULATION

An

Introductory Text

SECOND EDITION

YEAR BOOK MEDICAL PUBLISHERS   INCORPORATED

35 EAST WACKER DRIVE, CHICAGO

Reprinted, January, 1966
Reprinted, January, 1968
Reprinted, September, 1968
Reprinted, September, 1970
Reprinted, April, 1971
Second Edition, 1972

Library of Congress Catalog Card Number: 70-182003
Cloth: 0-8151-1363-3 Paper: 0-8151-1364-1

The author is grateful to one of the "Fathers of Biophysics," Ludwig von Helmholtz. He obviously considered that the behavior of living things was as much in the province of a Physicist as were the phenomena of the nonliving world.

The author is also very grateful to H. C. Bazett, his teacher, who showed him that Physiology is fun.

Preface to the Second Edition

THERE IS NO GUARANTEE that revision of a textbook which has been successful for the readers for whom it was designed (here undergraduate medical students) will result in any improvement. Yet a textbook must be revised periodically. Professors of physiology, rightly, will not recommend a textbook that is more than five or six years "out of date," since they believe that very significant advances in their subject have resulted from research in that period. When an author revises a textbook, he almost inevitably adds details of complicated phenomena which detract from the simplistic view and from the emphasis on general principles, which may have made the book successful in its original edition. An author seldom can bring himself to eliminate any of what he wrote before. Readability and stimulation of the interest of the student may suffer. From comments received from students (often written in pencil on scratch paper), these features were evidently why they liked the first edition. It is hoped that the revision retains their interest, without boredom with too much addition of details. One favorable factor is the advanced age of the author, which makes it likely that he has not learned too much in the intervening years, except of the researches in his own laboratory.

The usual minor errors and typographical mistakes that escape the most vigilant of proofreaders have been corrected as far as possible. Some new knowledge as to just how blood flows has been added. The chief addition is a new chapter (Chapter 8) devoted to vascular smooth muscle. There has been so much new information from research on this subject that the relevant paragraphs that were scattered through the text were collected, and information distilled from the numerous modern reviews was added. Another major change is the extension of the chapter on energetics (now Chapter 11) to include important new discoveries of how the flow of blood in the vessels, particularly if disturbed from the usual pattern (e.g., turbulence), can initiate pathological changes in the vessel wall. The short section on turbulence, which was in old Chapter 14 in connection with heart sounds and murmurs, is also now in Chapter 11, where it better belongs. Discussion of the mechanics of heart muscle has been added in Chapter 19.

New information on the role of increased oxygen tension concerning the stimulus to closure of the ductus arteriosus at birth has been added to the final chapter.

The over-all result is a longer book, including the addition of 17 new illustrations. Perhaps too many new references have been added, but, to prove the book is up to date, the most recent studies must be cited, although the older references are just as good as they were. The undergraduate student need not, and probably will not, read the original papers in most cases, but it is hoped that his teachers and the graduate students will verify that the author interpreted them correctly.

In making the revisions, I am indebted to Mrs. Vera Jordan for typing and secretarial work.

ALAN C. BURTON

Preface to the First Edition

MOST TEXTBOOKS OF PHYSIOLOGY claim to be written for the medical undergraduate (for the large market lies there); but many of them are, in reality, written more for the physiologist, or at least for the graduate student of physiology. The wealth of detail included in these texts is far beyond the possibility of being remembered by the medical student. This monograph will be quite inadequate for the graduate student in physiology, and possibly for the medical student, although if he were to remember most of the facts in it and to understand most of the ideas expressed, we would have to let him pass the examinations. By concentrating on ideas more than on facts, the author hopes to give more permanence to any value this monograph may have, for new "facts" of physiology are added and old "facts" amended so fast, by modern physiological research, that a purely factual monograph is out of date before it reaches print.

The more dogmatic the statements in a textbook, the more popular the text will be with the student, who is so harassed by simultaneous multiple courses on different subjects, each with its overwhelming load of information, that he feels he has no time to hear that "A found this but that experiments of B seemed to contradict it, and that the correct view might be this or that." He wants the "straight goods" so that he can memorize them and pass the examination. Yet how can one be dogmatic and at the same time right in physiology? The author has invented, hopefully, the device of being relatively dogmatic in the text and has asked the publisher to set off by a symbol (thus: [▶ . . . ◀]) those statements with which the author thinks other physiologists might disagree, or statements about which he himself is not really sure.

It is traditional that physiology texts on the circulation include a section on the blood, including a great deal about the development of the various types of blood cells and about clotting—subjects that are taught and written about much more competently in other disciplines to which the medical student is exposed. Since I was told I must, I have written a section on the blood but have emphasized only the aspects that are important to an understanding of the flow in the circulation. The section on the erythrocyte sprang from our very great interest in the biophysics of this cell, not from any detailed knowledge of its biochemistry and physiology.

Undergraduate textbooks of physiology ought to leave something to the professors of physiology; so the highly integrative aspects—for example, hemorrhagic shock, the physiology of exercise and hypertension, which are so important to the student of medicine—are not treated as such, but are mentioned merely in connection with some principle that is being discussed.

The use of references is consistent only in its inconsistency. Symposia, reviews or monographs are cited in preference to individual contributions to the literature. How many medical students read the references anyway? Specific papers are cited for one or more of three reasons: (a) a particular paper may substantiate an unorthodox view expressed in the text; (b) it is the latest reference available, in which the older work is also cited; or (c) it is from our own laboratory and, naturally, we think that it is worth more attention than has generally been given.

It will be seen (e.g., from the Table of Contents) that the organization of the material is much more according to principles of the circulation than according to specific topics. For example, instead of sections on the blood flow of special regions, muscle, skin and so on, these topics are worked in as examples of the particular principles of control that they may illustrate. This feature may not be convenient for the student preparing for an examination, but it seemed best to emphasize the principles rather than a mass of facts. Examples from human physiology are preferred to those from other animals, not because the latter are of less interest to a physiologist but because the human being interests the student much more.

The author is a biophysicist as well as, he hopes, a physiologist. Although considerable restraint had to be exercised not to scare the medical student by including too much physics and mathematics (to which medical students have a violent allergy), the point of view of the physicist is bound to taint the physiology. Perhaps the skepticism of the physicist about conclusions that are not based on quantitative considerations or on sound physics is needed in physiology.

The lapses into levity throughout the monograph may appear unseemly to some. Above all, my great teacher, H. C. Bazett, showed me that physiology was fun—and why should not the student learn that physiologists have a sense of humor? In our experience, students remember the things taught in a dramatic, exaggerated or amusing way, when they have forgotten everything else in the lectures.

Will Rogers had a favorite phrase: "All I know is what I read in the papers." This certainly applies to 90% of what is written in this monograph. I am greatly indebted to my colleagues in other departments, and to the graduate students of our department, for telling me which papers to read (or what radio or television programs to note) on the many subjects of which I was ignorant. My thanks are extended particularly to Drs. D. E. Busby, G. J. Cropp, R. H. Phibbs and Peter Rand; also, to J. J. Faber, who kindly wrote part of Chapter 14. Mrs. D. Elston helped greatly with the illustrations; Mrs. Olive Hayter patiently typed, retyped and retyped the manuscript; and my wife most patiently put up for so long with being a book widow. Thanks are due to the publishers for the very great patience they exercised when it took so long to finish the writing.

ALAN C. BURTON

Table of Contents

SECTION 4

THE HEART and ITS ACTION

SECTION 5

THE REGULATION of the CIRCULATION

Introduction

1

Why Have a Circulation?

"Begin at the beginning, and go on till you come
to the end; then stop."—LEWIS CARROLL, *Alice's Adventures
in Wonderland.*

The Celestial Committee on Control
of Mammalian Circulation

THE ABOVE ADVICE was that of the King to the
White Rabbit, who asked how he should act, as
defense counsel, at the trial of the Knave (for
stealing the tarts). However, as Gilbert Highet, in
The Art of Teaching, points out, while this may be
the best way to tell a story, it is definitely not the
best method to use in a lecture or a textbook. It is
better to start by explaining what the whole
subject is about, before going into detailed study
of each of the special topics within it. Let us look
at the woods before we examine each tree.

In this chapter, therefore, the following questions are asked about the circulation:

Purpose.—What are the normal functions of the
circulation; what has it to accomplish?

Priorities.—It is unlikely that this purpose can
be fulfilled in every respect and for every tissue.
If so, are there "priorities" (i.e., paramount functions that must be satisfied) for the benefit of the
whole organism, even if other functions may have
to be unsatisfied?

Possibilities.—How could these purposes best
be satisfied by proper design of a circulatory
system, in view of the answers to the questions
regarding purpose and priorities?

Problems.—Obviously, no design could be expected to function best in all of the circumstances
of the life of an animal to which it may occasion-
ally be exposed. The design must be best suited to
the "normal," or "physiological," conditions of
the animal. This sort of compromise inevitably
will result in special problems in the special
circumstances of unusual environments—for example, either external (altitude, high pressures,

heat, etc.) or internal (i.e., states of disease or
disturbed physiology). What are these problems?

Such an approach is frankly "teleological." In
connection with physiology, the doctrine of teleology* is very useful indeed; and although it is
officially condemned, the dangers of its use are
slight as long as the consideration in the preceding
paragraph on "problems" is emphasized. Someone, probably a Frenchman, said that "teleology
was a mistress that no biologist could live without,
yet he would be ashamed to be seen on the street
with her." Those who are squeamish about using
teleology may substitute, for the idea of "design"
for a specific function, the concept of "adapta-
tion" for best function through the evolutionary
process of natural selection. Either way of thinking will lead us astray unless it is realized that
arrangements for best function in the normal
circumstances of life for animals cannot possibly
be the best arrangement for all the abnormal
circumstances that may be encountered occasion-
ally, as when men leave the ground to fly, or eat,
smoke or drink too much. The student is invited to
join an imaginary group appointed by the Crea-
tor—that is, the Celestial Committee on Design of
a Mammalian Circulation (C.C.D.M.C.).

THE PURPOSE (FUNCTION) OF
THE CIRCULATION

Physiologists would be unlikely to agree on
details of any statement, but the following would
be given general approval: *The function of the*

---

*Teleology: "The fact or doctrine of final causes or design as
applied to the existence and development of individual beings or
the universe at large; the theory which assigns a definite end or
ends in explanation of the structure and behaviour of things. . . .
Its claims have been contested in the field of biology." (Funk &
Wagnalls Standard Dictionary 1913.)

3

circulation is to supply oxygen, metabolic fuels, vitamins and hormones, and heat, to every living cell of the organism, and also to remove metabolic end-products (e.g., carbon dioxide, water) and heat, from every cell. The amount of circulation should be in accordance with the individual needs of each cell.

The Committee (C.C.D.M.C.) considered carefully every word of this statement. In particular, it felt that the last sentence must be included in the interests of economy of the energy of the organism, since to pump blood to tissues in excess of their requirements would be wasteful. Since the requirements of some tissues, like muscle, would vary so greatly from time to time, according to the activity of the animal, the provision of a steady circulation, enough to meet the maximal needs of each tissue, would be uneconomical. These considerations convinced the Committee of the need for designing an effective distribution of circulation to the various tissues by a *control system* which would be responsive to the particular needs of the moment of individual tissues.

It was also recognized that there were several distinct functions of the circulation. One was concerned with nutrition of cells; another, with maintenance of heat balance of the whole organism. In some cases, these two functions would be only remotely related. For example, in the enormous tail fin of the whale, a large circulation is required to keep alive all the cells of the tail; yet the excessive heat loss of the whole animal that would result must somehow be prevented. (This was eventually met by the invention, by a member of the Committee, of a special device, namely, the "countercurrent heat exchanger" (Scholander [1].) Again, in the control of the circulation of the skin of the extremities in man, the requirements of regulating body temperature (thermoregulatory functions) might be very much more important than those of supplying the metabolic needs of the skin cells (2).

Also, in considering the requirements for circulation of organs with special functions, such as the kidney, the metabolic requirements of the tissues of that organ might not be the important consideration. The blood flow of the kidney is very much in excess of any metabolic requirements of its cells; it is related, instead, to the excretory function of the kidneys, which demands that a large volume of blood be "treated," or "cleared," by the kidneys every minute.

Oxygen Requirements of Different Cells and Tissues

Most metabolic processes ultimately require a supply of oxygen. Some indication of the requirements for blood flow of different tissues is given by the determinations of the oxygen consumed per gram of tissue (wet weight or dry weight) that have been made on tissue slices (in the Warburg manometric apparatus [3]). These values are usually expressed in "ml O_2/Gm wet weight of tissues/hour" (known as the Qo_2). Reservations as to the reliability of these values as indicating those of the living tissue in the intact animal are, of course, in order. However, it has been shown (Martin and Fuhrman [4]) that, when the values of Qo_2 (ml O_2/Gm/hour) for tissue slices, together with the relative weight of each organ and tissue in the body, are combined to estimate the total oxygen consumption of the whole animal, the agreement with actual measured values of total oxygen consumption is astonishingly good (72% in the rat; 105% in the dog). It seems worth while, then, to take the in vitro values, at least as an index of the wide variety of metabolic needs of tissues. Table 1–1 shows the Qo_2 for different tissues of a dog. Even if we allow a very large uncertainty in the figures (which vary greatly in the results of different workers), it is clear that kidney, liver and brain tissue are much more metabolically active per unit weight of tissue than

TABLE 1–1.—Oxygen Consumption as Qo_2 (Ml O_2/Gm Wet Weight of Tissues/Hour)*

High Activity		Moderate Activity		Low Activity	
Kidney	2.2	Spleen	0.8	Fat	0.2
Liver	2.0	Heart muscle	0.7	Skin	0.2
Brain	1.3	Skeletal muscle (at rest)	0.5	Bone	0.03
Intestinal mucosa	1.2	Smooth muscle of G.I. tract	0.4	Blood	0.006
		Lung tissue	0.4		

*Simplified from work of Martin and Fuhrman for the dog (4).

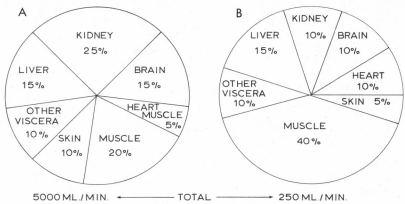

Fig. 1-1.—A, estimated percentage of cardiac output (supply). **B,** oxygen consumption to different organs of the body in a man at rest (demand). The estimates are very rough, from data taken from many sources and not very consistent. The kidney is greatly overperfused, and the muscles are underperfused. In exercise, the proportion of blood flow to muscle increases enormously, as it does for skin in hot environments.

skin and bone. We would, therefore, expect that these tissues would be much more vascular, with a richer network of small blood vessels between the cells and a greater blood flow per gram of tissue. The so-called "capillary count" (i.e., the number of capillaries visible in a cross-section of a tissue per square millimeter of area) has been made on the muscles of several animals; but comparable figures for brain, liver, etc., are not available. As far as available comparisons go, in the guinea pig and the dog, the count for cardiac muscle is about 2,500–3,000 per square centimeter, whereas for skeletal muscle it is 1,500. The expression "2,500 capillaries to the square centimeter" means that, on the average, no cell is more than 10 μ from a capillary.

When we multiply these Q_{O_2} values by the relative weights of the different tissues in the whole body (e.g., muscle forms 50% or more of the total body weight in the dog and in man), we get a different order of importance in the percentage of the total oxygen consumption required by the different organs (Fig. 1–1,*B*). About half, in the dog, is required by muscle. In the segments of Figure 1–1,*A*, are shown the estimated percentages of the total output of the heart that go to the different organs (data averaged from many sources). A convenient way of memorizing the data is that one fourth of the cardiac output goes to each of the four categories of kidney, liver plus viscera, brain plus coronary and skin plus muscle. There are, thus, considerable differences between the actual distribution of blood flow and the estimated requirements for oxygen. From the point of view of oxygen requirements only (Fig. 1–1,*B*), we would conclude that the kidney and

the skin are greatly "overperfused." This indicates, as I have just mentioned, the requirements for blood flow that are other than metabolic for the cells of these tissues (e.g., clearance by the kidney, temperature regulation). In contrast, muscle, particularly heart muscle, is underperfused. Also, it must be remembered that only about 25 or 30% of the content of oxygen in the arterial blood reaching cells is utilized (i.e., venous blood still has 75% of the oxygen content of arterial blood, as shown by comparing the total blood flow and total oxygen consumption in Figure 1–1). Each 100 ml of blood carries about 20 ml of oxygen; so a cardiac output of 5,000 ml per min carries a total of 1,000 ml of oxygen, of which only 25% is used (Fig. 1–1). This feature is described by the *extraction ratio*

$$\left(\frac{\text{Arterial O}_2 - \text{Venous O}_2}{\text{Arterial O}_2}\right)$$, and this may be very

different for the different tissues. Very little is known as to what governs how much oxygen can be "extracted." The extraction is much more complete for muscle than for the kidney.

Range and Variability of Requirements of Tissues

An important consideration for any committee designing the circulation, if blood flow has to be "in accordance with the needs of every tissue," is how these needs may vary for a given tissue from moment to moment. How much does the metabolic rate of tissues alter with circumstances?

Temperature universally changes the rate of all chemical and physical reactions. Its effect is described by the Q_{10}—that is, the factor multiplying the rate at one temperature to obtain the rate at a temperature 10° C higher. The Q_{10} for oxygen consumption of tissue slices, for organs in vitro, to some extent, and for the whole animal, has been measured. The general result is that the Q_{10} lies between 2 and 3; that is, a rise of 10° C increases metabolic activity, and therefore the requirements for blood flow, by between 2 and 3 times.

The relation is described by the famous law of Arrhenius, which in mathematical terms is:

$$\text{Rate} = A\, exp\,(-\mu/R_0 T)$$

where A is a constant, μ is the so-called activation energy in calories per mole, R_0 is the universal gas constant and T is the absolute temperature. It follows that a plot of the logarithm of the rate versus the reciprocal of the absolute temperature gives a straight line; that is, the logarithm of the rate decreases linearly with $1/T$. For, taking logarithms of the original equation:

$$\log\,(\text{rate}) = \log A - \frac{\mu}{R_0} \times \left(\frac{1}{T}\right)$$

Figure 1–2, *A*, shows how remarkably the metabolic rate of cells increases geometrically with the temperature. The graph is drawn assuming a Q_{10} of 2.3. Figure 1–2,*B*, shows the straight line obtained in the Arrhenius plot. The slope of this line enables the activation energy to be deduced. The law of Arrhenius has no firm thermodynamic basis, and it should be applied only to velocity constants of reactions. However, many over-all rates of biological activity are found to follow the law approximately over the limited range of temperatures of cells in biology. In applying this law to the range of requirements in vivo, the fact that the higher warm-blooded mammals regulate the temperature of their "core" tissues to within narrow limits (37.0° C ± 1° C for man) means that this factor is of no significance for the brain, the liver, the kidney, etc., except in the nonphysiological (but most important practical) conditions of hypothermia or of fever. The temperature of the peripheral "shell" of the body, however, is very variable. The skin of the extremities in normal physiological circumstances may have a temperature between a maximum of 36° C (65° F) in a warm environment to less than 10° C (50° F) in a cold one. The metabolic rate of skin, therefore, may change by a factor of some 5 or 6 times, according to the temperature of the skin. However, the metabolic rate of skin is very low, and the blood flow to skin is always greatly in excess of the requirements of cellular metabolism, being regulated, instead, by the needs of temperature regulation of the whole organism. Actually, the blood flow of the skin of the human digits is found to vary more than 50-fold (2).

For the tissues and organs of the core of the body, the range of requirement is due not so much to temperature differences as to the range of functional activity, the latter requiring different rates of energy turnover. At one end of the scale of variability of needs is the brain. Apparently the

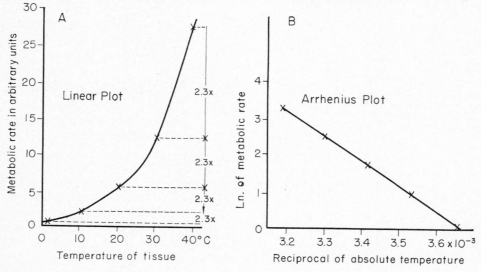

Fig. 1-2.—A, linear plot, showing the logarithmic increase of metabolic rate (oxygen consumption) with the temperature of tissues, for a Q_{10} of 2.3. **B,** Arrhenius plot, giving a straight line, the slope of which indicates the Q_{10}.

activity of the brain cells is not very variable, judging from the measurements of oxygen consumption and blood flow of the brain that are available. Certainly "mental activity," as of students writing examinations all day, does not involve an increased oxygen consumption of the whole student. (Benedict measured this in his human calorimeter and concluded that the extra calories required were less than the calories in half of one peanut [5].) Within the brain itself there is evidence of redistribution of blood when certain cells are active (e.g., motor cells of the cortex), but the total blood flow may not change. We should think of the brain as in continuous activity (the "brain waves," or electroencephalogram, suggest this), which is "organized," or channeled, into synchronized activity to control specific bodily activities, rather than that there is a change in the total activity of the brain. Some method, in the design of the circulation, that would ensure a relatively constant and adequate blood flow of the brain would thus be suitable.

At the other extreme stands skeletal and, to a lesser extent, cardiac muscle. Between the resting state of relaxation of muscle and its maximal contraction, the rate of oxygen consumption may change as much as 10 or 20 times. In fact, the oxygen consumption is closely proportional to the product of tension the muscle maintains and the time it is maintained (6). In the case of the heart muscle, we would expect that in heavy exercise, where the mechanical work of pumping blood is greatly increased (up to 5 times in heavy exercise), the oxygen consumption, and thus the circulation to heart muscle by the coronary vessels, would have to be correspondingly increased. However, it turns out that the change in total energy requirement is not so great as would at first sight be expected (at least in normal physiological circumstances), for physiologists, on heart-lung preparations, have found that the pumping work of the heart can be increased 20 times with only a few per cent increase in oxygen consumption, so long as the size of the heart, the heart rate and the blood pressure are not greatly altered (7).

The Committee (C.C.D.M.C.) therefore realized that a control of the circulation that increased or decreased the total circulation (cardiac output) in accordance with the over-all activity of the animal would not be enough. Specific control, acting automatically (reflexly) for distributing the blood flow to each organ or tissue in accordance with its specific individual needs, must also be devised. Doing this, it is true, would amount to giving parts of the organism some degree of local autonomy. The dangers were foreseen that such autonomy might, in unusual circumstances, such as diseased states, lead toward a state of anarchy. The local control of circulation by a given part might not be in the best interests of the whole organism. The best safeguards against such anarchy become clearer when the Committee considered the next point, the "priorities" of the circulation.

Priorities in the Circulation

Priorities in the circulation could be based on two considerations: (1) How ultimately essential are the different members of the organism? ("If thine eye offend thee, pluck it out . . .: it is better for thee to enter into life with one eye, rather than having two eyes to be cast into hell fire" [Matthew 18:9].) (2) Some members of the body might be essential but could temporarily be deprived of circulation (if not for too long) to provide circulation to some other essential members not having such a "reserve."

On the score of ultimate essentiality, it is clear that animals can, and have, lived without their limbs and without the function of much of the tissues of the viscera. (The surgeons count on this.) There are two of most organs; and the patient can live with only one kidney, one lung, only half his stomach and without large parts of his brain. This would suggest that there is a good deal of "functional reserve." However, we also have some experimental information on the survival of certain organs when they are deprived completely of their blood supply *(ischemia).*

A common experiment for medical students in the physiological laboratory is to inflate a cuff around the upper arm to a pressure greater than the maximal blood pressure (say to 200 mm Hg) so that the supply of blood to skin and muscles of the arm is completely prevented. While there is "ischemic pain" after several minutes, no irreversible damage results, certainly for periods of complete ischemia of 20 min or more. Moreover, the arm muscles can work during the ischemia. Skeletal muscle has the property of "anaerobic metabolism." Contraction of muscle and performance of work until there is a very considerable degree of "oxygen debt" is possible, although, of course, this debt must eventually be made up when circulation is once more available. An interesting example of this is the functioning of diving mammals. Seals have been observed by Irving (8) to remain under water, with vigorous use of their muscles in swimming after fish, for over 12 min. Study of the total reserve supply of oxygen in their blood showed that this would not suffice for more than a fraction of this time if it were circulating to anything but the heart, brain and lungs. There is evidently a reflex mechanism that shuts off the supply to the muscles of peripheral tissues during the dive, and the muscles are able to work anaerobically. A very large oxygen debt is acquired, which must be made up immediately on return to the surface.

As cited above, the metabolism of the cells of the skin is so low, especially if their temperature falls (as it does when circulation is cut off), that permanent damage (necrosis) does not result until after many hours of complete ischemia. Patients in profound hypovolemic shock (having a severe loss of blood volume) show almost complete lack of blood flow in the limbs, which appear quite cold and "lifeless"; yet permanent damage to peripheral tissues seldom results.

In contrast, neuroanatomists have been able to detect permanent damage to the cells of the brain after only 1 or 2 min of complete ischemia if the brain is kept at the normal body temperature. Realization of this fact is most important to a medical student, for if resuscitation is achieved after many minutes of arrested circulation (as in cases of drowning), serious and permanent deficiencies of brain function must be expected. The modern use of hypothermia (lowering of the brain temperature) by neurosurgeons has lengthened the time the brain cells can survive ischemia, but it remains relatively brief. The brain has evidently very little possibility of surviving a "blood flow debt."

In contrast to skeletal muscle, the cardiac muscle has much less "reserve," although it has some possibility of anaerobic activity. Arrest of the circulation to the heart muscle (the coronary supply) for over 5 or 10 min at normal body temperature is almost sure to result in permanent damage to cardiac muscle (infarcts). Here, again, the use of hypothermia in cardiac surgery has extended the limiting time to up to 30 min or more. Continuing the perfusion of the coronary circulation by artificial means is desirable, even with hypothermia.

With these considerations, the Celestial Committee decided that the highest priority for circulation belonged to the brain and the heart, both on the score of essentiality of their function to the organism and because they had so little ischemic reserve. This decision guided the Committee in their discussion of the next topic: how adequate systems of control could be set up.

Possibilities of Control of the Circulation

The job to be done by the Celestial Committee was divided into two categories:

a) There must be assurance of adequate circulation at all times to the organs of highest priority—brain, heart and lungs. In the case of the brain, the design was the simplest, since the needs for circulation were so constant. For the heart, provision for a considerable alteration in blood flow in accordance with cardiac activity was desirable. For the pulmonary blood flow, the greatest variability with the needs of general body activity (indicated by the oxygen consumption) would be needed. The needs of lung tissue itself (only, at most, a few per cent of the total oxygen consumption) were not important, particularly since these tissues could obtain oxygen directly from the air in the lungs.

b) There was need for specific, local control of blood flow to different organs and tissues in accordance with changes in their specific needs.

The Celestial Biophysicist clarified the discussion of possibilities of control greatly by pointing out that there was a general principle of hemodynamics, approximately true but modified in some details (see later chapters), that must be the basis of any control. This was the law of flow:

$$F = \Delta P/R$$

where the flow, F, depends on the driving force, ΔP, which is the "pressure drop" down the circulatory bed (i.e., from artery to vein), and R is the resistance to flow for the particular route of blood flow (i.e., of the vessels of that particular vascular bed). This resistance depends on the geometry of these vessels (i.e., their length and diameter), as well as on the fluid being driven through them (specifically its viscosity). Control of the distribution of blood flow therefore could be arranged in two ways: (a) by controlling the driving pressure (ΔP) and (b) by controlling the resistance to flow (R) of each vascular bed.

PROVISION FOR THE PRIORITIES

The highest priority, that of the brain, was easily satisfied by using this hemodynamic principle of flow. Let the arterial pressure at the portals to the brain (i.e., the aorta and carotid area) be controlled to a constant value by some reflex mechanism (the carotid sinus and aortic pressure reflexes). The resistance to flow of the vascular bed of the brain could then remain constant, or relatively so. This would ensure an adequate and relatively constant brain blood flow in all circumstances, as long as the reflex control of aortic pressure could still operate.

We now would also have a constant pressure of perfusion, from the aortic pressure, for the coronary circulation. Provision of some degree of local adjustment of the coronary resistance to flow would provide for the increasing needs of greater cardiac activity. (As pointed out earlier, the increasing need is not so great as the increase in the cardiac output in exercise would indicate.) How to provide the adjustment of coronary resistance was discussed later by the Committee, under the general consideration of mechanisms of local autonomy.

GENERAL INCREASES AND DECREASES OF THE TOTAL CIRCULATION

From the fundamental law of flow, since it had been decided to hold the driving pressure (ΔP), in general, to constancy, general increases in flow to every part must be achieved by a general lowering of the resistance to flow (R) (the "total peripheral resistance"). In addition, there could be some mechanism of overriding, in heavy exercise, of the homeostatic mechanism of the arterial blood pressure. (The mean blood pressure rises, but not proportionally to the increased cardiac output, which may increase 4 times in heavy exercise.) Two general mechanisms of lowering the total peripheral resistance offered themselves: (1) the sympathetic vasoconstrictor system and (2) humoral agents.

GENERAL NERVOUS CONTROL (SYMPATHETIC SYSTEM).—The first mechanism considered by the Committee was the use of a nervous control (the sympathetic vasoconstrictor system) to govern the caliber of the small vessels in all vascular beds. These small vessels offer the greatest item of peripheral resistance to flow. The controlling vessels are the *arterioles,* with rings of smooth muscle in their walls, under sympathetic nervous control. Characteristically, this sympathetic nervous system would discharge, from a brain center (the vasomotor center) en masse rather than differently to different areas, producing a general change in resistance everywhere. Inhibition of the system during heavy exercise would produce the desired fall in total peripheral resistance.

HUMORAL AGENTS.—Secondly, the Committee considered the use of agents, either hormones released from glands (e.g., adrenaline [also called "epinephrine"] from the adrenal gland [never called the "epinephrine gland"]) or products of metabolism, which would enter the blood and circulate everywhere to produce general changes of resistance by acting on the smooth muscles of the small blood vessels. Such agents are called *humoral agents* and, in particular, *vasoactive substances.* Those that produce vasoconstriction are called *pressor agents,* since they tend to raise the blood pressure. Those that dilate the vessels are *depressor agents.* As for products of metabolism in this role, carbon dioxide is a universal product of complete oxidation for energy and enters the blood from the tissues in proportion to their general activity. The action of excess carbon dioxide as a general vasodilator thus offers a convenient way of lowering the total peripheral resistance to flow in accordance with the needs of a particular tissue, as well as producing general increases in the total circulation.

CONTROL OF OUTPUT OF THE PUMP

If the reflex mechanism ensuring the priorities (i.e., that which kept the aortic pressure constant) was in operation, the changes in total peripheral resistance to flow would produce the desired general increases in total circulation. However, this pressure could only be kept up if there was a corresponding increase in cardiac output. The heart activity, although independently rhythmic, must therefore be correspondingly controlled by nerves (sympathetic and parasympathetic) and by circulating vasoactive substances. Both the rate of the heartbeat (i.e., of the pacemaker of the heart) and the strength of the beat (i.e., the force of contraction of the cardiac muscle) are affected by the same mechanisms as is the peripheral resistance—that is, by sympathetic and parasympathetic nerves and by humoral vasoactive substances. Cardiac output can increase both by increases in rate and by increases in the amount pumped out in each beat (the stroke volume). These are known as *"chronotropic"* and *"inotropic"* aspects of control. Increases in heart rate are the more important physiologically.

LOCAL AUTONOMY OF CONTROL

The obvious mechanism for giving some degree of local autonomy has already been mentioned —that is, by the universal product of aerobic metabolism, carbon dioxide. A more limited control, operating only when a given tissue (e.g., a muscle) is receiving inadequate circulation for its needs, would be by a specific product of anaerobic, rather than of aerobic, metabolism. Lactic acid in muscle is such a product of incomplete metabolism and produces vasodilation of the muscle vessels. This sort of local control of circulation, by the products of local metabolism, is in general described by the term *reactive hyperemia;* and it is most dramatically shown by the circulation to the skeletal muscles and, to a smaller degree, by the skin (9). [►It is not, however, exhibited by other tissues, such as those of some of the viscera, where lack of circulation may even lead to vasoconstrictor rather than vasodilator substances. The kidney is an example. After the circulation has been shut off for some minutes, there is often evidence of vasoconstriction rather than vasodilation.◄]*

Substances resulting from pathological physiology of tissues (e.g., in infection) can also cause local increases in circulation by vasodilation. This sort of local autonomy is described by the general term *inflammatory reaction.*

While the sympathetic system is one that usually discharges en masse to all the target areas, the parasympathetic system seems to be much more specific in its activity, seldom discharging en masse. This latter system, therefore, provides a mechanism of specific local changes in circulation (although not autonomous changes). The parasympathetic nerves are characteristically vasodilator rather than vasoconstrictor.

A quite different means of providing highly specific control of circulation of different organs, although making use of the general control by humeral agents and mass discharge of sympathetic nerves, was suggested by the Celestial Pharmacologist on the Committee. He pointed out that the responses of the blood vessels of different organs and tissues to the same circulating agent, or to, say, mass discharge of sympathetic nerves, could be quite different. For example, in heavy exercise the circulation to the working striated muscles must be increased, whereas that to the skin need not be so increased. Why not have the

vessels of striated muscle (and of the coronary vessels) dilated by circulating adrenaline (discharged into the blood in heavy exercise by the adrenal gland), in contrast to the vasoconstriction of skin vessels by this same circulating agent? Similarly, sympathetic nerve impulses might produce dilation in some vessels (e.g., the coronary vessels) but vasoconstriction in others (e.g., the skin, kidney vessels).

At this point, the Celestial Committee felt that the various schemes of control, both general and local, were becoming so complicated that it should draw up a scheme of the general principle of control. Below is the only existing copy of this, from the minutes of the Committee:

HEAVEN, Aeon Zero

OFFICIAL PLAN OF THE C.C.D.M.C. FOR CONTROL OF THE DISTRIBUTION OF THE CIRCULATION

1. *General Rule:* Flow = Pressure drop/Resistance.
2. *Priorities:* Brain, heart. Control driving pressure in aorta to constancy, by special reflexes. Keep resistance to flow of brain relatively constant; change resistance of coronaries somewhat by local and nervous control.
3. *General Control: (a)* By mass action of sympathetic nerves; *(b)* by circulating hormones; *(c)* by universal aerobic metabolite (carbon dioxide).
4. *The Heart* shall be independently rhythmic, but controlled by nerves for general control of circulation.
5. *Special Local Control: (a)* Different vessels can respond differently to the same circulatory hormones. *(b)* Special (parasympathetic) nerves to special organs.
6. *Local Autonomy of Control: (a)* By local metabolites (carbon dioxide, lactic acid, pH)—that is, reactive hyperemia. *(b)* Inflammatory reactions to disease and pathology.

This scheme will in general be followed in original design, and by evolutionary processes of selection.

(Signed) GABRIEL, *Secretary*

Problems of Control of the Circulation

The problems that such a scheme would generate were, of course, foreseen by the Celestial Committee, in their Infinite Wisdom and Foreknowledge. The problems arose chiefly from the inevitable conflict, in unusual circumstances of the animal, between the interests of individual parts of the organism, provided for in part by the degree of local autonomy of circulation that had been granted, and the interests of the whole organism. A good example is the situation where the animal is exposed to a cold environment, below freezing temperatures. For the thermal

---

*The device of being relatively dogmatic has been used in this text; but wherever other physiologists might disagree, or the author is not really sure of what he says, the passage in question is enclosed by special brackets: [►. . .◄]. There is certainly an advantage in letting the student know how much in physiology is still debatable, while still giving him some definite ideas with which to work.

economy of the whole animal, the maintenance of an intense vasoconstriction in the exposed limbs is desirable to reduce the total heat loss. However, the consequent fall of temperature of the peripheral tissues will endanger the cells if ice crystals form. A local autonomous reaction, in the rabbit ear and the human digits, was discovered by Sir Thomas Lewis (10). This is an abrupt local vasodilation with a rise in temperature of the exposed parts. This is known as the "hunting reaction of Lewis," or as "cold-induced vasodilation." The vasodilations are interrupted by periods of constriction. The mechanism of this local protective reaction is still obscure, but it is largely independent of central control. Yet these vasodilations increase the heat loss of the whole animal and may lead to its eventual death in hypothermia. Here there is a conflict of interest between the whole organism and the individual cells.

Another example is in the field of disease states. Goldblatt (11) discovered that, if the blood flow to the kidney was restricted (by a Goldblatt clamp on the renal artery), the kidney will put out into the circulation a substance or substances (renin, angiotonin) that tend to raise the central blood pressure to levels far above normal, overriding the reflex control of the aortic blood pressure and creating a condition called *renal hypertension.* This rise of blood pressure may well protect the tissues of the affected kidney by increasing its blood flow toward normal, for it is found that the cells of the clamped kidney are much less affected by the ischemia than would be expected. But the cells of the remainder of the body (e.g., those of the retina) may eventually suffer pathological changes because of the general hypertension. Again there is the conflict between central control and local autonomy.

Conclusions

The foregoing examples serve to show how dangerous, although useful, teleological thinking may be unless caution be used. The mechanisms of functioning and control of the circulation are astonishingly well "designed" or "adapted" to the normal circumstances of the life of animals. Physiological research reveals living devices and ways of accomplishing desired ends that are usually far better than the achievements of our engineers. For example, if a man's heart beats, on the average, 70 beats per min and he lives 70 years, the heart has completed 26 billion (2.6×10^{10}) beats before it stopped. How does this compare with the endurance of a piston and cylinder of an automobile four-stroke engine? Taking 3,000 revolutions per min at cruising speed, 60 miles per hour, this means 1,500 power strokes per mile. Twenty-six billion strokes would correspond to over 17 million miles. Very few engines could attain this even with continual repair (and this is the secret of normal physiological endurance).

Physiologists have to agree with the verdict of the first chapter of Genesis: "And God saw that it was good." We must congratulate the Celestial Committee on Design of a Mammalian Circulation and freely admit that we could not have done the job any better.

REFERENCES

1. Scholander, P. F.: The wonderful net, Scient. Am. 196:197, 1957.
2. Burton, A. C.: Physiology of Cutaneous Circulation: Thermoregulatory Functions, in *The Human Integument* (American Association for the Advancement of Science Publ. No. 54) (Washington, D. C.: 1959), pp. 77–88.
3. Warburg, O. H.: *The Metabolism of Tumors* (New York: Richard R. Smith, 1931).
4. Martin, A. W., and Fuhrman, F. A.: The relationship between summated tissue respiration and the metabolic rate in the mouse and dog, Physiol. Zool. 28:18, 1955.
5. Benedict, F. G., and Benedict, G. B.: *Mental Effort in Relation to Gaseous Exchange, Heart Rate, and Mechanics of Respiration* (Washington, D. C.: Carnegie Institution of Washington, 1933).
6. Sarnoff, S. J.; Braunwald, E.; Welch, G. H.; Stainsby, W. N.; Case, R. B., and Macruz, R.: Hemodynamic Determinants of the Oxygen Consumption of the Heart, in Rosenbaum and Belknap (eds.): *Work and the Heart* (New York: Paul B. Hoeber, Inc., 1959), Chap. 3.
7. Burton, A. C.: The importance of the shape and size of the heart, Am. Heart J. 54:801, 1957.
8. Irving, L.: Respiration in diving mammals, Physiol. Rev. 10:112, 1939.
9. Patel, D. J., and Burton, A. C.: Reactive hyperemia in the human finger, Circulation Res. 4:710, 1956.
10. Lewis, T.: Observations upon the reactions of the vessels of the human skin to cold, Heart 15:177, 1930.
11. Goldblatt, H.: *The Renal Origin of Hypertension* (Springfield, Ill.: Charles C Thomas, Publisher, 1948).

The Circulating Fluid, Blood

"Blood is a truly remarkable juice."—GOETHE,
Mephistopheles to Faust.

2

Composition of Blood

Scope of the Chapter

DETAILS OF THE "formed elements" of blood and their life history are to be found in textbooks of hematology and of histology. The biochemical mechanisms of the clotting of blood are today taught in courses in biochemistry, and the serological aspects in pathological chemistry. For these reasons, only those aspects of the topic of blood which bear directly on the circulation of blood are here treated in any detail. The all-important function of the circulation of blood—that is, the transport of oxygen and carbon dioxide between lungs and the cells of tissues—is discussed in more detail in the monograph on respiration* in this series, and the exchange of water, electrolytes and other plasma constituents, in the volume on kidney and body fluids.†

Fractions of Blood: Plasma, Cells and Serum

Blood is a soupy-thick suspension of cellular elements (which occupy about 50% of the total volume) in an aqueous solution of electrolytes and some nonelectrolytes. By *centrifugation*, the blood is separated into the two categories of *plasma* and *cells;* the overwhelmingly greatest proportion of the cells are *erythrocytes*, or *red cells*, with *white cells* of various categories making up less than 1/600th of the total cellular fraction. The third fraction of blood is *serum*, which is the result of allowing blood to clot. When the clot then spontaneously "retracts" (contracts on itself), a straw-colored fluid is expressed into the

*Comroe, J. H., Jr.: *Physiology of Respiration* (Chicago: Year Book Medical Publishers, Inc., 1965).

†Pitts, R. F.: *Physiology of the Kidney and Body Fluids* (2d ed.; Chicago: Year Book Medical Publishers, Inc., 1968).

plasma. Serum is similar in composition to plasma, but with one of the important colloidal proteins, *fibrinogen*, removed in forming the clot. Most of the *platelets* are also enmeshed in the contracting clot.

Separation of Cells and Plasma: Sedimentation and Centrifugation

The specific gravity of red cells is about 1.10, whereas that of plasma is 1.03. The small difference (0.07) will lead cells to settle out of suspension at a very low rate, called the *sedimentation rate*, which normally is only a few millimeters per hour, unless this is prevented by the motion of the blood. The physical principle involved is *Stokes' law*. Sir George Stokes (1845) showed that a sphere of radius a cm, falling through a viscous fluid of viscosity* η poises, would experience a drag force of F_η dynes, which was proportional to the velocity (v cm per sec) of its fall, given by:

$$F_\eta = 6\pi\eta v a \text{ dynes} \qquad (1)$$

Initially there is an acceleration; but when this drag force has increased (as v increases) to equal the force of gravity on the sphere, a steady *terminal velocity* will be reached. The gravitational force is given by:

$$F_g = 4/3 \ \pi \ a^3 g \ (\rho_1 - \rho_2) \text{ dynes} \qquad (2)$$

where ρ_1 and ρ_2 are the densities (g) of the particle and the medium, respectively (here of the red cells and of the plasma). Equating the two forces, F_η *and* F_g, when the terminal velocity, v_t, is reached gives:

$$v_t = 2/9 \ a^2 \ \frac{(\rho_1 - \rho_2)g}{\eta} \qquad (3)$$

Thus the terminal velocity is proportional to the

*For full discussion of viscosity, see Chapter 5.

square of the radius of the particles. Other things being considered constant, *the sedimentation rate is therefore a measure of the effective size of the particles or aggregates that are sedimenting.*

The red cell is not normally spherical, but discoid, so that modifying numerical factors have to be applied to Stokes' law *(eq. 1)* for the shape and for the relation of volume to shape, as indicated by equation 2. The orientation of the cells in falling, which apparently is random when blood is sedimenting, also matters. In addition, the interaction of the cells upon each other when the concentration is high must be considered. The result of all this modification of the theory is that a red cell sediments at about the rate of a sphere of equal volume of diameter 6μ instead of the 8.5μ maximal diameter of the cell. In the standard determination of the *erythrocyte sedimentation rate* (ESR), a vertical tube of narrow bore (2.5 mm) is filled with blood to a height of 10 cm or more. The blood is diluted with anticoagulant (e.g., sodium citrate), otherwise clotting would supervene long before sedimentation had proceeded far. At the end of an hour, a clear zone, relatively free from cells, can be seen at the top of the column of blood. In normal blood, this zone is only 1–3 mm deep in men and 4–7 mm in women; but in many acute infections and some chronic diseases (e.g., tuberculosis), the sedimentation rate rises to 100 mm or more per hour. It is a most useful clinical indication. To the physiologist, the important point is to know which of the several factors of equation 3 can have changed, in disease, to increase the sedimentation rate manyfold. There is no doubt that, while changes in red cell shape and size, changes in viscosity of plasma and changes in densities of cells and plasma could have minor effects, the change in effective size of the sedimenting cells or aggregates by *clumping and rouleaux formation* is the factor responsible. *The sedimentation rate is, therefore, a measure of the tendency of red cells to stick together.* The normal low sedimentation rate indicates very little such tendency in normal blood. A change in sedimentation rate is to be considered as indicating a change in the surface properties of the membrane of the red cell. The plasma proteins, such as those present in diseased states as antibodies, are the potent agents in changing the red cell surface. Of the normal plasma proteins, fibrinogen increases the sedimentation rate.

[►The standard method for ESR has an "all or nothing" character. The top of the cloud of sedimenting cells only is observed, and this will consist of the smallest (and therefore the slowest) aggregates, i.e., single cells if any exist. Larger aggregates will have passed more rapidly below the top of the cloud. An increased ESR in disease thus indicates that the tendency to aggregate is so great that very few cells remain single. We may be missing the full clinical information as to aggregation of cells because of this.◄]

Sedimentation of cells occurs in vivo in the blood vessels when flow is prevented, and in death (Gospel of St. John 19:34), and is observed by those who study the circulation by the microscope.

The Hematocrit

The percentage of the total volume of blood occupied by the cells is called the *hematocrit;* normally this is from 45 to 50%. The determination of hematocrit depends on an extension of Stokes' law, as applied in the erythrocyte sedimentation rate, with increased values of *g* in equation 3 produced by centrifugation. It is important to realize the arbitrariness of the absolute value of the hematocrit. The cells are thrown to the bottom of the hematocrit tube to form a layer of packed cells (Fig. 2–1). Above this lies a thin layer of white cells, whose specific gravity, although greater than that of plasma, is less than that of the red cells. This is the *buffy coat* of historic note. The volume of cells, as a percentage, is read off the tube. At a given speed of rotation, the apparent volume of cells will decrease with time (Fig. 2–1,*A*) but will eventually reach a constant value. However, this does not mean that the cells have reached a maximal closeness of packing, for spinning at higher speeds will produce a lower constant volume (Fig. 2–1,*B*), as shown by Millar in 1925 (1). Thus the endpoint depends on the speed of the centrifuge. The size and shape of the hematocrit tube used and the nature of the anticoagulant alter the result, and one of the several standard methods (e.g., Wintrobe) must be followed (tube bore, 5 mm; 3,000 rpm, or 1,500 G, for at least 15 min*).

---

*What matters in centrifugation is, not the speed of rotation of a particular apparatus, but how many times the acceleration of gravity it produces. This depends on the radius at which the cells lie in the centrifuge tube, as well as on the speed. The acceleration in centimeter-gram-second (cgs) units is $\omega^2 r$, where ω is the angular acceleration in radians per second and r is the radius. Translated into practical units and in terms of G (980 cm per sec²), this becomes:

$$G = (rpm)^2 \times r \times 11.2 \times 10^{-6}$$

where r is in centimeters.

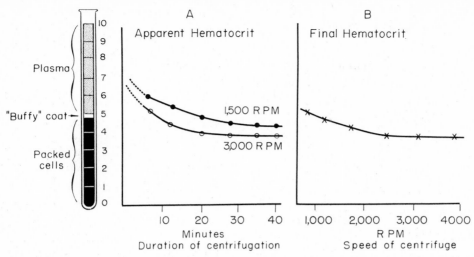

Fig. 2-1.—Measurement of the hematocrit, showing (**A**) how, at a given speed of centrifuge, the packing reaches a constant final value, yet (**B**) the final value at a higher speed may be less. (After Millar, 1925.)

The amount of *trapped plasma* after such procedures has been measured by adding radioactive plasma protein to blood and observing the activity in the packed-cell fraction. The amount is less than 5%, and a correction of this amount is often made in determining the hematocrit.

The normal hematocrit of 45–50% represents a very close packing of the erythrocytes, as will be discussed under the viscosity of blood in Chapter 5. In *polycythemia*, where the number of red cells is excessive, hematocrits of 60–70% are found, and there is then considerable interference with the free movement of blood in the circulation.

Red Cell Count and Mean Corpuscular Volume

Next to the determination of the hematocrit, the measurement of the number of red cells per cubic millimeter of blood is the clinical test that most often has been made. Although its use has been declining, because of the difficulty in determining it visually with sufficient reliability, the new electronic methods for counting particles (e.g., the Coulter or the Celloscope counter) will undoubtedly revive its use (2). If we combine the count with the hematocrit, the *mean corpuscular volume* of the cells is calculable, by the simple rule:

Mean corpuscular volume in μ^3 =

$$\frac{\% \text{ Hematocrit} \times 10}{\text{Red cell count in millions/mm}^3} \qquad (4)$$

The standard value for the *red cell count* is 5 million per mm³ of blood. Inserting this in equation 4 gives a mean corpuscular volume for the

red cell of $\dfrac{45 \times 10}{5} = 90\,\mu^3$. This agrees fairly

well with the red cell volume calculated from the average dimensions and shape of the red cell (see later [p. 22]).

The classic determination of the red cell count is by means of the hemocytometer (Thoma-Zeiss). A counting chamber with a rectangular space 0.10 mm in depth, covered with a specially ruled cover slip, is flooded with blood (diluted 200 times). The number of cells seen in each of a great number of the squares is then recorded. The distribution of the cells, coming to rest at random on the slide, follows the Poisson distribution (where the standard deviation equals the square root of the mean), not the Gaussian normal error curve, so that the coefficient of variation V associated with a total number of n cells counted is given by:

$$V = \pm \frac{100}{\sqrt{n}}\% \qquad (5)$$

Thus, if a total of 600 cells is enumerated, the error is ±4%. If the technician records the number of cells in each of 80 squares of the hemocytometer by the standard method, the standard error on the normal count of 5,000,000 per mm³ is ±350,000 (Ponder). Statistically, then, two red cell counts could not be considered different (to the 95% level of confidence) unless they differed by at least 14%. In addition to this "field error," there are errors in the use of the pipet, and it requires considerable skill to flood the chamber so that a really random distribution is achieved. All of these sources of error are greatly reduced, however, by the electronic counter, where the blood is very greatly diluted and drawn through a narrow orifice, so that one cell passes at a time. As each cell passes through, it trips a scalar counter, such as is used in making radioactivity counts. A hundred times as many cells can be counted in a fraction of the time, with a corresponding increase in accuracy of the mean count.

Other Cellular Elements of Blood; White Cell Count

The hemocytometer or the modern counting techniques are also used to give the *white cell count.* The blood is diluted 1 part in 20, instead of 1 in 200, with a fluid which destroys the red cells and stains the white cells. The normal white cell count is considered to be from 5,000 to 8,000 per mm³ (red cells are 5 million per mm³). This is only 1/600th of the population density of erythrocytes. Thus, while the function of the white cells (leukocytes) in maintaining resistance to infection is of the greatest importance (see textbooks of medicine), from the point of view of the circulation their presence has little effect. Figure 2–2 shows how unlikely it would be that an observer stationed in the wall of an artery, vein or vessel, watching the cells go by, would happen to see a leukocyte. Leukocytes are about as relatively rare as the "traffic cop" on our arterial highways. Similarly, the platelets, which are vital to hemostasis (e.g., clotting), although they are much more numerous than the white cells (the normal platelet count is 250,000–500,000 per mm³, a concentration about 1/20th of that of the red cells), are so small (about 2.5µ diameter) as to have negligible effect on the flow of blood.

There would be little point for one more incompetent author of a text on the physiology of the circulation to plagiarize the excellent accounts in books on histology and hematology, with their expensive colored illustrations of the different types of white cells *(differential count)* or of the origin, life history and function of either red or white cells. The function of platelets is mentioned in the chapter on hemostasis (Chapter 4). Another justification for omitting details of the leukocytes of different kinds from a monograph on circulation is that many of the functions of these cells are performed, not in the circulation, but in the tissue

Fig. 2-2.—Diagram indicating relative populations of cells in the blood. The black dots represent 1,200 erythrocytes; with these are associated only 2 white cells and 60 platelets (the latter shown as small irregularly shaped fragments). The dots representing the red cells should, truly, be much larger and should occupy 50% of the volume. (Compare Fig. 5–4, B.)

spaces outside the blood vessels. In the *inflammatory reaction,* when tissues are injured or infected, the leukocytes, instead of rolling along the wall of the small blood vessels as they do normally, become more "sticky," pause and then pass with remarkable ease through the capillary wall. The process is called *diapedesis;* and it is astonishing to view in micromotion pictures, for the cells migrate through the endothelial lining where there was apparently no "hole" previously, often in the form of an hourglass with the cytoplasm flowing from the "bulb" in the vessel through the narrow "waist" into the "bulb" outside the wall. As soon as the cells are through the wall, they move off to the injured area, presumably under *chemotactic forces,* the nature of which is not yet understood, although we conceal our ignorance by using this jargon.

The leukocytes, of course, have functions in the blood stream. *Monocytes* play a role in the transport of antibodies and possibly in producing serum globulins. *Basophilic granulocytes* contain *heparin*, an anticoagulant important in preventing intravascular clotting. *Neutrophils* and *monocytes* take part in phagocytosis (the engulfing and transport of foreign particles) in the circulation, as well as in the tissues to which these leukocytes migrate in the inflammatory reaction.

Composition of Plasma

Plasma is about 90% water by weight, most of the solid content being plasma protein (7%), the remainder inorganic (1%) and organic substances (1%). There are enough "free" molecules and ions to give a total osmotic pressure of about 8 atmospheres (atm), equivalent to a sodium chloride solution of 0.9% by weight (physiological saline). Since the ions of the electrolytes in plasma are so much smaller than the large protein molecules that make up the bulk of the weight of solids, there are a great many more of the small molecules, and these are the important contributors to the total osmotic pressure. However, the total osmotic pressure would be relevant only if we were concerned with membranes which permitted water to pass but held back all other species of molecule present. The membranes of the wall of the blood vessels, particularly the capillaries, are freely permeable not only to water but to electrolytes and small organic molecules (e.g., sugars) and are impermeable only to the larger protein molecules. The relevant osmotic pressure governing the exchange of water between the circulation and the tissues is therefore the *colloidal osmotic pressure*, due to the plasma proteins. This amounts normally to only 25 mm Hg, in contrast to the 8 atm (more than 6,000 mm Hg) of total osmotic pressure.

INORGANIC CONSTITUENTS OF PLASMA

The medical student is required to memorize the standard values of the important cations (Na^+, K^+, Ca^{++}, Mg^{++}) and the important anions (Cl^-, HCO_3^- and phosphates $HPO_4^=$ and $H_2PO_4^-$) in plasma or serum. The values in serum may be slightly less than in plasma, for the protein fibrinogen, which is removed to obtain serum from plasma, tends to absorb some of the ions. The requirement of memorization is justified because in health the concentration of these ions is regulated by special hormonal and other feedback mechanisms, to a narrow range of normality. Small deviations from this narrow range are therefore significant indicators of diseased states.

Frustration for the student in memorizing the standard values is due to the many different units—milligrams per 100 ml (mg/100 ml), milliequivalents per liter (mEq/L), millimoles (mM), milliosmols (mOsm), etc.—used in different books (sometimes without self-consistency in the figures, more than one set of units being used). Of the two sets of numbers worth remembering—that is, mg/100 ml and mEq/L—the second is by far the most logical choice, since the total mEq/L of the cations must equal the total mEq/L for anions (these totals are each about 155) ([see Table 2–1]) (3).

The concentration in mg/100 ml may be calculated from the mEq/L by multiplying by the molecular weight, then dividing by the valency and finally dividing by 10 (to turn from "per litre" to "per 100 ml"). There is some uncertainty about what valency to take for the phosphates, since they provide some of the buffers of the blood, and the proportion of bivalent ($HPO_4^=$) and monovalent ($H_2PO_4^-$) phosphate alters with the pH. At normal blood pH, this proportion is about 80% bivalent to 20% monovalent; so an average valency of 1.8 is used. The calcium is only partly ionized, about half being bound to plasma proteins.

Table 2–1 probably represents the minimum of memorization with which a medical student can manage to pass his examinations. The aim of the practicing pathological chemistry laboratories should be, eventually, to establish firmly, statistically, the mean deviation around the accepted

TABLE 2–1.—CONCENTRATIONS OF ELECTROLYTES IN PLASMA*

	CATIONS				ANIONS			
	Na⁺	K⁺	Ca⁺⁺	OTHERS†	Cl⁻	HCO₃⁻	Phos.	OTHERS†
mEq/L	140	4	5	6	103	29	2	21
S.D. (or range) in mEq/L	±5	±0.5	±1.0	±5	±0.5		±1.0	
Total		155 mEq				155 mEq		

*The figures are rounded off.
†Others include Mg^{++} cations, and plasma protein anions.

mean for healthy populations, so that it would be possible to report that a given patient's serum potassium was, say, $+1.8\sigma$ (two thirds of healthy persons would be within 1σ of the mean; only 5%, outside 2σ), without giving the actual numerical value, the absolute value of which is not important. It would then not be necessary for the student to memorize the standard values. The information that this patient's K^+ is $+1.8\sigma$ is really all that is essential.

Plasma Proteins

Since the wall of the blood vessels, particularly the capillaries, is quite freely permeable to all but the larger molecules, the plasma proteins are the constituents which are important in governing the exchanges of water between blood and tissues, and the "colloidal osmotic pressure," rather than the "total osmotic pressure," is what concerns us in a treatise on the circulation.

Figure 2–3, a diagram produced many years ago by workers in the Department of Physical Chemistry of Harvard University, shows the relative shape and size of the important proteins of the blood. It is not to be thought that the proteins are actually ellipsoidal. The fact is that the only shape, other than a sphere, which lends itself to reasonable mathematical treatment by the physical chemists is an ellipsoid (cigar shape), of which the ratio of major to minor axes appears in the theory of birefringence, viscosity and so on. What

is true is that the molecules are longer than they are broad, in some such ratio as that indicated in the drawings in Figure 2–3. Study of the figure at once raises some interesting questions. The capillaries of the kidney evidently have pores large enough to allow the passage of hemoglobin, since, when this exists in plasma because of hemolysis, it appears in the urine. The smaller diameter of the albumin, globulin and fibrinogen molecules appears to be the same or less than the diameter of the hemoglobin molecule. Why, then, do not these plasma proteins leak steadily from the blood stream via the kidney? [►If they presented themselves "narrow-end-on" to the pores, they might do so. The answer may well be in the phenomenon of *orientation by streaming* (4), very adequately studied by the physical chemists. In a flowing liquid, ellipsoidal particles are oriented, so that the probability of their having their long axis parallel to the direction of flow is much greater than at right angles (Fig. 2–4). This is particularly true near the wall of a blood vessel, where the velocity gradient is maximal. The flow of blood thus prevents the leakage of protein that might occur if the flow were stopped, when the protein molecules would be randomly oriented, so that a fraction might offer themselves at right angles to a pore (Fig. 2–4). In support of this theory, there is abundant evidence that stasis of blood flow in kidney glomeruli leads to the appearance of plasma proteins in the urine, which disappear when renal blood flow is once more normal. Examples

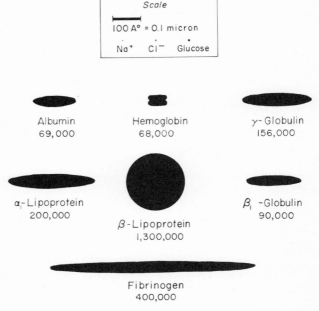

Fig. 2-3.—Relative shape and size of various proteins of the blood. The ellipsoidal shapes are not to be taken too seriously; they simply mean that the molecules are longer than they are thick. (Redrawn from a diagram supplied through courtesy of the Department of Physical Chemistry, Harvard University.)

Scale

100 A° = 0.1 micron

Na⁺   Cl⁻   Glucose

Albumin
69,000

Hemoglobin
68,000

γ-Globulin
156,000

α₁-Lipoprotein
200,000

β-Lipoprotein
1,300,000

β₁-Globulin
90,000

Fibrinogen
400,000

Flow stopped

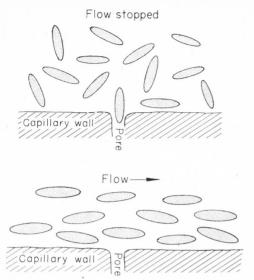

Fig. 2-4.—Diagram showing how orientation by streaming, when blood is flowing in capillaries, may prevent the escape of ellipsoidal protein molecules, which otherwise would enter pores in the wall.

are the "benign albuminureas," noted in heavy exercise, and with the upright posture, in some healthy individuals.◄]

The plasma proteins fall into four classifications—albumins, globulins, fibrinogen and lipoproteins, making a total of 7 Gm/100 ml. Albumin and globulin make up nearly all of this. These are synthesized by the liver, and the ratio of albumin to globulin in the plasma, *the A/G ratio,* is an index of liver function. The normal A/G ratio is considered to be from 1.5:1 to 2.0:1. The standard values depend on whether the proteins are separated by electrophoresis or by differential precipitation.

The functions of plasma protein are several:

1. The *albumins and globulins* are essential to maintaining the *osmotic balance,* which controls the movement of water from the blood stream to the tissues. Although the concentration of albumin is only a little greater than that of globulins in Gm/100 ml, since its molecular weight (69,000) is considerably less than that of globulins (90,-000–160,000), there are considerably more albumin molecules than globulin molecules in plasma. The albumin is therefore more important than globulins in providing colloid osmotic pressure.

2. *Globulins,* particularly γ-globulin, are concerned with *antibody reactions,* in protection against disease.

3. *Fibrinogen* is intimately concerned with the *clotting of blood.*

4. *Lipoproteins* are probably all-important in the carriage and provision of lipids to the cell. Figure 2–3 shows lipoproteins as if these could be considered to be definite molecules, with the molecular weight shown—this is not so, for the protein is merely associated with the lipid in these particles *(chylomicrons),* very likely as a surface layer over a lipid interior. [►The preferential fuel of skeletal muscle in vivo is probably lipid (5, 6), not carbohydrate as the biochemists seem to emphasize from the results of study of tissue slices in vitro; so the lipoproteins in plasma serve a very important transport function.◄]

5. It has been suggested that the plasma proteins provide a *reserve of protein for nutrition.* While it is true that in extremes of starvation the concentration of plasma proteins declines, this may be due to lack of synthesis, plus excessive loss by excretion, rather than loss by metabolism. However, plasma proteins might provide amino acids, after breakup in the liver, for resynthesis into new proteins in the tissue cells. The total plasma protein (350 Gm) would provide, if completely metabolized, only about 1,400 kilocalories (Cal), hardly enough for the total metabolism of a man for one day.

6. The proteins take part in the maintenance of blood pH *(buffering).* Since proteins are "zwitter ions," capable of acting as both anions and cations, serum proteins combine with hydrogen and other cations to assist the other buffer systems (carbonate, phosphates, hemoglobin) in keeping the pH of blood within very narrow normal limits (mean value 7.4).

REFERENCES

1. Millar, W. G.: Observations on the hematocrit method of measuring the volume of erythrocytes, Quart. J. Exper. Physiol. 15:187, 1925.

2. Maltern, G. T.: Determination of number and size of particles by electrical gating: Blood cells, J. Appl. Physiol. 10:56, 1957.

3. Gamble, J. L.: *Chemical Anatomy, Physiology, and Pathology of Extracellular Fluid* (6th ed.; Cambridge, Mass.: Harvard University Press, 1954).

4. Peterlin, A.: Streaming and stress birefringence, Ztschr. Physik. 25:615, 1956.

5. Andres, R.; Cader, G., and Zierler, K. L.: The quantitatively minor role of carbohydrate in oxidative metabolism by skeletal muscle in the basal state, J. Clin. Invest. 35:671, 1956.

6. Zierler, K. L., and Andres, R.: Carbohydrate metabolism in intact skeletal muscle in man during the night, J. Clin. Invest. 35:991, 1956.

𝟛

The Erythrocytes

Introduction

No BIOLOGICAL OBJECT, except possibly the heart, has been the object of such careful, and so many, measurements as the adult red cell. Excellent books, such as those by Ponder (1, 4) and Prankerd (5), have been devoted to the erythrocyte. The easy availability and ease of storage of red cells make them the ideal object for research for anyone who can afford a really good microscope. Yet many features of the morphology of the red cell remain mysterious.

Above all, the function of the red cell is the carriage of the respiratory pigment, *hemoglobin*. While biochemists recognize many more metabolic functions of the red cell than the taking-on and giving-up of oxygen and of carbon dioxide, most of the physiological functions are related to these phenomena. This explains the remarkably great content of hemoglobin in the erythrocyte.

Dimensions of the Red Cell

The biconcave discoid shape of normal red cells (Fig. 3–1) makes it difficult, if not impossible, to measure accurately the dimensions other than the maximal diameter because of microscopical or microphotographical errors due to refraction and to focusing through other layers; but Table 3–1 (taken from a more complete tabulation by Pon-

der [1]) gives mean values based on a very large number of direct microscopic measurements. The dimensions, of course, have a biological variation. The distribution of diameters has been most studied, since this dimension can be measured most easily by a variety of methods. The distribution is normally symmetrical; and since the standard deviation is about $\pm 0.5\mu$, two-thirds of the cells have diameters between 8.0 and 9.0μ.

Table 3–1 shows the considerable variation in a normal population of red cells, of both size and shape. We need an index of shape that does not involve size, so that two cells of very different volume but of the same shape will have the same index of shape. This is the *sphericity index* (2),

$$\text{Sphericity index} = \frac{4.84 \, (\text{Volume})^{2/3}}{\text{Area}}$$

TABLE 3–1.—THE DIMENSIONS OF THE NORMAL RED CELLS WITH THE STANDARD DEVIATIONS*

	MEAN	±S.D.	
Diameter	8.1	± 0.43	μ
Greatest thickness	2.7	± 0.15	μ
Least thickness	1.0	± 0.3	μ
Area	138	± 17	μ^2
Volume	95	± 17	μ^3

*The original table of Ponder (1) has been modified in view of more modern data from various sources, by P. B. Canham, including our own statistical geometrical studies (2). There would not be complete agreement among the experts, but the figures represent reasonable compromises.

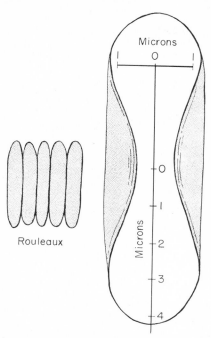

Fig. 3-1.—The shape of the normal red cell, with the mean values of the dimensions according to Ponder. **Left**, illustrating rouleaux.

lating blood represents a population that has already been "screened" by such geometrical criteria; those cells that have inappropriate combinations of size and shape have been eliminated. An increase of sphericity index with age (3) of the red cell probably accounts for the 120-day life span, although other factors such as change in electrical charge are undoubtedly involved.◄]

The shape, which is shown with the mean values of the dimensions in Figure 3–1, is far from constant even in the same animal, since the coefficient of correlation between the diameter and least thickness is only about 0.4. There is, therefore, considerable uncertainty as to the surface area, which is calculated from the shape by use of theorems of geometry applying to solids of revolution. There is no doubt that the surface area is very much greater than it would be for a sphere of the same volume as the red cell. If the figures in Table 3–1 are used, the sphere of the same volume would have a diameter of 5.6 μ and a surface area of 101 μ^2, only about 73% of that of the red cell, as emphasized in later paragraphs. As to the mean volume (95 μ^3), a calculation of this from mean dimensions agrees well with the values of mean corpuscular volume derived from hematocrit and red cell counts.

Reason for Shape of the Red Cell

The main function of the red cell is the transport, and the oxidation and reduction, of the hemoglobin it contains. Since the respiratory gases may have to reach the hemoglobin by diffusion through the contents of the red cell, a shape which allows diffusion to the innermost parts in the shortest time is advantageous. It has often been pointed out that the discoid shape provides this far better than a sphere. This is, of course, no explanation of the existence of that particular shape, and a flatter disk of larger diameter would permit even faster diffusion. Moreover, it is probable that actual mixing of the content of a red cell occurs during the passage of red cells, one at a time, through the smallest capillaries. Even when flowing in the large vessels, the red cells are being continuously deformed by collision with their fellows and probably hardly ever of the "normal" shape when in the circulation! The process of exchange to all of the red cell contents is therefore not dependent on diffusion alone.

Ponder emphasizes that the normal shape is only one of many shapes a red cell may take when conditions are changed (e.g., disk-sphere trans-

which is dimensionless. The factor 4.84 is included so that for a sphere, which is the shape that has a maximal volume for a given surface area, the index is unity. All other shapes have lower sphericity indexes, down to zero for an infinitely thin disc. The sphericity index for a population of normal red cells ranges from 0.72 to 0.86, with a mean of 0.77 ± .025 S.D.

Results from photographing hundreds of cells at random from a sample of blood reveal that shape and volume are not independently variable; cells with greater than average volume are significantly "thinner," with a lower sphericity index; those of smaller volume than the mean tend to be "spherocytic," with a higher index. (Interestingly, the same is true of mercury droplets of different size. Why?) [►The basic reason for this is that while the membrane of the red cell is easily bent (very flexible), it cannot suffer a stretch that increases its area by more than a small percentage (5–10%) without hemolysis of the cell (see later in this chapter), which becomes rigid. Thus, spherocytic cells can be deformed very much less than cells that are less spherocytic, before their surface area is increased. Consequently, cells of large volume survive passage in the circulation only if their sphericity index is lower. A sample of circu-

formations discussed below). We must regard the shape as in equilibrium, under the existing physical forces on the cell. When some of these forces change, as by changes in adsorbed molecules on the surface membrane, or of the membrane itself, the shape at once changes.

[►Electron micrographs have not clearly revealed structure within the red cell, although the inside of the membrane surface does show attached filamentous material (probably protein fibers). However, studies of individual red cells with polarized light, using crossed polarizer and analyzer, give evidence of the type of birefringence ("form birefringence") that occurs when fibers are lined up, across the dimple region of the red cell, where the opposite membranes are closest (6). There is no evidence of such bridges across the cell in the rim region. A force of attraction between the two membranes across the inside of the cell is postulated. This could correspond to the attractive force between the membrane of one red cell and the membrane of another, which leads to rouleaux formation. This (outside) force is known to depend on the mediation of long-chain molecules (normally fibrinogen in plasma). So may the attractive force inside the cell. Away from the dimple region, where the membranes are farther apart, the polarized light studies indicate a palisade of oriented fibers on the membrane surface but not linked across the cell in "long chains." With osmotic swelling of the cell, the indication was that the links were broken across the dimple. This leads to the view that a mosaic pattern of electrical charges on the membrane surfaces, inside and outside, leads to those attractive forces and that if the surfaces are brought close enough together chain linkages are formed. Perhaps the structure of the membrane is not different at the dimple region from that at the rim, and if we first swelled and then shrank a red cell, its dimple and rim might exchange places. This phenomenon has not yet been recorded with certainty. Another view is that the biconcave shape for a given value of the volume and area of a red cell represents the shape in which the total energy of bending of the membrane is least (7).◄]

Disk-Sphere Transformations

The addition of very small concentrations of a number of agents, called *sphering agents,* such as *saponin, digitonin, lecithin, rose bengal,* and of *anionic detergents,* such as glycocholate and taurocholate, causes a reversible change from the discoid to a spherical shape without any significant change in volume of the red cell. These agents in higher concentration are "lytic" (i.e., they disrupt the cell membrane); but if the cells are removed at an early stage and resuspended in saline, to which a small amount of plasma has been added, they revert to their original biconcave form. There is, therefore, a protein in plasma which preserves the discoid shape. *Chloroform, ether* and *some alcohols,* like this plasma factor, will act as *antisphering agents.* Ponder points out that some sphering agents can produce the transformation when they are present in such exceedingly small concentrations that they could not cover the surface of the cells, even with a monolayer. However, in the case of the most active agent *(tetradecyl sulphate),* it has been noted that the effective minimal concentration corresponds to one molecule of this agent per protein molecule of membrane (i.e., protein of the fixed framework, excluding hemoglobin). [►All this supports the concept of the shape depending on the organization of structural proteins in the membrane and of proteins adsorbed on the surface.◄]

Variations of Red Cell Shape

As has been already mentioned, even in health there is a wide variation in shape of the red cells in the blood of a single animal. In abnormal physiological conditions and in disease, a number of different forms are recognized by pathologists. After splenectomy, unusually flat cells (with the ratio of diameters to thickness 6.6:1, instead of the usual 3.5:1), called *leptocytes* or *platycytes,* may predominate. *Ovalocytes* are biconcave but are slightly elliptical instead of circular in cross-section. *Spherocytes,* which are biconvex but by no means spherical, are often reported in disease. In conditions where there has been a shrinkage of the cells, as in hypertonic media, *crenation,* where the membrane is "crinkled" or "bumpy" instead of smooth, is common. All of these may be metastable states of the adult red cell, which will revert to the normal discoid shape when conditions in the blood are changed to normal.

A well-known variation of shape, of a different character, is that of *sickle cell anemia,* an inherited abnormality that is practically confined to the Negro race. Here a large percentage of the cells look like crescent moons in profile and are called *meniscocytes.* Again, it should be noted that this shape represents a metastable state, for, if the oxygen tension of the blood is sufficiently increased (above about 50 mm Hg oxygen tension), the cells become discoid and indistinguishable in shape from the normal cells. [►One of the recent achievements of biochemistry has been the proof that in sickle cell anemia the hemoglobin molecule is slightly different from the normal (different in the globin part of the molecule only), and it is thought that this change in the molecular force field enables the closely packed hemoglobin molecules in the red cell to be organized into a semicrystalline state (tactoid) which somehow imposes the sickle shape on the whole cell.◄]

Osmotic Swelling of the Red Cell and Hemolysis

The red cell contains a very high concentration (340 Gm/100 ml) of hemoglobin, and really little else, in terms of weight per liter. For example, the concentration of glucose in the cell is only 75 mg/100 ml, which is only about 1/5,000th of the concentration of hemoglobin. As Drabkin pointed out, the picture is very different when we consider the number of molecules involved, for the glucose molecule is so very much smaller than the hemoglobin molecule. There are 3.4×10^8 molecules of hemoglobin per red cell, and 2.2×10^8 molecules of glucose (a comparable number). The total osmotic pressure depends on the sugar and ions (mostly sodium and chloride) in the red cell as much as on the content of hemoglobin molecules. However, while the membrane of the red cell is fairly permeable to water and to many smaller molecules (e.g., sugars), it is normally quite impermeable to hemoglobin. Thus the hemoglobin mainly determines the behavior of the red cell as an osmometer.

When red cells are placed in distilled water or a hypotonic solution, water enters and the cell swells. An interesting series of changes in shape occurs (Fig. 3–2). The biconcavities of the original biconcave cell fill out until, after the volume has increased about 30%, the cell is spherical, although the surface is less than originally; cells may show crenation. Swelling as a sphere then occurs until a critical point is reached, at which point the membrane abruptly becomes permeable to hemoglobin, which leaves it almost completely and enters the external medium *(hemolysis)*. The membrane is still intact, for the cell persists as a *red cell ghost*, which usually soon reverts to the discoid form. [►This is proof that the shape depends on the membrane, not the contents.◄] It is possible, by placing "ghosts" in a strong solution of hemoglobin, to cause some hemoglobin to enter once more, and subsequent exposure to hypertonic saline will shrink the cell back toward the original volume.

[►The explanation of this sudden dramatic "increase of permeability" so that the hemoglobin can leave the cell is still obscure. It has been suggested that at the critical point in the swelling process the surface of the erythrocyte, which decreased when it became spherical, reaches the original surface area which it had in the initial discoid shape. "Holes" then develop in the membrane when it is further stretched (8). Data on the surface area, initially and at the moment of hemolysis, which have been available only statistically for populations of red cells in experiments on hemolysis by swelling, cannot settle the question whether it is a critical surface area or a critical increase in volume that determines the point of hemolysis. The "stretching theory" is

Fig. 3-2.—Stages in hemolysis by swelling: **A,** original discoid cell; **B,** the concavities become convex; **C,** when the volume has increased by 30%, the cell is a "rough sphere"; **D,** the cell continues to swell as a sphere; **E,** when the volume is increased by about 100% and the surface area (*S. area*) is the same as in **A,** hemoglobin leaves the cell; **F,** the resulting ghost may revert to the discoid shape; **G,** hemolysis without swelling (by sphering agents) results in a rough or crenated sphere with much reduced surface area.

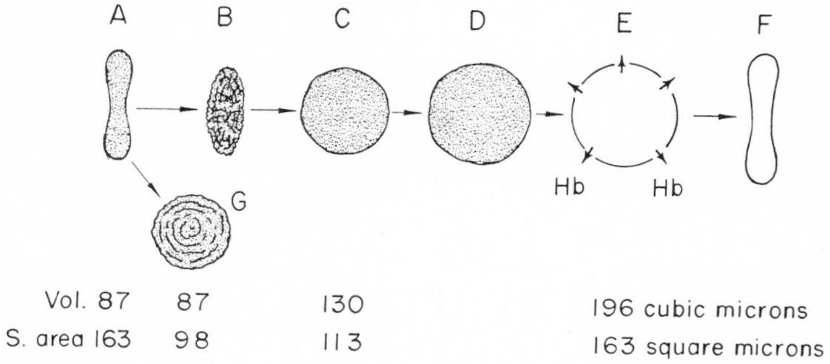

	A	B	C		E	F
Vol.	87	87	130		196 cubic microns	
S. area	163	98	113		163 square microns	

attractive, together with a more sophisticated view that a monolayer of molecules of some protein from the plasma, coating the surface of the cell, was responsible for the normal impermeability to hemoglobin. If the area exceeded the original surface area of the membrane, such a monolayer would no longer cover the surface, which would be full of "holes." This sort of behavior is seen in work on Langmuir surface trays, with monolayers of protein on buffer solutions. Support for the monolayer theory is provided by the fact that hemolysis is accelerated by many surface active agents, such as *saponin* and *bile salts,* and inhibited by components of plasma, such as *cholesterol, serum globulin, lecithin* and *albumin.*◄]

Hemolysis in Vivo; Hemolysins

In health, there is a continual hemolysis, which relates to the life span of the red cells in the circulation (details in Chapter 4). In disease, this normal hemolysis may be greatly accelerated, as in *hemolytic jaundice* (bile salts in the plasma are responsible). Since free hemoglobin is just small enough to pass through the pores of the membrane of the kidney glomeruli, excessive hemolysis is detected by the presence of hemoglobin in the urine as well as in the plasma *(hemoglobinuria* and *hemoglobinemia).*

Hemolysis by osmotic swelling may not be of any significance in vivo (certainly not in health), since the osmotic pressure of blood is controlled by homeostatic mechanisms *(osmoreceptors)* to stay within narrow bounds. Mechanical trauma of red cells bumping each other and into the walls of vessels may be a significant factor limiting the life span of red cells, but small quantities of hemolysins are probably the main factor.

An interesting rare disorder involving excessive hemolysis is *paroxysmal nocturnal hemoglobinuria.* The rate of hemolysis of normal red cells is not greatly affected by changes in blood pH. The cells of patients with this disorder appear to have a normal fragility (see below) in tests at normal pH, but hemolysis is greatly increased when the blood is more acid than normal. The accumulation of carbon dioxide because of the changed breathing (alveolar ventilation) in sleep is enough to cause the hemoglobinuria. Keeping the patient awake, or having him take sodium bicarbonate, can reduce the hemolysis.

Tests of Erythrocyte Fragility

The test of fragility depends on hemolysis by osmotic swelling. Blood is diluted with distilled water to different tonicities of the plasma, or red cells are resuspended in buffered sodium chloride of various tonicities. Usually, a tonicity of 0.5 that of normal plasma is used, with steps of more dilute solutions down to a tonicity of 0.1. After 15 min or so, the cells are centrifuged to the bottom of the series of test tubes used, and the degree of hemolysis is judged visually or measured colorimetrically by the amount of hemoglobin in the supernatant. This gives the *percentage hemolysis curve* (Fig. 3–3). Normal cells are 100% hemolyzed in solutions of sodium chloride of less than 0.3% (tonicity, 0.35). Half of the normal cells will be hemolyzed at a tonicity of 0.44. In some diseased states, the fragility is greatly increased and complete hemolysis occurs in stronger solutions than this. It has been shown that the original shape of the red cells greatly affects their osmotic fragility. Cells (e.g., spherocytes) which are more spherical than the average (i.e., have a lower ratio of maximal diameter to minimal thickness) hemolyze at a much less increase of volume than normal. Old cells are more "fragile" than young cells.

Cytochemistry of Red Cell Membrane

There have been many analyses of the red cell ghost to indicate the composition of the fixed framework of the red cell. In man, only 3.3% of

Fig. 3-3.—The percent hemolysis and frequency distribution curves of normal human erythrocytes. Half of them will hemolyze in sodium chloride solutions of tonicity 0.44. (Redrawn from Ponder [1].)

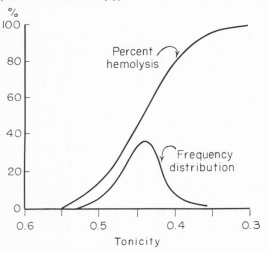

the mass of the red cell is accounted for by the membrane plus any internal fixed structure, if this exists. The chemical analysis shows that more than 90% of the original lipids of the cell are left in the ghost. The weight of protein is about twice that of the lipids; but on the other hand, there are about 90 lipid molecules for each molecule of protein. The protein is called *stromatin*, although there is more than one protein present (other than hemoglobin).

[►On the basis of the dry weight, and assuming a density of 1.0, if all this material were in the membrane, with no internal stroma at all, the thickness of the membrane would be about 180 Å, with a variation of ±60 Å, corresponding to a 1% uncertainty in the percentage dry weight. Optical methods (the leptoscope) and the electron microscopic pictures agree that the thickness in human red cells is between 150 and 200 Å.◄]

Examination of the membrane of red cell ghosts with the polarization microscope (Schmitt, Bear and Ponder [9]) indicate a surface ultrastructure similar to that of the axon sheath of invertebrate nerve. Such studies have suggested a model (Davson and Danielli [10]) consisting of three organized layers: a central lipoid layer with radial orientation, covered by a layer of protein molecules, tangentially oriented, on each side, with the lipid layer sandwiched between. The evidence from the special permeability of the membrane, which was the lifetime study of Jacobs* and his students of the University of Pennsylvania, compels us to think of the red cell surface as a mosaic of many different areas. Probably we should think of the surface as like that of a ball loosely wound with bundles of string (the "stromatic patterns"), with specific polar groups of the proteins sticking out at many key points. Jacobs found that the pattern of specificity of permeability for different substances was astonishingly different for red cells of different mammalian species—so much so that he could identify the species, among a great number, by a kind of stepwise permeability analysis (similar to high-school inorganic chemical analysis). The forces causing the "stickiness" of

red cells (rouleaux formation, agglutination) probably depend on such patterns, associated with variations in electric charge over the red cell surface.

Contents of the Red Cell

The most striking feature of the contents of the red cell is the remarkable closeness of the packing of the hemoglobin molecules. About 25% of the available volume is occupied by these molecules, 70% by water and only 5% by all the other constituents. Assuming spherical hemoglobin molecules and hexagonal packing (which is the closest arrangement possible), a hemoglobin molecule would have a radius of about 28 Å and a "shell," around each, of radius 38 Å. The contents of the red cell are therefore very close to the state of "gelation" and the "paracrystalline state" (Fig. 3–4). The ions (mostly K^+, Cl^- and Na^+) between the hemoglobin molecules are therefore in conditions very different from those of dilute solution, and it would be expected that there would be evidence that the red cell does not act as a "perfect" osmometer.

The ionic contents of the human red cell are similar to those of living cells in general, for the K^+ concentration is high and the Na^+ low. Table 3–2 shows a few of the items present.

[►No satisfactory theory of how this disparity in ionic concentration between inside and outside of the red cell can exist is as yet available. The

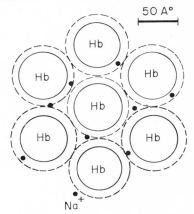

Fig. 3-4.—Showing how closely packed the hemoglobin molecules are in the red cell. The broken-line circles represent shells of 10 Å thickness surrounding each hemoglobin molecule. The small dots represent Na^+ ions, in about their relative numbers. There are four or five times as many K^+ ions and three times as many Cl^- ions. (Modified from Ponder [1]).

---

*Merkel Jacobs worked out a very complete analysis of the kinetics of swelling and shrinking of red cells when different penetrating substances were added to the medium. When the substance penetrates the red cell, it may be followed by water, so that there is first a shrinking and then eventual swelling. We may owe this very sophisticated body of knowledge to the accident that Jacobs, in his youth, was confined to his cot for some weeks by a broken leg when camping in remote woods and that all he had to read was a textbook of calculus and differential equations.

TABLE 3–2.—STANDARD VALUES OF
IONIC CONCENTRATION*

IONS	SERUM (mM/L)	RED CELLS (mM/L)	RATIO OF CELLS TO SERUM
Na+	135	18	1:7
K+	5	81	16:1
Cl−	104	52	1:2
HCO−	26	19	1.3:1
Protein	2	5	2.5:1
Water (Gm/L)	935	707	
Total	290	205	

*Adapted from Peters (11).

view that active transport mechanisms of ion accumulation have operated in the premature stage of the red cell when it was metabolically very active (with a functioning nucleus like other cells) and that the results are perpetuated in the impermeable nonnucleated cells is quite untenable, for, while the permeability of the mature cell to cations is much less than to anions, it is sufficient to produce equilibration in a short time. In time, in solutions other than those equivalent to plasma, Na+ and K+ are exchanged across the membrane. We do not know enough about active ion transfer, of the "binding" of ions in the interior, of the internal pH, even of the hydrostatic pressure within red cells (which may not be equal to the outside because of tension in the membrane), to know whether or not a steady state maintained by the very low continuous metabolic activity of the mature red cell could account for the curious disparity of ionic concentrations. The years of concentrated research on the subject have not yet given satisfactory answers.◄]

It should not be assumed that mammalian red cells of different species universally concentrate K+ and exclude Na+. While horse and human red cells concentrate K+, the red cells of cats and dogs contain much sodium but little potassium. A remarkable case is that of sheep, where Tosteson (12) has shown that one genetic type has high potassium inside the red cell, another rather low concentrations, although the Na+ and K+ concentrations in the plasma are identical. The type with high K+ was found to have over 100 times as great a concentration of the enzyme adenosine triphosphatase in the red cell membranes as the type with low K+. Significant understanding of the role of the "metabolic pump" in ionic transport may come out of this sort of research.

Metabolism of the Red Cell

The oxygen consumption (Qo_2) of suspensions of red cells is so low that the question may be raised whether it might not be due to the metabolic contamination by a small number of white cells and of nucleated immature erythrocytes. The Qo_2 is only 1/100th or less than the Qo_2 for liver and kidney cells. However, if the oxygen consumption is expressed in terms of the fixed framework only of the red cell, since this is only about 1% of the dry weight, the respiration of the red cell is appreciable and comparable to that of other living cells. The respiration of *reticulocytes* (nucleated immature red cells) is some 50 times greater than that of the mature nonnucleated red cell.

[► *Glycolysis* (metabolism without oxygen consumption) takes place in the red cell but is likewise very small, on the basis of the weight of the whole cell. The oxidative fraction of the total metabolism (oxidation plus glycolysis) is large (about 60%) compared with other cells. The metabolism of the red cell, small as it is on a weight basis, may be important in maintaining the cell membrane in its normal state of selective permeability. The cells of blood in storage deteriorate unless the proper nutrients are provided, as a series of papers by Denstedt and his co-workers (13) have shown. The metabolism is sufficient to be considered as maintaining a steady state, based on a metabolic pump and "active transport" (14).◄]

REFERENCES

1. Ponder, E.: *Hemolysis and Related Phenomena* (New York: Grune & Stratton, Inc., 1948).
2. Canham, P. B., and Burton, A. C.: Distribution of size and shape in populations of normal red cells, Circulation Res. 22:405, 1968.
3. Canham, P. B.: Difference in geometry of young and old human erythrocytes explained by a filtering mechanism, Circulation Res. 25:39, 1969.
4. Ponder, E.: Red Cell Structure and its Breakdown, in *Protoplasmatologia*, Vol. 2 (Vienna: Springer-Verlag, 1955), pp. 1–123.
5. Prankerd, T. A. J.: *The Red Cell: An Account of Its Chemical Physiology and Pathology* (Springfield, Ill.: Charles C Thomas, Publisher, 1961).
6. Shrivastav, B. B., and Burton, A. C.: Evidence from studies of birefringence of structure across the dimple region of red cells, J. Cell. Physiol. 74:101, 1969.
7. Canham, P. B.: The minimum energy of bending as a possible explanation of the biconcave shape of the human red cell, J. Theoret. Biol. 26:61, 1970.

8. Burton, A. C.: The Stretching of "Pores" in a Membrane, in Bolis, D., *et al.* (eds.): *Permeability and Function of Biological Membranes* (Amsterdam: North-Holland Pub. Co., 1970).

9. Schmitt, F. O.: Bear, R. S., and Ponder, E.: Optical properties of the red cell membrane, J. Cell. & Comp. Physiol. 9:89, 1936; 11:309, 1938.

10. Davson, H., and Danielli, J.: *Permeability of Natural Membranes* (London: Macmillan & Co., Ltd., 1943).

11. Peters, J. P.: *Body Water* (Springfield, Ill.: Charles C Thomas, Publisher, 1935).

12. Tosteson, D. C.: Active transport, genetics and cellular evolution, Fed. Proc. 22:19, 1963.

13. Denstedt, O., *et al.:* Studies of the preservation of blood: VII, Canad. J. Biochem. & Physiol. 37:69, 1959. (One of a series of similarly entitled articles published in this journal.)

14. Stein, W. D.: *The Movement of Molecules across Cell Membranes* (New York and London: Academic Press, 1967).

4

Homeostasis of Composition of Blood: Hemostasis, Clotting, Agglutination

"La constance due milieu interieur est la condition de la vie libre."—CLAUDE BERNARD (1813–1878).

Constancy of the Circulating Fluid

THE PRESERVATION of the "status quo" in blood may be considered in the following several aspects:

MAINTENANCE OF THE CHEMICAL CONSTITUTION OF PLASMA.—The concentrations of Na^+, K^+ and Ca^{++} in health are kept within very narrow limits, as is the concentration of sugar. These limits are so constant that relatively slight deviations are good indexes of diseased states. The homeostatic mechanisms that achieve this constancy are remarkable examples of the reflex and endocrine feedback that distinguishes the living organism. These controls, as well as the control of plasma volume, are discussed elsewhere in this series in the texts on endocrinology* and on kidney and water balance.†

HOMEOSTASIS OF THE FORMED ELEMENTS.— The concentration of red cells, white cells and platelets are also so well controlled to constant levels in health that counts of these elements give most important indexes of disease. The constancy in each case represents a steady state, in which the rate of production in the hemopoietic tissues balances the rate of removal or deterioration from the blood by trauma, toxic agents and the reticuloendothelial system.

HOMEOSTASIS OF THE VASCULAR BED.—A wound in the vascular bed would lead to loss of blood unless there was a hemostatic mechanism that was at once triggered into violent action (in local vascular reactions and in the clotting mechanism) to prevent further hemorrhage and to initiate repair of the blood vessel wall.

As Waugh (1) points out, the hemostatic system must be capable, not only of abrupt, almost explosive, activity to deal with massive hemorrhage, but also of well-controlled mild activity in repair of the continual damage to capillaries, which might lead to very slow but steady, and eventually serious, loss of blood.

The latter two aspects—homeostasis of the formed elements and homeostasis of the vascular bed—are discussed below, in principle only. Details regarding homeostasis of the formed elements are to be found in textbooks of histology and of pathology, and of homeostasis of the vascular bed (the biochemistry of clotting) in textbooks of biochemistry.

Life Span of the Red Cell

A simple equation aids in thinking about the steady state of the population of red cells in the blood:

$$\frac{dn}{dt} = P - Q$$

where $\frac{dn}{dt}$ is the rate of increase in the number of red cells in the blood, P is the rate of production by hemopoietic tissues and Q is the rate of destruction or elimination. In the steady state, there is no change with time; so:

$$\frac{dn}{dt} = 0 \text{ and } P = Q$$

---

*Tepperman, J.: *Metabolic and Endocrine Physiology* (2d ed.; Chicago: Year Book Medical Publishers, Inc., 1968).

†Pitts, R. F.: *Physiology of the Kidney and Body Fluids* (2d ed.; Chicago: Year Book Medical Publishers, Inc., 1968).

The problem for physiological research has been to determine P and Q separately in health and disease. Three general categories of methods have been available for this.

First, however, it is necessary to discuss what we mean by the term *life span*, as applied to the red cells. Whether or not the term is appropriate depends on how the rate of destruction of individual red cells varies with their "age," i.e., the time since they first appeared in the blood stream. To justify speaking of a true biological life span, the probability of the destruction of the red cells must be slight until a certain age is reached, and then greatly increased at later ages, as the cumulative effects of wear and tear *(aging)* reach a critical level. Of course, the resistance to aging may differ between individual cells, in some kind of normal distribution, so that the life span will be a mean of a population of individual life spans, having a distribution similar to that of Figure 4–1 *(top).* In contrast, if the destruction of the red cells, as by hemolysis in the blood, were *indiscriminate*, so that young cells were destroyed as readily as were old cells, we ought not to speak of

a true life span. Instead, we should use the term *half-life*, familiar in study of radioactive decay. The two views have been variously described (first by Schoidt [2]) as the *theory of longevity* versus the *theory of destruction*, or as the *intrinsic theory of destruction* (i.e., aging or longevity) versus the *extrinsic theory of destruction*. As explained later in this chapter, the two kinds of destruction would lead to very different shapes of curves of rate of change of number of red cells. Modern methods of investigation have allowed a decision to be made between the two views. The general conclusion is that, in normal physiology, *probability of destruction is, indeed, a function of age of the cell*; so it is justifiable to speak of the "life span." *In diseased states, however (e.g., hemolytic anemia), the increased rate of destruction is largely independent of the age of the cell*, and the curves follow the extrinsic theory. In this case, the results ought really to be expressed in terms of half-life rather than of life span. Differences in the two types of kinetics are pointed out after the three categories of methods are described.

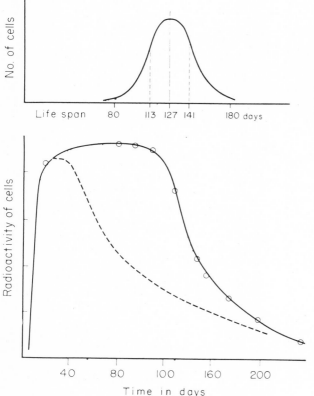

Fig. 4-1.—**Top**, distribution of life spans of cells deduced mathematically from the curve shown below. **Bottom**, *solid curve*, experimental results on labeled red cells in the blood after ingestion of radioactive glycine for 3 days. *Broken curve*, the exponential curve expected if the destruction of red cells is independent of their age (as in the case of hemolytic jaundice). (Redrawn from Shemin and Rittenberg [4].)

Methods of Measuring
Life Span of Red Cell

DISTURBANCE OF THE STEADY STATE

The oldest method of measuring the life span of red cells was to study a disturbance of the steady state. The red cell count was increased by a physiological stimulus (e.g., anoxia) to extra production or by a transfusion of packed cells of the same blood group. Alternatively, the red cell count might be reduced by bleeding or by the injection of a hemolytic agent. The rate of return of the red cell population toward normal was then taken to represent, in the case where the count had been *increased*, the normal rate of destruction of cells in the blood stream. In the case where the count had been *decreased*, the rate of return was taken as the normal rate of production and supply of cells to the blood stream. These two rates of production and of destruction are equal in the normal steady state.

These classic methods gave values of P and Q that would correspond to a life span of about 30 days only, much less than the value now accepted for the normal life span, which is 120 days. The reason for this very great discrepancy is that *disturbance of the normal red cell count at once calls into action the homeostatic control mechanisms*. A decrease in red cell count results in a stimulation of hemopoiesis, so that P is far greater than the normal rate. Similarly, an increase in red cell count suppresses hemopoiesis, and may possibly increase the rate of hemolysis Q. Indeed, it is the discrepancy between the results for the life span obtained by methods which disturb the steady state and those described below which is the best evidence for the existence of the control mechanisms. The mechanism of the stimulation or inhibition of hemopoiesis is still a subject of research (hemopoietins).

RATE OF EXCRETION OF END-PRODUCTS OR OF TURNOVER OF PRECURSORS

A second group of methods uses the rate of excretion of such end-products of red cell destruction as bilirubin, iron or urobilinogen in urine and feces. Results of these methods indicate values for the life span which do not agree at all for different end-products—for example, 20–40 days for bilirubin excretion, 54–200 days for urobilinogen excretion and 170 days for iron excretion. The fault in the methods is that, on the one hand, the breakdown of red cells is not the only source of these substances in the urine, and, on the other hand, a large proportion of the iron resulting from red cell destruction may be utilized again, rather than being excreted.

ADDITION OF IDENTIFIABLE (TAGGED) RED CELLS

Before modern methods of radioactive tagging of molecules, the *Ashby technique* (3) was ingeniously devised. In this technique, red cells from a donor, of compatible but different blood type, are injected into the blood of the recipient (e.g., O cells into an AB recipient). The number of the "foreign" cells surviving after different periods of time can be followed by *agglutination tests* with serums which will agglutinate the cells of the recipient but not the donor cells. When the ratio N/N_0 of the surviving cells to the number originally transfused is plotted versus time, a straight line results—that is, an equal number of cells is destroyed each day (since equal numbers of the injected population reach their life span) until the destruction is almost complete, when there is a tailing-off of the curve. The Ashby technique gave values for the life span of the red cell of the order of 120 days, the presently accepted value. The increase in total red cell count could be so slight that the control mechanisms changing P and Q were not stimulated.

The methods of radioactive tagging are much more easily used; they are free from the objection that the cells being followed are, after all, in an environment different from their own, for red cells taken from or made by the same subject may be "tagged." Two methods of tagging are used: (1) the subject synthesizes the tagged molecules by his own hemopoietic processes, from a radioactive precursor such as radioactively labeled glycine, which is fed for a few days; (2) cells are removed from the blood, labeled in vitro with radioactivity (usually by cromium) and reinjected. In both cases, the changes of radioactivity in the blood are followed by counts on samples withdrawn day after day. The curves are different in the two cases, as explained below, but the life span may be determined from either method. The second method can be criticized if it is not certain that the radioactivity incorporated in vitro is not completely immobilized (i.e., if it could leave the cells by diffusion exchange). *These methods agree on a normal life span of 120 days for human red cells*, with a distribution such that half of the cells reach their life span at between 113 and 141 days, the remainder lying outside these limits (Fig. 4–1, *top*).

KINETICS IN THE EXTRINSIC VERSUS INTRINSIC THEORIES

The curves of disappearance of the identifiable cells (either radioactive or serologically distinct) will be different according to whether the added cells are all of much the same age (as when the subject synthesizes them) or from a population of cells labeled outside the body, in which case cells of all ages up to the maximum will be represented. We have to consider, then, the curves to be expected in these two types of test, on the basis of the rival theories of extrinsic destruction (independent of age) and intrinsic destruction (dependent on senescence).

Let us suppose that the "longevity" or "senescence" theory applies and that all the cells are approximately the same age, with a moderate scatter about a mean age. When the subject is fed a labeled precursor, the rise of radioactivity in the blood is rapid and reaches a maximum in a very few days (Fig. 4–1, *bottom*). There will be no fall of radioactivity below this maximum until some of the cells reach the end of their life span (80–90 days, from Figure 4–1). After that, more and more of the cells will arrive at this point each day; so the fall will become steeper. Finally, as the higher age limit of the distribution of life spans is reached, the rate of fall will become less (the tail of the curve of Figure 4–1). This was exactly the shape of the curve found by Shemin and Rittenberg (4), and this proved conclusively that the senescence theory applied to the normal blood, which they were investigating. By mathematical analysis, a correction can be made for the fact that the cells were not all synthesized at the same time, but over a few days, and the true distribution curves (Fig. 4–1, *top*) of life span can be deduced.

If the senescence theory did not apply, but the theory of extrinsic destruction did, we would expect the number of cells to decline immediately after the maximum was reached; that is, when the synthesis was complete. As the total number of tagged cells declined, the rate of fall would decrease proportionately; that is, we would expect the exponential curve shown in the broken curve in Figure 4–1 *(bottom)*. Thus, when the added cells are all about the same age, the shape of the curve clearly indicates which theory is applicable.

Similarly, when blood is withdrawn, labeled and reinjected (or in the Ashby technique), different curves will result on the two theories. In this case, the reinjected sample will contain presumably equal numbers of cells of all ages up to the maximal age. On the senescence theory, the same number will reach senescence (or the end of their life span) each day. There will thus be a *linear* decline of radioactivity, tailing off only at the end because of the distribution curve of life spans (Fig. 4–2). If, however, there is destruction independent of age, the curve will again be exponential. (If age does not matter, the distribution of ages in the added cells cannot matter; so the two methods of experiment must give the same result—that is, the exponential curve.) In health, the curves are linear rather than exponential. Both methods of test, therefore, leave no doubt that in normal physiology the susceptibility to destruction of red cells depends on their age and that there is truly a "life span."

On the other hand, when similar experiments were made in states of hemolytic anemia, curves of the exponential type were found (by both methods of test), indicating that age does not influence the susceptibility to abnormal hemolytic agents very much. In this case, we can modify our original equation to

$$\frac{dn}{dt} = P - qn$$

where q is the rate of destruction, n being the number of cells. This will reach a steady state $\left(\frac{dn}{dt} = 0, \right.$ where the number of cells is given by $n = \frac{P}{q} \left. \right)$. The approach to the new

Fig. 4-2.—The decline of identifiable red cells in the blood when a sample of blood is withdrawn, labeled and reinjected (or when serologically identifiable cells are injected). *Solid curve,* linear fall (as in normal blood) in the senescence theory. *Broken curve,* exponential curve if destruction is independent of age (as in hemolytic jaundice).

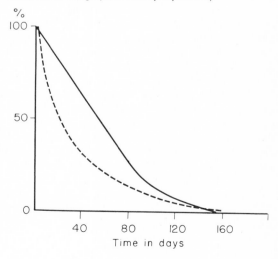

steady state will give an exponential curve (which is the solution by integration of the equation above). If the disturbance of normal conditions does not elicit the compensatory homeostatic mechanism of increased rate of production (P), the steady state value of n will be lower than normal, as it is in hemolytic anemia.

It was studies of this kind that led to the discovery of the importance of the *intrinsic* and *extrinsic factors* of hemopoiesis (e.g., liver therapy in pernicious anemia), for which Whipple, Murphy and Minot shared the Nobel prize in Medicine of 1946.

In addition, the techniques of injection of tagged red cells allow us to determine whether a case of accelerated destruction of red cells is due to an intrinsic factor (i.e., an increased fragility of cells) or to an extrinsic factor in the plasma (e.g., hemolysins), for the cells of a patient may be injected into the blood of a normal recipient, or normal cells into the blood of the patient.

Hemostasis: Bleeding Time and Clotting Time

It is important for the medical student to realize that the preservation of the integrity of the circulation involves more than just the clotting of the blood. Patients may have prolonged *bleeding time* yet a normal, or almost normal, *clotting time*. Trauma to small vessels (as of the skin, in a "nick" during shaving) results in constriction of the vessels so that the oozing soon ceases. The platelets seem to play the major role in this process, for prolonged bleeding time from small cuts is associated clinically with *thrombocytopenia* (low platelet counts). In distinction, patients who have real disturbances of clotting mechanism, as in *hemophilia* of various kinds, may have a normal bleeding time* when slight injuries to the skin occur but they cannot deal adequately with massive hemorrhage from damage to large vessels. Also, a marked reduction in platelet count is consistent with a normal clotting time.

The mechanism of the arrest of oozing from small vessels is not fully understood. [►Presumably, the platelets release a vasoconstrictor substance when in contact with injured tissue. Contact with blood proteins, particularly fibrinogen, fibrin and with muscle protein, also obvi-

ously assists in the hemostasis (e.g., use of fibrin in surgery).◄]

Mechanism of Clotting

Casual comments only will be made here in regard to the mechanism of clotting; texts on biochemistry should be consulted for details.

So many biochemical factors—enzymes, cofactors, accelerators and inhibitors—released from platelets, in the tissues or in the plasma, are now known to contribute to the mechanism of blood clotting that it is very difficult for the medical student to remember that the "backbone" of the process still depends on five stepwise reactions, each of which is the trigger for the next. The first is *physicochemical,* the next two *enzymatic* and the last two again *physicochemical.* David Waugh (1) has pointed out that the added complexity is probably made necessary by the two distinct functions required of the system. On the one hand, very well controlled clotting activity at a low level must be provided for the process of continual repair of small leaks in the vascular system. On the other hand, the system must be capable of being triggered into intense activity to deal with major crises of hemorrhage and trauma. Moreover, checks and balances must be provided so that this massive, rapid response may be confined to the area of trauma and does not lead to general intravascular clotting.

In spite of the very many complications, the backbone of coagulation is the sequence of reactions shown in Figure 4–3 and described below:

1. *The first physicochemical reaction: release of thromboplastins* (from platelets and from injured tissue). [►This takes place on the injured surface of the blood vessel wall, for it has been shown that there is a migration of platelets from the center of the blood in a beaker to the interface between the blood and the glass wall, and to the blood-air interface. If the glass of the beaker is coated with hydrophobic material, such as wax or silicones, this migration to the wall is not seen and clotting is much delayed.◄] The thromboplastins are enzymes that, once released and activated, catalyze the next step, which is the first in a chain of two biochemical reactions.

2. *The first biochemical reaction: prothrombin to thrombin.* Prothrombin, manufactured by the liver, is a protein always present in the blood in quantities large enough to clot the whole blood volume if it were converted to thrombin. The amount that is actually converted depends on the

---

*To obtain "bleeding time," a needle prick is made in the ear lobe; the oozing blood is removed every 20 sec by a swab, so that clotting is not involved; and the time is observed before bleeding ceases.

degree of trauma to the vessels, since this determines how much of the enzyme thromboplastin is released from damaged tissues and from the platelets that have migrated to the site of injury. Thrombin is the enzyme necessary to catalyze the next biochemical reaction.

3. *The second biochemical reaction: fibrinogen to fibrin.* Fibrinogen, a normal blood protein, does not form long fibrous threads, as does the fibrin into which it is converted. Calcium ions, as well as the enzyme thrombin, are necessary to the reaction.

4. *Another physicochemical reaction: condensation, or polymerization, of fibrin.* The fibrin forms long threads which link with each other to form the structure of the clot, enmeshing within it the red cells, plasma and platelets.

5. *The final physicochemical reaction: retraction of the clot.* A few minutes after the clot is

Fig. 4-3.—The backbone of clotting. Diagram shows the essential three physicochemical and two chemical reactions in blood coagulation. At the left are indicated the all-important accelerators and inhibitors which play a part in the autocatalytic activation and in the shutoff mechanisms (i.e., positive and negative feedbacks).

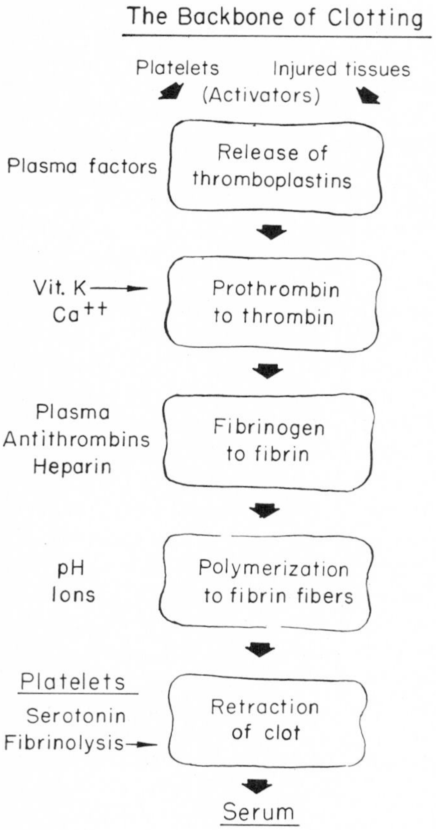

The Backbone of Clotting

formed, it begins to retract. [►The fibrin threads become folded or kinked, adhering to each other, squeezing the clot into a smaller volume and expressing the serum. The platelets probably play the key role in clot retraction, by releasing some activating substance, very likely *serotonin.*◄] Thus, by their control of the initiation of the whole chain in the release of thromboplastin, and of the clot by release of serotonin, the platelets are essential to the whole process. They are the "alpha and the omega" of clotting. The fibrin threads play a second role in hemostasis: by adhering to the walls of vessels and by retraction, they help to close a wound in the wall. This property has made fibrin preparations of very great assistance to the surgeon in controlling oozing of blood from cut surfaces.

The above five reactions are the essential ones in the mechanism of clotting, as depicted in Figure 4–3. To this skeleton, the student must add the many controlling systems of each step, described in textbooks of biochemistry or in review articles on the coagulation of blood. A few of these control systems are as follows:

a) The level of *prothrombin* in the blood depends on *vitamin K,* which controls the synthesis of prothrombin in the liver. The anticoagulant *Dicumerol* is antagonistic to this synthesis.

b) Platelet thromboplastin is not active until it is activated by a number of factors in the plasma, called *plasma cofactors.* Absence of these will prevent clotting, as in the congenital diseases *hemophilia* and *Christmas disease. Tissue thromboplastin* seems to be already primed to act when released from damaged tissues.

c) There are powerful *antithrombins* in the blood which inhibit its action in catalyzing the fibrinogen to fibrin reaction. *Heparin* is one of these, but it requires the cofactor *plasma antithrombin.*

[►The explosive features of massive clotting depend on "positive feedbacks," or "autocatalysis." Thrombin is probably the main substance contributing to this, for thrombin, itself formed by the action of thromboplastin, is said to activate thromboplastin. Since thrombin is an enzyme, it is not used up in its action in catalyzing fibrinogen to fibrin. One wonders, therefore, why, once the level of thrombin in the blood reaches some critical level, all of the fibrinogen in the blood is not converted to fibrin and the whole of the blood coagulated. Here is where the antithrombins present in plasma play their part. As long as the blood is free flowing, outside the area of the clot, thrombin will be checked by the supply of these antithrombins. Also, the fibrin threads of the clot may adsorb thrombin and so limit the coagulation to the place where it is required.◄]

Nomenclature of Clotting

The discovery and naming of many new factors in clotting led to such confusion that the International Committee for the Standardisation of Blood Clotting Factors was established in Basel in 1954 (Irving S. Wright, Chairman). Its most useful work has been published in many places (e.g., Canad. M. A. J. 80:659, 1959*). The factors are grouped into nine categories, with the many names that the various discoverers, or others, originally used for what may, in many cases, be identical substances. Factor VI is left vacant, evidently as a recognition that all is not known at the present stage of research. The International Committee's listing follows:

Factor I.—Fibrinogen

Factor II.—Prothrombin

Factor III.—Thromboplastin (tissue)

Factor IV.—Calcium

Factor V.—Synonyms:
Factor V (Owren)
Proaccelerin (Owren)
Labile factor (Quick)
Plasma Ac-globulin (Ware and Seegers)
Thrombogene (Nolf)
Proprothrombinase (Owren)
Prothrombokinase (Milstone)
PPCF—Plasmin prothrombins—conversion factor (Stefanini)
Component A of prothrombin (Quick)
Prothrombin accelerator (Fantl and Nance)
Co-factor of thromboplastin (Honorato)

Factor VII.—Synonyms:
Factor VII (Koller)
Proconvertin (Owren)
SPCA—Serum prothrombin conversion accelerator (deVries, Alexander)
Co-factor V (Owren)
Serozyn (Bordet)
Kappa factor (Sorbye and Dam)
Co-thromboplastin (Mann and Hurn)
Prothrombinogen (Quick)
Serum accelerator (Jacox)
Prothrombin conversion factor (Owren)

Prothrombin converting factor (Jacox)

Factor VIII.—Synonyms:
Factor VIII (Koller)
Antihaemophilic globulin (Patek and Taylor)
Antihaemophilic globulin A (Cramer)
AHF—Antihaemophilic factor (Brinkhous)
PTF—Plasma thromboplastic factor (Ratnoff)
Plasma thromboplastic factor A (Aggeler)
TPC—Thromboplastic plasma component (Shinowara)
Facteur antihemophilique A (Soulier)
Thromboplastinogen (Quick)
Prothrombokinase (Feissly)
Platelet co-factor (Johnson)
Plasmokinin (Laki)
Thrombokatilysin (Lenggenhager)

Factor IX.—Synonyms:
Christmas factor (Biggs and Macfarlane)
Factor IX (Koller)
PTC—Plasma thromboplastic component (Aggeler)
Antihaemophilic globulin B (Cramer)
Plasma thromboplastic factor B (Aggeler)
Plasma factor X (Shulman)
Facteur antihemophilique B (Soulier)

Agglutination of Red Cells, the Blood Groups and Transfusion

The surface of the red cell carries specific proteins, called *agglutinogens*, which, when brought into contact with other "foreign" proteins in the plasma, called *agglutinins*, combine to form protein attachments which will irreversibly cement red cells together, as shown by electron micrographs (Fig. 4–4). This clumping of cells together is called *agglutination*.

Each of the four main types of human blood—types O, A, B, AB—contains a specific kind of agglutinogen on the red cells, with its companion agglutinin in the plasma* (see Table 4–1). No reaction occurs between these in the normal combination found in any one type of blood, but plasma of another blood type will agglutinate the cells of the given type.

As originally discovered by Landsteiner in 1901, there are four main blood types in humans, each with a different combination of these factors. The combination of A and α, or B and β, will each react to cause agglutination. A plus β and B plus α (as in blood of types A and B) give no agglutination. Knowledge of the blood type of the donor's and recipient's blood is thus essential to a safe transfusion. The *important principle is that the*

---

*Long before this edition is published, there will certainly be more candidates for the list of factors advanced by those who discover them. Let us hope the International Committee periodically will review the list and tell the student just how many factors to remember and what to call them.

---

*The agglutinogens (A, B) are genetically inherited; but it is probable that the agglutinins, or antibodies (α, β), are not inherited but are elicited in early life as an antibody reaction to foreign proteins in food, etc.

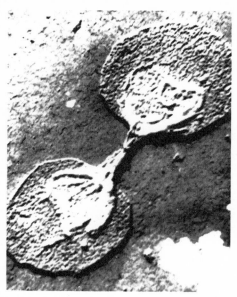

Fig. 4-4.—Electron micrograph of two red cells of type A blood agglutinated by anti-A serum, showing the protein fibers connecting the cells. (From Bessis and Bricka: Rev. hémat. 5:396, 1950.) From an original photograph kindly supplied by Professor Bessis.

donor cells must not, when introduced into the recipient's plasma, meet an agglutinin which would cause them to agglutinate and form thrombi, blocking the circulation. There is far less concern whether or not the plasma of the donor might agglutinate the cells of the recipient, for the agglutinins of the donated plasma will be very much diluted by the volume of recipient plasma, *unless the transfusion is massive.* Since O cells contain neither A nor B factors, agglutination of O cells is unlikely to occur when these cells are transfused into a recipient of any of the other types. In this sense, type O is called the *universal donor.* Similarly, since type AB has no agglutinins in the plasma capable of agglutinating with either A or B cell factors, persons of this type can, with moderate safety, receive transfusions of any type blood. Type AB individuals are therefore said to

be *universal recipients.* On the other hand, transfusions between type A and type B will certainly result in agglutinations. Type O, although the universal donor, can safely receive transfusion with only type O blood.

The interaction between the four main blood groups can easily be understood by studying Figure 4–5, invented by the author when a student. Blood of the same group should always be used, if possible, and the use of compatible but different bloods is for emergency only. *Cross-matching,* by incubating the donor cells with the serum of the recipient, to be sure that no agglutination will occur, is the only really safe precaution.

While the identification and separation of the four main blood groups involved a great deal of tedious and clever research, now that it is done, the *typing* of blood is a simple routine. Red cells of the patient whose blood is to be typed are mixed with serums known to be of type A and of type B. If there is no agglutination with either, the patient's blood is of type O. If there is agglutination with both, the blood is of type AB; if with type A serum alone, the blood is of type B; if with type B serum alone, it is of type A.

Not until 1940 was a second antigenic factor of great importance, the *Rh factor* (the name derived from the Rhesus monkey), discovered by Wiener and Peters. Before this discovery, unknown thousands of fetuses, and a smaller number of mothers, may have died from Rh incompatibility of the parents. Since the Rh factor has at least six important subtypes, and the Rh typing is, accordingly, complicated, the student is referred to textbooks of hematology and of medicine for details, as also for discussion of the inheritance of Rh factors. Knowledge of Rh factors is important, not only in questions of transfusion, but also in marriage counseling and in obstetrical management (since the blood of mother and fetus may come in contact by "leakage" past the placental barrier). About 85% of the white population is Rh-positive.

TABLE 4–1.—FACTORS IN BLOOD CAUSING AGGLUTINATION

BLOOD TYPE	SERUM FACTORS (AGGLUTININS)	RED CELL FACTORS (AGGLUTINOGENS)	% IN WHITE POPULATION
O	α, β (anti-A and B)	None	46
A	β (anti-B)	A	42
B	α (anti-A)	B	9
AB	None	A and B	3

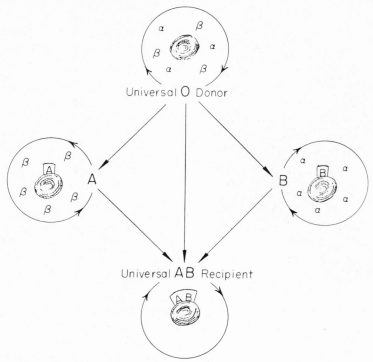

Fig. 4-5.—Diagram explaining the importance of blood groups in transfusion. The arrows show the permissible transfusions of blood (if not too massive) of the donor blood type (at the tail of the arrows) to the recipient (at the point). The circular arrows emphasize that transfusion with the identical group is the safest of all. Within the circles are shown the responsible cell factors (agglutinogens A and B) and the serum factors (agglutinins α and β).

REFERENCES

1. Waugh, D.: Blood Coagulation, A Study in Homeostasis, in *Biophysical Science: A Study Program* (New York: John Wiley & Sons, Inc., 1959), pp. 557–562.
   Also in *Reviews of Modern Physics*, April, 1959.
2. Schoidt, E.: On the duration of life of the red blood corpuscles, Acta med. scandinav. 95:49, 1938. Results of historical interest only; analysis good.
3. Ashby, W.: The determination of the length of life of transfused blood corpuscles in man, J. Exper. Med. 29:267, 1919.
4. Shemin, D., and Rittenberg, D.: The life-span of the human red blood cell, J. Biol. Chem. 166:627, 1946.

5

Viscosity and the Manner in which Blood Flows

"A lack of slipperiness between adjacent layers of a moving fluid."—SIR ISAAC NEWTON.

Laminar Flow

COHESIVE FORCES (forces of attraction) between blood and the blood vessel wall prevent the infinitesimally thin layer of plasma that is in contact with the wall from moving, even when the blood farther away is flowing. In other words, in blood, as in most aqueous fluids in contact with the walls of tubes, there is no "slip" at the wall, as there is in the case of some plastic fluids. It follows that when blood is forced through the blood vessels by the gradient of pressure, generated by the action of the heart, there must be a *gradient of velocity* across the vessel, with the highest velocity of flow along the axis of a cylindrical vessel (Fig. 5–1, *B*). The successive cylindrical "shells," or laminae, of blood, as one proceeds from the axis, move with decreasing velocity, until at the wall the velocity is actually zero. It is, therefore, a great mistake to think of the resistance to flow of blood as due in any way to a friction between blood and the wall of the blood vessel. The resistance is due, rather, to the friction between adjacent laminae of blood (i.e., the *inner friction*, or *viscosity*, of blood) as these laminae have to slide over each other with different velocities. The cases of flow in pipes that are usually dealt with in textbooks or handbooks of engineering are of *nonlaminar flow* (e.g., turbulent flow), and here the friction with the wall is a factor and the roughness of the wall may affect the resistance to flow. Not so with the normal flow of blood in the blood vessels, except in special places, as in the aorta, and near the heart valves, where flow may be nonlaminar at times.

Coefficient of Viscosity

The reason for the inner friction of a fluid, or, as Sir Isaac Newton brilliantly put it, for this *lack of slipperiness*, between the adjacent laminae, is that, although in laminar flow there is no gross exchange of fluid from one lamina to the next, molecular random motion, as well as motion of the particles in a suspension like blood, does take place from one layer to the next, transferring energy. The faster layer tends to speed up the slower layer in contact with it, and vice versa. The bigger the difference of velocity between the layers (i.e., the greater the "velocity gradient"), the greater the energy transfer. The degree to which this transfer takes place is measured by the *coefficient of viscosity* of the fluid.

Newton first formulated the equation of viscosity by which the coefficient of viscosity, η, is defined (see Fig. 5–1, *A*). This equation is in fundamental centimeter-gram-second (cgs) units; so the tangential force, F, is in dynes. The equation states that the tangential, or "drag," force (F) between the laminae is proportional to the area of contact between laminae and to the velocity gradient (i.e., the increase in velocity in centimeters per second for each centimeter distance at right angles to the direction of laminar flow). The unit of viscosity is the *poise*,* so named in honor of Poiseuille, the French physician who made the pioneer measurements of viscosity of water and other liquids (*ca.* 1820). A liquid of 1 poise vis-

---

*"Poiseuille" is pronounced "Pwas-ai-ye," but in English we do not pronounce the unit as "pwas," but as "poise" to rhyme with "boys."

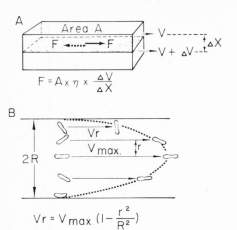

$$F = A \times \eta \times \frac{\Delta V}{\Delta X}$$

$$Vr = V_{max} \left(1 - \frac{r^2}{R^2}\right)$$

Fig. 5-1.—A, illustrating the fundamental definition of viscosity formulated by Sir Isaac Newton. The two *F*s are the tangential (drag) forces. The upper lamina is urged forward by the lower lamina with higher velocity, while the lower lamina is held back by the upper lamina. **B,** the parabolic distribution of velocity across the blood vessel that results from applying the Newtonian law (given below **A**) to the case of laminar flow of a Newtonian liquid in a cylindrical tube.

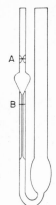

Fig. 5-2.—An Ostwald viscometer. The large bulb is filled with the test liquid through its vertical tube. Liquid is then sucked up into the narrow limb until the meniscus reaches a point above *A* then allowed to fall under its own hydrostatic pressure head. The time for the meniscus to pass between *A* and *B* is measured, first for the test liquid and then for the water, at the same temperature. The ratio of these times gives the relative kinematic viscosity (viscosity divided by density). If, as usually with aqueous fluids, the densities are the same, the ratio of times gives the relative viscosity.

cosity would have a force of 1 dyne per cm² of contact between layers, when flowing with a velocity gradient of 1 cm per sec per cm.

Since the commonest liquid encountered (i.e., water) turns out to have a viscosity of only about 0.01 poise at room temperature (21° C), the practical unit is the *centipoise* (equal to 0.01 poise). Water at room temperature has a viscosity of about 1 centipoise.

Measurement of Viscosity—
Viscometers

The measurement of viscosity has become very important in the control of industrial products (e.g., in the oil industry), as well as in basic physical chemistry. Special apparatus is used (e.g., the Couette viscometer), based on a different principle (rotating coaxial cylinders) from the original experiments of Poiseuille, where the flow was through cylindrical tubes. To assist in understanding the viscosity of blood, and the flow of blood in the circulation, only the *Ostwald viscometer* need be discussed here. This is nothing but a simple apparatus (Fig. 5–2) by which the time is measured for the flow of a fixed volume of liquid under a standard gradient of pressure through a length of glass capillary tube.

It is a simple matter, by the use of calculus, to proceed from the simple basic equation of Newton (given under Figure 5–1, *A*) to the prediction of the volume flow (milliliters per second) through a cylindrical tube under a given pressure difference (Δ*P*) between the ends of the tube (of radius *r* cm and length 1 cm) if the flow is laminar. In the first steps of this calculation, made first by Hagen, it is shown that for a *Newtonian fluid* (i.e., one that obeys the basic law of viscosity) the distribution of velocity across the tube must be *parabolic*, with the equation given under Figure 5–1, *B*. A third step of integration yields the famous Poiseuille formula:

$$F = \Delta P \times \left(\frac{\pi}{8}\right) \times \left(\frac{1}{\eta}\right) \times \left(\frac{r^4}{l}\right)$$

The term $\frac{\pi}{8}$ may be called the "numerical factor"; it arises in the course of the integrations of the calculation. The next term, $\frac{1}{\eta}$, is the "viscosity factor"; the last is the "geometrical factor," $\frac{r^4}{l}$. The surprise is that the radius enters to the *fourth power,* which means that the amount of flow depends very much on the size of tube. Halving the radius will reduce the flow to 1/16th of what it was, for the same pressure drop. Poiseuille established the law empirically, with quite remarkable accuracy.

Relative Viscosity

The measurement of absolute viscosity by a viscometer is very difficult to make accurately, particularly because the precision of the measurement of the radius of the tube is so important. It is much more convenient to "calibrate" the viscometer by timing the passage of water through it and to report the viscosity of the test liquid (e.g., blood) as the "relative viscosity," which is the ratio of its viscosity to that of water at the same temperature. (This will equal the ratio of the two

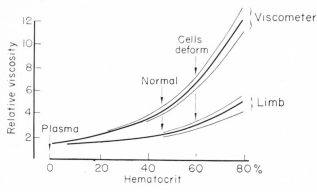

Fig. 5-3.—The increase of relative viscosity of blood with increasing hematocrit: *upper curve,* when a viscometer with diameter of tube greater than 1 mm was used; *lower curve,* when the vascular bed of the hind limb of a dog was used. (Redrawn from Whittaker and Winton: J. Physiol. 78:331, 1933.)

times—for the test with liquid and with water if the densities are the same).

Fortunately, although there is a large change in the viscosity of water with change in temperature (an increase of $2\frac{1}{2}$ times between 37° C and 0° C), the change (with temperature) of many aqueous fluids, including blood, is almost the same as that with water. As a consequence, the relative viscosity changes very little with the temperature at which the measurement is made. The relative viscosity of blood is between 3 and 4 for a normal

hematocrit of 45–50%. The high value is mostly due to the presence of the red cells, for the relative viscosity of plasma, due to the plasma proteins, is only about 1.8.

Dependence of Viscosity of Blood on Hematocrit

The relative viscosity of blood increases very greatly with increasing hematocrit; for example, if the hematocrit were 80%, the relative viscosity

Fig. 5-4.—**A,** illustrating the closest packing of red cells in the blood that is possible without deforming the red cell. This is hexagonal packing in sheets. It corresponds to a hematocrit of only 63%. (The dimensions in the drawing have been slightly altered to modern estimates in calculating this 63%.) **B,** a cross-section, 5 μ thick, of the blood in the femoral artery of a rabbit, quick-frozen in less than 0.1 sec as it rushed through the artery and subsequently prepared by freeze-substitution. Note: (1) Most of the cells are "on

edge," oriented by the shear; (2) they tend to be oriented with the major diameter parallel to the wall; (3) many of them are deformed by the crowding; (4) the cell-free layer at the wall is irregular and very thin. The hematocrit was 34%. *a,* Smooth muscle of arterial wall; *b,* internal elastic membrane; *c,* erythrocyte; *d,* nuclei of endothelial cells. (From unpublished work of R. H. Phibbs, Department of Biophysics, University of Western Ontario.)

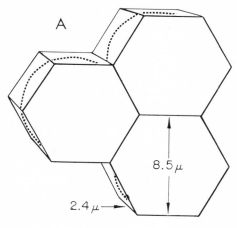

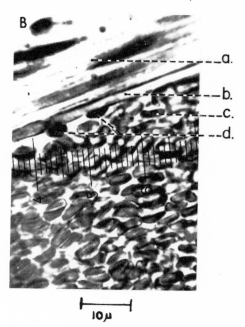

A

8.5 μ

2.4 μ →

B

a.
b.
c.
d.

10 μ

would reach 12 (Fig. 5–3, *upper curve*). At such hematocrits, we can hardly think of the blood as liquid rather than as solid. Even at normal hematocrits, the crowding of erythrocytes is great. To see the true picture, let us calculate how high a hematocrit would be possible before the cells would have to be deformed from their normal biconcave discoid shape. Each red cell could be enclosed as in a hexagonal prismatic box (Fig. 5–4, *A*), and the boxes could be laid side by side to make a sheet, and then the sheets piled on top of each other. No closer packing, *without deformation*, would be possible. With the values of Table 3–1 for the dimensions of the red cell (i.e., maximal diameter, 8.1μ; thickness, 2.7μ), the volume of each box would be 152μ³. The volume of the standard red cell is 95μ; so the hematocrit in this arrangement would be 95/152 × 100 = 63%. We learn, then, that *hematocrits of more than about 63% are not possible, even for blood at rest, without deformation of the cells*. With blood of normal hematocrit in motion, there must be a very great deal of bumping and deformation of the red cells (Fig. 5–4, *B*). In diseases such as *polycythemia vera*, hematocrits up to 70% are reported. In such cases, the cells cannot be of normal shape, and it is to be expected that obstruction of blood flow in the smaller vessels will occur.

The Optimal Hematocrit for Transport

Physiologists are accustomed to discovering cases where the prevailing conditions in living things are the best possible for function, i.e., biological adaptations that indicate how well the

Celestial Committee of Chapter 1 (or the process of evolution) has worked. One of the most remarkable is that the normal hematocrit differs in different species, e.g., camel 27%, goat 33%, sheep 32%, dog 46%, man 47%, and that in each case this is the *optimal value for transporting the most oxygen per unit time* in the circulation, assuming that the driving pressure (arterial B.P.) in a given species were kept constant. Increasing the hematocrit will allow more O_2 to be carried for a given rate of blood flow, but the viscosity will be increased so that the flow for a given driving pressure will be reduced. The optimal combination of these two factors corresponds to a maximal value for the ratio of hematocrit/viscosity. The increase of viscosity with hematocrit is different for blood of different species, since it depends on size, shape and flexibility of the red cell. Figure 5–5, redrawn from Stone *et al.* (1) shows the curves of η vs. hematocrit for the camel and for man, and the measured flow of blood, in terms of hemoglobin, through a tube, with constant driving pressure. The very sharp maxima for this correspond very well indeed with the normal levels of hematocrit in the two species. This is true for the other three species listed. (If we are given the curve of η vs hematocrit, we may draw a tangent from the origin to the curve. The point of contact is at the optimal hematocrit, since the slope of the line is the lowest value of η/Hct possible.)

Thus the transport of O_2 to the tissues is effected with the minimal expenditure of cardiac energy. However, in chronic anoxemia (decreased O_2 per ml blood), due to anemic disease or condi-

Fig. 5-5.—A, relative viscosity vs hematocrit for human blood and camel blood. **B,** the transport of oxygen through a glass tube vs hematocrit, with a constant driving pressure.

See text for explanation. (Redrawn from data of Stone, Thompson and Schmidt-Nielson [1].)

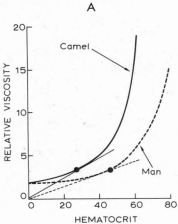

A

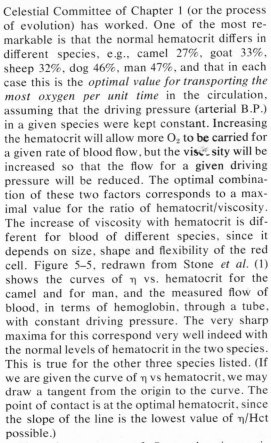

B

tions of high altitude, the hematocrit increases as a physiological compensation. The optimal conditions have to be sacrificed, and extra work of the heart is required.

Anomalies in the Viscosity of Blood

EFFECT OF SIZE OF TUBE

As long as the diameter of the capillary tube used in a viscometer is more than 1 or 2 mm, the relative viscosity of blood is the same, whatever the size of tube used. When, however, tubes of narrower diameter are used, the value for relative viscosity found is less (Fig. 5–6). This is because the absolute viscosity of water is the same however small the diameter of the tube, but that of blood decreases to less than half the value found when large tubes are used.

This has long been known as the *Fahraeus-Lindqvist effect.* [▶Although two different explanations have been offered, neither alone is really satisfactory for the results over a wide range of hematocrits. The first explanation is that "plasma skimming" occurs—that is, that next to the wall of the tube there is a relatively cell-free layer, which has a lower viscosity (that of plasma) than the rest of the blood. The smaller the tube, the greater the proportion of the whole that would consist of this cell-free or cell-poor "sleeve," and so the total effective viscosity would be less. The other explanation is that in the calculation by

which Poiseuille's law is deduced, we should not "integrate" as if the laminae were infinitely thin, unless the tube were large compared with the diameter of the red cells, which actually limits the thinness of the laminae. Instead of an "integration," we should, where there are only, say, 5 laminae across the tube, make a "summation" of five terms. The result would differ from Poiseuille's law.

We have, therefore, two theories, each quite plausible, for the Fahraeus-Lindqvist effect. One is based on a cell-free zone of given thickness (t) at the wall (no one really thinks that there is a marginal zone actually free of all cells); the other is based on the finite thickness (δ) of the thinnest laminae that could exist in blood. Haynes (2) has shown that neither theory is acceptable as the only explanation, over the whole range of hematocrits. For example, to explain the data, the minimal lamina thickness would be 30μ for hematocrits of 70%, 16μ for normal hematocrits and only 2μ for 20%. The last value does not seem plausible. In contrast, the thickness (t) of the marginal zone would be 1.8μ for 70% hematocrit, 2.8μ for normal hematocrit and 4.7μ for 20% hematocrit. A proper combination of the two theories would be plausible over the whole range.◀]

Whatever the explanation, the decrease of effective viscosity of blood with size of blood vessel is a real physiological factor. In the original work of Whittaker and Winton (Fig. 5–3), they

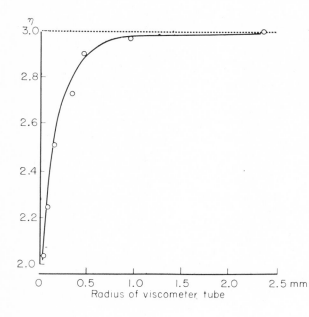

Fig. 5-6.—The decrease in relative viscosity of blood (η) when viscometers of very small-bore tube are used. The data are those of Kumin, analyzed by Haynes (2). For tubes of more than 1 mm radius, there is no further change in relative viscosity.

used not only an Ostwald viscometer of large bore *(upper curve)* but also the hind limb of a dog as their viscometer *(lower curve)*. The relative viscosities from the limb experiments were, at all hematocrits, less than half of those found in the glass viscometer. From the curves of Figure 5–3, this would be explained if the average diameter of the "resistance vessels" in the leg was about 55μ, which is about right for the arterioles, known to be the vessels offering the greatest resistance.

EFFECT OF VELOCITY OF FLOW; AXIAL ACCUMULATION

There has been a great deal of argument by physiologists about the fact that blood does not behave (even in rigid glass tubes) as a Newtonian fluid, but as one having *anomalous viscosity* (i.e., blood is a *non-Newtonian fluid*). The apparent viscosity decreases as the velocity of flow increases. The explanation undoubtedly involves the phenomenon of *axial accumulation of red cells*. As the velocity of flow increases, there is a greater and greater tendency of the red cells to move toward the axis of the tube, increasing the hematocrit there, while lowering it near the wall. Physical reasons for the force causing this axial drift have been advanced. They are much more complicated than the simple application of Bernoulli's principle that some textbooks suggest. [▶The matter need not be pursued further here, since, fortunately, it is now certain that the phenomenon of axial accumulation reaches a "saturation value"—that is, results in a maximal reorganization of the cells in the blood, at a velocity which is very low compared with the physiological velocities of blood flow in all types of vessels (3). Between blood that is still and blood that is flowing with a very small velocity, axial accumulation occurs and reduces the effective viscosity in the vessels, but further increases in velocity produce very little further change. Thus, in spite of this anomaly in the viscosity of blood, we are justified in using, as an approximation, an almost *constant viscosity coefficient in the physiological range of blood flow.*◀]

Axial accumulation has other consequences besides lowering the effective viscosity of flowing blood. A most interesting anatomical peculiarity of the arteries which leave the main trunk of the uterine artery has been described. The opening of the small artery, in adult female rats and other species, has an *arterial cushion* (Fig. 5–7), so that blood is withdrawn, or "sampled," from the axis

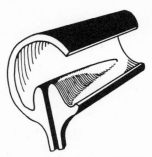

Fig. 5-7.—Drawing illustrating an arterial cushion where a side artery leaves its parent artery. (Adapted from Fourman and Moffat [4].)

rather than near the wall. In contrast, the mesenteric arterial branches have no such cushions. Fourman and Moffat (4) found that for the arteries with "cushions" the hemoglobin concentration (as an index of the hematocrit) was greater than in the parent artery, whereas for those without "cushions," the hemoglobin concentration was less than in the parent artery. Arterial branches of the kidney are said to have the same type of "arterial cushions." [▶It may be that axial accumulation of red cells makes possible, by such anatomical devices, some degree of selection of the relative "richness" of blood flowing to different organs.◀] Also, it has long been known that the hematocrit of capillary blood (obtained by needle prick of a finger) may be quite different from that of blood withdrawn from a vein. In calculations (e.g., of blood volume) which require the hematocrit, this may introduce considerable uncertainty.

Motion of Red Cells in Flow

The motion, even of a sphere, in the "shear gradient" of a flowing liquid is complicated, and that of nonspherical deformable particles is even more complicated. There is no doubt, on experimental evidence, that a very small degree of flow of blood results in an over-all *orientation of the cells*, where they have room to be oriented. For example, it is a very old observation that there is a marked change in the reflection of red light by blood between stagnation and a slight degree of flow. Müller (5) made a large-scale model of blood flow in an artery, pumping a fluid full of small rubber discs (to imitate erythrocytes) down a transparent tube. The orientation and continual rotation of the discs in the stream was obvious, and when the flow was speeded up, there was axial accumulation of the rubber discs. In general, there is continuous, but not uniform, rotation of particles in a shear gradient, which Mason and Bartok (6) cleverly photographed by using a Couette viscometer, in which the inner cylinder rotates in opposite direction to the outer cylinder. In this setup, there is a cylindrical layer in the fluid between, which is at rest relative to the observer, so that the motion of particles in this zone can be followed by cinematography. [►Results have been quite remarkable; they suggest that a good deal of the inexplicable behavior of particles in living cells, as well as in the blood stream, may be the result of "shear physics." As with axial accumulation, orientation effects soon reach a saturation value, at even lower velocities of flow than those that give saturation of axial accumulation.◄]

As intimate knowledge as to just how blood flows in the circulation increases, it is clear that, although it may be laminar flow on the macroscopic view, on a smaller scale there is nonlinear "microturbulence" with motion of plasma between the cells in all directions, and motion of the contents of the red cell within its membrane.

Importance of Flexibility of the Red Cells

At normal hematocrits, the blood is so crowded with cells that their flexibility (deformability) greatly affects the ease of flow. Goldsmith and Mason ingeniously invented methods of studying the motion and deformation of particles in very dilute suspension when flowing, by rendering the relative motion of an individual particle and a cine-camera zero. However, in blood of normal hematocrit, only the cells on the outside of the flowing column would be visible. By using suspension of biconcave ghost cells, up to high hematocrits, with a few "marker" cells containing hemoglobin, they have given us a picture of what happens to a red cell flowing down an artery or vein (Fig. 5–8). There is continued and quite marked deformation with constant collisions with other red cells. (An excellent review has been published [7].)

The relative viscosity of blood of 50% hematocrit is about 4. The cells of normal shape can be made rigid by treatment with glutaraldehyde, or other means. The relative viscosity of normal blood is reached at only 20% hematocrit with the rigid cells, and at 50% hematocrit the relative viscosity reaches 100 compared with 4 with normal cells. It is not known whether decreased flexibility of cells of normal shape occurs in disease, increasing the viscosity to pathological levels, but, in sickle cell anemia, the cells, if anoxic, sickle and show a relative viscosity many times that of normal cells. Sickle cell anemia cells, when oxygenated, have normal viscosity.

In normal physiology, there are many "feedback" mechanisms that operate to maintain constancy of conditions (homeostasis). The mechanisms work by *"negative feedback";* a deviation from normal results in a process which returns it toward normal. In disease, however, we may encounter *"positive feedback,"* leading to disastrous instability. The case of the blockage of peripheral vessels in sickle cell anemia is such an example. If there is a (normally temporary) stasis of red cells in the small vessels, the oxygen tension of the cells is reduced, they "sickle," viscosity increases greatly and the blockage tends

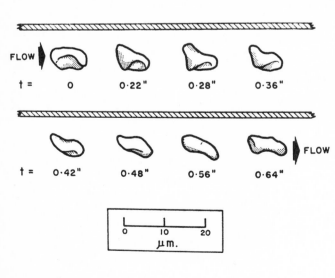

Fig. 5-8.—Tracings of photomicrographs showing the distortion of the shape of a human erythrocyte flowing in a 70% ghost cell suspension contained in a tube, radius 47 μ, from left to right at 200 μ/sec. (From Mason and Goldsmith [7].)

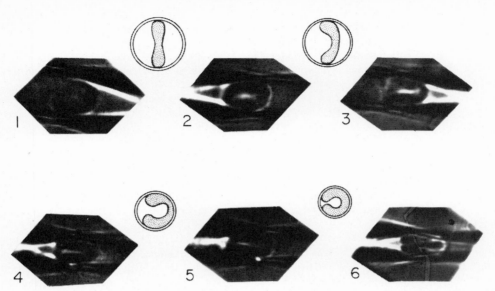

Fig. 5-9.—Phase contrast micrographs showing the way in which a red cell can be forced, with a very low pressure of less than 1 mm H₂O, through a micropipet with a diameter at the tip of only about 3 μ. In *1*, there is room for the cell to be the normal shape. In *2–6*, it reaches successively narrower parts of the pipet and a folding (like an apple turnover) occurs. The diagrams indicate what the cross-sectional view would be at different stages. (From work of P. Rand, Department of Biophysics, University of Western Ontario.)

to become permanent. The markedly "episodic" character of peripheral vascular troubles in sickle cell anemic patients is consistent with this "positive feedback."

How Blood Flows through Capillaries

The smallest blood vessels (i.e., the capillaries) are comparable in diameter with the erythrocytes themselves, and many capillaries are a good deal smaller, perhaps down to 5μ diameter, or less. The picture of blood flow in capillaries should be that of red cells passing one at a time, in tandem, with segments of plasma trapped between them. It is obvious that all the discussion above—as to a parabolic distribution of flow across the stream, Poiseuille's law, axial accumulation of cells and orientation of cells—has no real meaning when applied to this part of the vascular bed.

There has been a preliminary exploration of the physics of capillary flow (8), in which this kind of motion, called *bolus flow,* has been observed in large-scale models, and in actuality by forcing red cells themselves through micropipets. The normal red cells are quite astonishingly deformable into an over-all sausage shape and are able to pass through pores (of millipore filters) down to 3μ diameter under a very low head of pressure (less than 3 cm of water), emerging intact, unhemolyzed and resuming their normal shape.

Work on the deformability of red cells with high-power microscopy and a micromanipulator (by Rand) has dramatically shown the remarkable deformability of the normal red cells and possibly how they pass through the small capillaries. Figure 5–9 shows how a red cell can be forced, with a pressure drop of less than 1 mm of water, out of a micropipet of only about 2μ bore at its end. The cell curls, or folds, about a diameter, like an apple turnover, and so enters the narrow bore. In addition, cells may be sucked into the mouth of such a pipet, also with a very low pressure gradient; in this case, they appear to develop a sausage-shaped pseudopod that advances into the pipet. Changes in rigidity of the membrane, which no longer permit such deformations, occur on swelling the cell (stretching the membrane).

The motion of the plasma trapped between successive red cells proceeding in tandem through a capillary is also of interest (Fig. 5–10). The plasma on the axis moves forward at about twice the velocity of transport of the cells, catches up to the red cell ahead, turns sideways to reach the wall and there waits for the following cell to catch up. As a result, to an observer traveling down the tube with the red cells, the motion of the "interbolic plasma" is circus-like, and there are at least 10 circuits in the length of a capillary. [►By the use of models and "modeling theory," which allow predictions for the actual case of the small

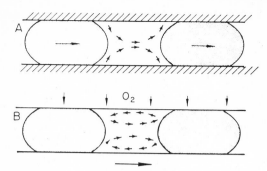

Fig. 5-10.—Illustrating the motion in the plasma between the red cells in bolus flow. **A,** the actual motion, that is, there is not an actual backward flow at the wall. **B,** the mixing motion as seen by an observer moving with the red cells. This mixing motion greatly facilitates the equilibration with the blood of gases coming through the wall, as in the pulmonary capillaries. (Adapted from Prothero, J., and Burton, A. C.: The physics of capillary flow, Biophys. J. 1:566, 1961.)

dimensions of the capillary, it has been shown that this curious mixing motion of the plasma significantly speeds up the equilibration of gases between the blood and the tissues, or in the lungs with the alveolar gases.◄] In addition, the motion described involves changes in direction and flow, which are equivalent to accelerations and decelerations, involving energy dissipation. Research as to the energy involved, and thus the equivalent value for viscosity that should be employed if a Poiseuille-like formula were used for the flow-

pressure relation, has shown that the energy losses are neglibible (because of the exceedingly slow velocity of blood flow, about 1 mm per sec in capillaries). Experimentally, with blood forced through micropipets, it has been shown that a relative viscosity of only about 2 applies, and this includes all the losses—that is, the energy to deform the red cell, the friction between the cell itself and the capillary wall, as well as the viscous dissipation in the mixing motion of the trapped plasma. Evidently the Celestial Committee on Design of the Circulation, referred to in Chapter 1, knew of devices to accomplish their purpose of which modern engineers have been unaware. It is interesting that engineers who work on transport of substances by pipe lines have belatedly rediscovered the Fahraeus-Lindqvist (or Scott Blair) effect (Fig. 5–6). Ore or coal may be carried as a "slurry" of powder in water, in small or large lumps or in special capsules. Jensen and Ellis (9) report, "Experiments showed the most favorable (least energy required for a given flow) cylindrical or spherical capsules were those large enough to fill 90 to 95% of the pipe diameter. The driving of a slurry calls for a greater consumption of pumping power."

The picture (Fig. 5–10) of red cells proceeding through capillaries in "bolus flow" that has been given should probably be modified for the smallest vessels of the pulmonary vascular bed. Both light and electron microscopic pictures show

Fig. 5-11.—Illustrating the sheet-flow nature of the pulmonary capillary flow. Photomicrographs of the cat lung, perfused with a transparent silicone elastomer, displacing the blood and then hardened for sectioning. **A,** in "plan," and **B,** in elevation. *P,* "posts" separating the two alveolar-

capillary membranes. *V,* the vascular space between the "posts." (Unpublished.) (Kindly supplied by S. Sobin of University of Southern California, School of Medicine, Los Angeles, and Y. C. Fung, Professor of Engineering, University of California, San Diego.)

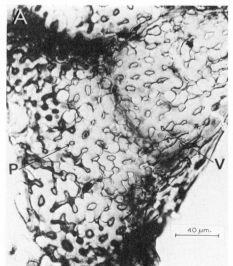

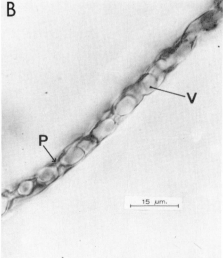

these to be larger in diameter, sometimes capable of accommodating two red cells abreast. Instead of thinking of a tube down which cells flow, we might better visualize two bedsheets, joining together in spots (quilted) that were quite widely spaced. The blood flows in the extended spaces between these places of contact, so that as much as 70% of the inner surface membrane of alveoli may be in contact with blood (Fig. 5–11). Perhaps "pulmonary sinusoids" would be a more appropriate term than "pulmonary capillaries." Sobin *et al.* (10) measured, by injection, the volume of the alveolar vascular channels of the cat's lung and found it to be 91% of the total tissue volume. Their data corresponded to a model of connected hexagonal chambers, each with a post or column (4μ diameter) in the middle (distance apart of the posts 9μ), separating the "floor" and "roof" of the chamber by 8μ (i.e., the sheet thickness).

Summary

A realistic picture of how blood flows in the circulation reveals the variety and complexity of what is occurring in vessels of different sizes, and of the motion of the blood itself. This picture is very far removed from that of the ideal simple liquids that are treated by simple physical laws based on normal Newtonian viscosity. Nevertheless, by fortunate circumstances, the actual laws of blood flow—at least in the range of physiological rates of flow—approximate sufficiently the simple laws (e.g., Poiseuille's law) for us to apply those laws with caution, using the appropriate value for the effective viscosity rather than that obtained in viscometers of large bore.

REFERENCES

1. Stone, H. O.; Thompson, H. K., Jr., and Schmidt-Nielson, K.: Influence of erythrocytes on blood viscosity, Am. J. Physiol. 214:913, 1968.

2. Haynes, R. H.: Physical basis of the dependence of blood viscosity on tube radius, Am. J. Physiol. 198:1193, 1960.

3. Haynes, R. H., and Burton, A. C.: Role of the non-Newtonian behavior of blood in hemodynamics, Am. J. Physiol. 197:943, 1959.

4. Fourman, J., and Moffat, D. B.: The effect of intra-arterial cushions on plasma skimming in small arteries, J. Physiol. 158:374, 1961.

5. Müller, A.: Abhandlungen zur Mechanik der Flüssigkeiten mit besonderer Berücksichtigung der Hämodynamik; Ströme in Röhren; Strömung von Suspensionen in Röhren, Arch. Kreislaufforsch. 8:245, 1941.

6. Mason, S. G., and Bartok, W.: The Behavior of Suspended Particles in Laminar Shear, in *Rheology of Disperse Systems* (London: Pergamon Press, 1959), pp. 16–48. (See also a long series of papers by Mason *et al.* in Colloid Science, the latest of which is in 17:448, 1962.)

7. Mason, S. G., and Goldsmith, H. L.: The Flow Behaviour of Particulate Suspensions, in Wolstenholme, G. E. W., and Knight, J. (eds.): *Circulatory and Respiratory Mass Transport* (London: J. & A. Churchill, Ltd., 1969), p. 196.

8. Prothero, J., and Burton, A. C.: The physics of capillary flow: I. The nature of the motion, Biophys. J. 1:566, 1961; II. The capillary resistance to flow, 2:199, 1962; III. The pressure required to deform erythrocytes, 2:213, 1962.

9. Jensen, E. J., and Ellis, H. S.: Pipelines, Scient. Am. 216:62, 1967.

10. Sobin, S. S.; Tremer, H. M., and Fung, Y. C.: Morphometric basis of the sheet flow concept of the pulmonary alveolar microcirculation in the cat, Circulation Res. 26:397, 1970.

The Vascular Bed

Arrangements of the Many Vessels

"A mind, nimble and versatile enough to catch the resemblances of things, and at the same time steady enough to fix and discern their subtle differences."—FRANCIS BACON (1650).

Introduction

A SENSIBLE MAN, if he were appointed to be a member of a river conservation authority, would make it his first task to become thoroughly acquainted with the whole of the river bed, the sources of the rivulets, their successive confluences, the depth and width of the contributing streams, the volume of water, the volume flow and the fall in height in all the branches and in the final river. So it should be with the student of the circulation. The first requirement is thorough familiarity with the vascular bed.

Routes from Arterial to Venous System

We first consider the large number of routes by which blood may flow from the high-pressure side of the circulation (i.e., the aorta) to reach the low-pressure side (i.e., the vena cava). These routes are *in parallel;* that is, the flow through each of them is not directly affected by the presence of the other routes (although there is an indirect effect), but only by the driving pressure, namely, the difference between the high aortic pressure (about 100 mm Hg mean pressure) and the low venous pressure. There are thousands of such parallel routes, which can be divided into different categories, according to their patterns, as depicted in Figure 6–1 (originally devised by H. D. Green [1]). These categories are:

A. Simple routes, where a single capillary bed is perfused in each route. Most of the routes in the body are of this type—for example, the circulation of the head and limbs, the coronary circulation, the hepatic circulation (the liver has a double circulation).

B. Routes where two capillary beds are arranged *in series*. The example here is the kidney, where the glomerular capillaries are in series with the capillaries surrounding the tubules.

C. Even more complicated routes, where more than two capillary beds are perfused. The example is the portal system, where the capillaries of the spleen are in parallel with those of the mesentery and both are in series with the capillaries or sinusoids of the liver.

D. The pulmonary circulation is, of course, different, in that it is a route from the high-pressure side of the right heart to the low-pressure side of the left heart, not a route from aorta to vena cava.

E. The bronchial circulation is unique, in that it constitutes a route, or shunt, across the left heart only.

Another difference is the location of "control points" (X in Fig. 6–1)—that is, the vessels which by their constriction, from the smooth muscle contraction in their walls, can control the flow through vascular beds. These control points are the *arterioles*, for reasons that will become apparent. Thus, in category A, there is a single set of control points, before the single capillary beds. In categories B and C, there are multiple sets. Both the mesenteric and splenic vascular beds are controlled by their arterioles, and there is evidence that arterioles, or their equivalent, control the flow in the liver also. The renal circulation, with its two capillary beds in series, also has two sets of arteriolar controls in series—namely, the preglomerular *(afferent)* and the postglomerular *(efferent)* arterioles. The variety of effects on pressures, and on flow, that is possible by the independent constriction of these is obvious.

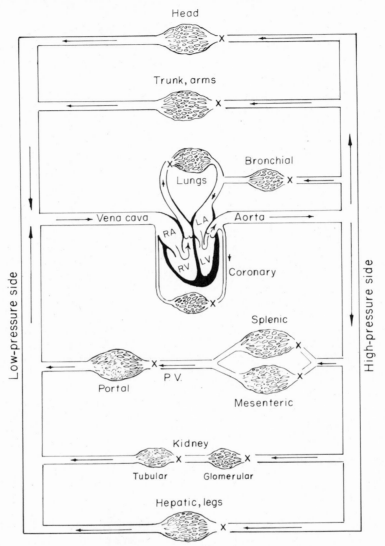

Fig. 6-1.—Arrangement of the parallel routes by which the circulation passes from the aorta to the vena cava. Representatives of the different categories of route discussed in the text are indicated. The *X*s indicate the location of control points where arterioles may control the flow. *RA*, right atrium; *LA*, left atrium; *RV*, right ventricle; *LV*, left ventricle; *PV*, portal vein. (From Green [1].) (Original illustration kindly furnished by H. D. Green.)

Category E, the bronchial circulation, although not an important route as to volume of flow, is unique in that it represents a route from the aorta to the "venous" side of one side of the heart only (from aorta to pulmonary veins), while all the other routes (except the pulmonary) are across both sides of the heart. The functional significance of this is discussed later, in Chapter 16.

[►Modern evidence shows that we must consider that here there are physiological control points in the pulmonary circuit—that is, the small pulmonary arteries—although how much control these exercise in health is not yet clear.◄]

Elements in Series within Each Route

Within each of these main routes there are many elements in series, each element consisting of many similar vessels in parallel with one another. The blood proceeds from a main artery, through many parallel distributing arteries and many more arterioles, to millions of capillaries. From these it converges from venules, collecting veins, to a main vein, emptying finally into the vena cava. Our quantitative knowledge of the details of the successive branching and of the dimensions of the different vessels is based on some painstaking work of a German histologist on the mesenteric vascular bed of dogs (Mall, 1888). Physiologists have come to rely on this data, hoping that the main features are typical of vascular beds in general. The figures are given in Table 6-1.

It will be noted in Table 6-1 that every time there is branching in the system into a larger total number of vessels in parallel, the total cross-sectional area of the vascular bed increases, until at the level of the mesenteric capillaries it has reached some 800 times that of the aorta. From that point on, the vessels converge, and the total cross-sectional area decreases until that of the vena cava is only 50% more than that of the aorta (Fig. 6-2). The great increase in area at the capillaries is due to the fact that, although each is so very small, there are over a billion (U.S.)* of them in parallel.

---

*A British billion is a million million (i.e., 10^{12}), but in the United States a "billionaire" has only a thousand "megabucks" (i.e., 10^9). This ensures that there are more billionaires in the United States than in the United Kingdom.

Volume of Blood in Different Vessels

From the same data (Table 6-1) the distribution of volume in the circulation may be calculated. It appears that the great proportion of the volume in the mesenteric bed is on the venous side, 80% being beyond the capillaries. It is a fact that by far the greatest part of the total blood volume of an animal is in the veins, venules and capillaries. Again, although the volume in each capillary is minute (of the order of 5×10^{-8} ml), there are so very many capillaries that the total capillary volume is 10% of the whole (500 ml for man). In *fainting,* there is a remarkable dilation of the capillaries of the muscles (which constitute 50% of the total body weight), and the capacity of the capillary bed then becomes a very significant proportion of the whole blood volume. It is fair to say that, in a faint *(syncope),* one bleeds into one's own capillary bed, and the fall in blood pressure results from this. The increase in volume of the arm muscles in a faint can easily be demonstrated by plethysmographic studies (the arm is placed in a volume-measuring plethysmograph).

Bazett collected data on blood volumes in man from many sources. The results of his work are given in Table 6-2.

The total blood volume is distributed between the greater, or systemic, circulation and the lesser, or pulmonary, circulation in the ratio of about 2 to 1.

TABLE 6-1.—GEOMETRY OF MESENTERIC VASCULAR BED OF THE DOG*

KIND OF VESSEL	DIAMETER (Mm)	No.	TOTAL CROSS-SECTIONAL AREA (Cm²)	LENGTH (Cm)	TOTAL VOLUME (Cm³)	
Aorta	10	1	0.8	40	30	
Large arteries	3	40	3.0	20	60	
Main artery branches	1	600	5.0	10	50	
Terminal branches	0.6	1,800	5.0	1	25	
Arterioles	0.02	40,000,000	125	0.2	25	
Capillaries	0.008	1,200,000,000	600	0.1	60	
Venules	0.03	80,000,000	570	0.2	110	
Terminal veins	1.5	1,800	30	1	30	
Main venous branches	2.4	600	27	10	270	740
Large veins	6.0	40	11	20	220	
Vena cava	12.5	1	1.2	40	50	
					930	

*Data of F. Mall.

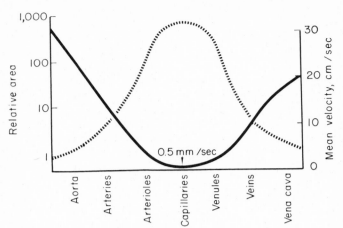

Fig. 6-2.—Schematic graph showing: *broken line*, the changes in relative total cross-sectional area (on a logarithmic scale) of the vascular bed; *solid line*, the mean velocity in the different categories of vessel.

In health, this ratio is remarkably constant, and it is evident that important control mechanisms exist that keep it so. The striking feature of cardiovascular disease, particularly *heart failure*, is that this regulation no longer seems to operate, and the partition of volume between the two systems may be grossly abnormal, with much greater proportion in the pulmonary bed. This leads to rise of pressure in the pulmonary circulation and left heart. Pulmonary edema rapidly results from the rise in pulmonary capillary pressure. (A discussion of some of the reflex controls that normally keep the volume partition accurately will be given in later chapters.)

Table 6–2 also shows that, while the veins

TABLE 6–2.—APPROXIMATE ESTIMATES OF BLOOD DISTRIBUTION IN VASCULAR BED OF A HYPOTHETICAL MAN, AGE 30, WEIGHT 63 KG, HEIGHT 178 CM, BLOOD VOLUME (ASSUMED) 5.2 L*

PULMONARY	VOLUME (Ml)	SYSTEMIC	VOLUME (Ml)
Pulmonary arteries	400	Aorta	100
Pulmonary capillaries	60	Systemic arteries	450
Venules	140	Systemic capillaries	300
Pulmonary veins	700	Venules	200
		Systemic veins	2050
Total pulmonary system	1,300	Total systemic vessels	3,100
Heart 250 ml		Unaccounted 550 ml	

(Probably extra blood in reservoirs of liver and spleen)

*Data from H. C. Bazett.

should be thought of as the important *reservoir* of the vascular bed, other reservoirs exist. The chambers of the heart can act as reservoirs, for normally they are never completely emptied at the end of each heartbeat; in fact, as much or more volume is left at the end of each beat (end diastolic volume) than is ejected in each beat (stroke volume). The liver and spleen are also reservoirs of blood volume.

Volume Distensibility of Vascular Bed

The term "reservoir" implies the capacity to accept a very great increase in blood volume without much rise in blood pressure (just as a city's water reservoir can accommodate much increase in quantity of water without much rise in level). The veins have a very great *volume distensibility*, compared with the arteries (Fig. 6–3); consequently, the volume of blood can increase in them many times with a rise in pressure of only a few millimeters of mercury (mm Hg). The fact that the large veins are normally almost closed (they collapse like surgical drainage tubing) is largely responsible for their very great volume distensibility, which is defined as follows:

$$\text{Volume distensibility} = \frac{\% \text{ increase in volume}}{\text{Increase in pressure (mm Hg)}}$$

As the pressure within the veins increases, they become more circular in cross-section. After they are cylindrical, the distensibility is very much reduced (Fig. 6–3), so that much more pressure is required to increase the volume still more. This is because the wall of veins contains a strong "jacket" of relatively unstretchable collagen fibers.

As a consequence of the very great relative

volume distensibility of the veins, where blood volume is lost by *hemorrhage,* or increased by *transfusion,* the decrement or increment of blood volume is lost or taken up by the venous system. Similarly, when the pressure within veins is changed by changes of posture (the pressure in the veins of the legs greatly increases when one stands up), there tends to be a very great shift of blood into the dependent vessels. This would seriously embarrass the circulation were it not for compensatory reflexes that are elicited (Chapter 21).

Mean Velocity of Flow in Vascular Bed

The mean velocity of flow in different parts of the vascular bed may easily be deduced from the geometry of the vessels, given in Table 6–1. A common-sense law of flow, called the *equation of continuity,* states that the product of the total cross-sectional area and the mean velocity must remain the same throughout the vascular bed. For (as in Figure 6–4) let the cross-sectional area be A cm² (whether of a single vessel like the aorta or the total area of the billion capillaries in parallel), and the mean velocity be v cm per sec. Then in 1 sec the volume that will have passed a fixed cross-section is obviously $A \times v$ ml. Unless blood is lost by leakage outside the system somewhere on the way, this product, $A \times v$, must be invariant, and equal to the total volume flow, V (i.e., the cardiac output). It follows that:

$$v = \frac{V}{A}$$

The human aorta is about the diameter of one's thumb—say 2 cm. Its cross-sectional area is thus about $\pi \times 1^2$, or 3 cm². Since the cardiac output of a man at rest is about 5L per min, or 83 ml per sec, the mean velocity in the aorta is given by:

$$v \text{ aorta} = \frac{83}{3} = 28 \text{ cm/sec } (\textit{Remember 30 cm/sec})$$

This will be the *mean* velocity. Actually, the flow is pulsatile, with a much higher velocity than this (perhaps 3 times) in systole and much less in diastole.

We deduced this mean velocity in the aorta purely from knowledge of the cardiac output and the geometry of the aorta. The value agrees well with velocities that have been measured, in anesthetized animals, by the use of special devices—for example, electromagnetic flowmeters, or the hot-wire anemometer, placed on or in the aorta. In exercise, the cardiac output may be increased up to 4 times the resting value, and the mean velocity is proportionately increased, to more than a meter per second.

From this estimate, we may easily deduce the mean velocity elsewhere than in the aorta, by multiplying by the ratio of the cross-sectional areas. For example, the cross-sectional area of the vena cava is 50% more than that of the aorta. The mean velocity in the vena cava is then about two-thirds that of the aorta (i.e., about 20 cm per

Fig. 6-3.—Comparison of the distensibility of the aorta and of the vena cava. The way in which the cross-section of the vessels changes in the two cases is also indicated.

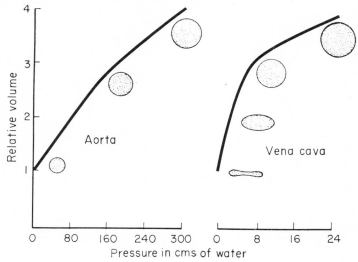

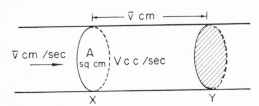

Fig. 6-4.—A glimpse of the obvious. A cross-section of the blood which will be at *X* at one moment and then will be at *Y*, $\bar{v}$ cm down the tube, 1 sec later (where $\bar{v}$ is the mean velocity of flow). The volume that has passed *X* in 1 sec is, therefore, $V = \bar{v} \times A$ (the cross-sectional area). The same applies if *A* is the total cross-sectional area of many tubes in parallel instead of a single tube.

sec for the resting state). This is a fairly high velocity and contradicts any naïve idea that the flow in veins is sluggish. Such an idea might result from mistakenly thinking of the slow bleeding from a cut vein, compared with the spurting of a cut artery. The velocity of escape of blood in a hemorrhage is governed, not by the velocity of flow in the vessel, but by the gradient of pressure from the vessel to the atmosphere. This is only a very few mm Hg in the case of veins, 100 mm Hg in the case of arteries. The velocity of flow in veins is, in fact, comparable to that of arteries.

Figure 6–2 illustrates the different mean velocities in different parts of the whole vascular bed, deduced from the geometry, and verified as to order of magnitude, in many cases, by experiment or observation.

Mean Velocity, Circulation Time and Flow in Capillaries

Similarly, since at the capillary bed the cross-sectional area has increased to 800 times that of the aorta, the mean velocity must have fallen to 1/800th of that in the aorta—that is, to about 0.4 mm per sec *(Remember 1 mm/sec)*. This agrees with direct microscopic observation of capillaries, where they are visible (as in the sclera, or mesenteric membranes of animals) and where one can time the progress of red cells across the reticule of the microscope.

Capillaries vary greatly in length, but the average is of the order of 1 mm. On the average, therefore, if the velocity is from 0.5 to 1 mm/sec, it takes red cells of the order of 1–2 sec to traverse capillary beds. This is all the time that is available for the exchange of respiratory gases between the blood and the tissues, or, in the case of the pulmonary capillaries, with the alveolar spaces. The small size of the capillaries (which gives a

very high ratio of wall area to volume), the mixing motion of bolus flow (described in Fig. 5–10, Chapter 5) and the presence of special accelerating enzymes (such as *carbonic anhydrase*) in the blood and the red cell make this short time quite adequate.

The fantastic number of capillaries in parallel in the body is emphasized if the volume flow in a single capillary is calculated. Let us take the estimates already made. The cross-sectional area of a single capillary will be, if the diameter is 8μ, about $\pi \times (4 \times 10^{-4})^2$, or about 5×10^{-7} cm^2. Multiplying this by the mean velocity of 0.4 mm per sec, we obtain for the volume flow about 2×10^{-8} *ml/sec*. At this rate, for 1 ml of blood to pass through a single capillary takes 5×10^7 sec, which amounts to about 1 year and 8 months. For 1 mm^3 of blood, it takes about 14 hours. Yet the heart manages to push at least 5L/min through the whole capillary bed. This is possible because of the billion or so of capillaries in parallel. No wonder the fact of the actual circulation of blood so long escaped detection by the early physiologists, until the genius of Harvey conclusively proved it by logic, even though he was unable to see the capillary bed.

Measurement and Meaning of Circulation Time

Formerly, the measurement of the *circulation time* between two points in the vascular bed was a popular one. It is still an interesting measurement, but it has been realized that the interpretation of a circulation time, without additional information, is very limited and that it cannot be used as an index of volume flow of blood.

The *total circulation time*, or *recirculation time*, is measured by injecting rapidly an identifiable marker, such as a dye, a radioactive tracer or a fluid of different electrical conductivity, into a peripheral vein (arm or leg) and detecting the moment at which it comes around the circuit once more, by serial samples of blood from the vein or by a device (e.g., photocolorimeter, radioactivity or electrical conductivity detector) mounted over the vein. The time before the marker recirculates is usually of the order of 1 min. In conditions of exercise, the time tends to be reduced, but need not be less. The time to traverse a shorter part of the whole circuit may also be measured. For example, a substance which gives a sensation of taste or smell when it reaches the receptors of the tongue or nose may be injected, the subject reporting the first sensation. Injection may be in the arm vein, with detection of arrival made from samples of an artery in the arm, in which case the time is from that through the main veins, the right heart, lungs, left heart, aorta and peripheral artery. By the modern use of catheters inserted in peripheral veins or arteries and pushed to desired spots, circulation times may be measured for various routes or parts of the circuits.

The shortest circulation time is probably that for the coronary circulation. This may be as little as 10 sec. Other routes from aorta to vena cava may take as long as several minutes. As a result of the great differences in time required for the many parallel routes, the "wave" of indicator substance arrives, not with a sudden onset, but spread out over a wide interval of time, so that only the shortest time can be measured with accuracy.

It is of great importance to realize that the time between any point, A, in the vascular bed and another point, B, is given by the simple equation:

heart very greatly reduces the volume of blood by lowering the venous pressure and draining a large volume from the veins; yet the volume flow may be little changed. In these circumstances, the circulation time would greatly decrease. It is a pity that more simultaneous measurements of circulation time—with measurements of either the changes in volume of a limb or its volume flow—have not been made, for the two measurements would tell the whole story, where one will not.

A knowledge of the circulation time remains important to the physiologist because the recirculation of a marker substance limits the methods (dye dilution, cardiac output methods, see Chapter 19) used for measurements to flow in the cardiovascular system. The recirculation of blood via the coronary circuit in as little as 10 sec is a severe limitation.

The above simple relation at once tells us the relative intervals of time that the blood flow spends in various parts of the series of vascular

$$\text{Circulation time (in sec)} = \frac{\text{Volume of vasc. bed between } A \text{ and } B \text{ (in ml)}}{\text{Volume flow, } A \text{ to } B \text{ (in ml/sec)}}$$

Figure 6–5 reveals this obvious relation. However, every physiological change in the volume flow in a vascular bed, due to a change in caliber of the "resistance vessels" (due to vasomotor tone or to a change in the blood pressure distending them), is necessarily accompanied by a change in the volume of blood in the vessels, so that both numerator and denominator of the fraction change. The effect on the circulation is unpredictable without measurement of more factors. This is why early work on the circulation time from artery to vein in limbs sometimes gave the seemingly paradoxical result that vasoconstriction, which undoubtedly caused a decrease in volume flow, might actually decrease the circulation time, presumably because the volume of the vascular bed (the numerator) decreased more than the volume flow (the denominator). The most striking example is that which occurs with change of posture of a limb, for elevating the limb above the

elements in any one route. If the total volume flow in the route is the same everywhere, the time interval must be proportional to the volume of the vascular bed in the given part. Referring to Tables 6–1 and 6–2, we deduce that most of the circulation time is spent in the venous side of the circulation, very little in the arterial side. Circulation time is, therefore, much more related to what is happening in the veins than in arteries or arterioles.

Architecture of the Terminal Vascular Bed

It is convenient to consider the distributing arteries and the arterioles, capillaries, venules and veins as systems in series with one another. Actual observations of the microcirculation reveal much more complexity than this. Terminal vascular beds differ greatly in different regions of

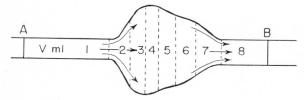

Fig. 6-5.—Another glimpse of the obvious. The profile represents the change in the cross-sectional area of a vascular bed between points A and B. Let the volume flow be V ml per sec. The broken lines represent the successive positions of the V ml each second. The volume of blood between A and B is obviously 8 V, and the circulation time is 8 sec.

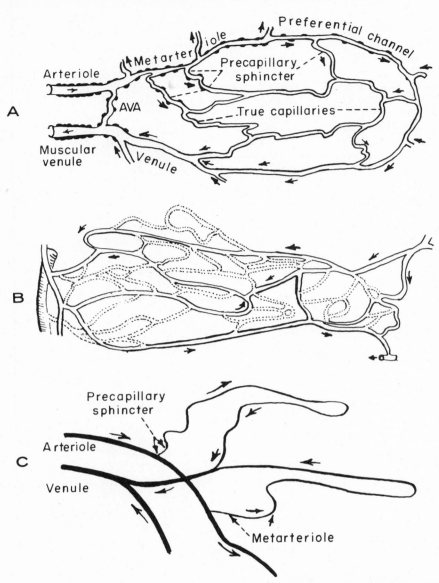

Fig. 6-6.—Three types of pattern of terminal vascular beds. **A,** muscle, with the preferential channels. The location of smooth-muscle control vessels is indicated. **B,** the mesentery. The true capillaries are shown by the dotted lines. **C,** the unique hairpin capillary loops of the human nail bed. (According to Zweifach, *Transactions of the Third Conference on Factors Regulating Blood Pressure* [Josiah Macy Foundation, 1950].)

the circulation. Microscopic observation of the living microcirculation, as by Zweifach and his colleagues (2), and modern methods of injection of plastic material, which give casts of the small vessels, have begun to give us the true picture (Fig. 6–6). Photographs made with soft x-rays and special point sources (x-ray projection microscopy) also reveal the fantastic complexity of the microcirculation (Fig. 6–7).

Groups or "tufts" of capillaries are supplied by terminal arterioles (or *metarterioles*), but in general the capillary bed is more like a "fish net" of interconnecting vessels than a simple parallel arrangement. Again, watching a living vascular bed under the microscope reveals that the flow in capillaries is not steady, or even uniform in direction. Instead, there is *vasomotion*, in which individual capillaries are seen to close completely

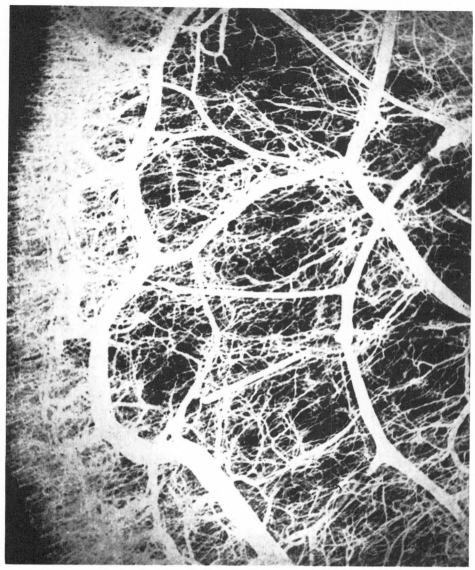

Fig. 6-7.—Microangiogram of the margin of a rabbit ear obtained by x-ray projection microscopy. The small arteries are united by arterioarteriolar arcades to form a macromesh, or coarse network, within which lies the capillary bed, or micromesh. At the left, venules drain into the marginal vein of the ear. (From Saunders, R. L. de C. H.: J. Anat. Soc. India 8:1–6, 1959.)

and then reopen. [▶Whether this is due to independent active constriction in the capillaries or is the result of constriction of arterioles outside the field of observation is controversial, although the consensus is that capillaries are not contractile.◀] As a result, the flow is intermittent, and it often proceeds in the reverse direction when the vessel reopens. This to-and-fro, intermittent, capillary flow serves as a sort of periodic "rinsing" of the blood. The contents of a capillary are immobilized for a few seconds, while diffusion and exchange of gases and materials can proceed. Then the capillary is flushed through with fresh blood once more. Although this is so, it does not invalidate the consideration of capillary exchange based on the idealized picture of continuous flow of blood through a capillary *(Starling-Landis hypothesis).*

Shunts—The Arteriovenous Anastomoses

A feature of many vascular beds that has not received the attention it deserves, at least in textbooks, is the existence of direct connections between terminal arteries and veins, called arteriovenous anastomoses (AVAs), which short-circuit, or act as a shunt, around the capillary system fed by their arterioles. Arteriovenous anastomoses were first noted in the rabbit ear (Grant [3, 4]) and in the fingers and toes of man. It has since been found that they are present in the vascular beds of the stomach and mesentery, and they are suspected to exist in many organs (e.g., the kidney).

Figure 6–8 shows the structure of AVAs. A long tortuous vessel leaves an end-artery just before the controlling metarteriole of the capillary bed. In its course there is a "glomus body" (where there is abundant smooth muscle, arranged circularly, and also special contractile epithelioid cells). The shunt empties by a long tortuous vessel into the venous system. Study of the function of these shunts in the vessels of the stomach by perfusion with spheres of different sizes (Walder [5]) reveals that the shunts are either completely open or closed and that, in general, they open when the capillary metarteriole closes, and vice versa. The physiological function of the AVAs in the extremities of man and the ears of such animals as

the sheep and rabbit is easily seen. They provide a way of greatly increasing the flow of blood to the extremities for increasing the loss of heat, in the temperature regulation of the body. In contrast, the function of AVAs in the stomach vasculature can have nothing to do with temperature regulation. Possibly they act as "safety valves," preventing too great a rise of blood pressure if the capillary beds close down, due to vasoconstrictor agents acting on the metarterioles, or to mechanical obstruction.

Another type of shunting that has also been suggested is that in the vascular bed of skeletal muscle. Zweifach (6) describes what he calls "through thoroughfares," or "preferential channels" (Fig. 6–6), confined to the superficial layers of the muscles, by which blood can pass without supplying the smaller deep arteries that feed capillary beds. It is important to remember the existence of capillary shunts (or shunts of other types), or AVAs, because this means that the total blood flow of regions which possess them may greatly increase (e.g., in response to drugs) without a corresponding increase in "nutritive flow," that is, flow which, by perfusing capillary beds, supplies oxygen and removes carbon dioxide, etc., from the tissues. A case in point is the attempt by surgeons to supply new blood vessels to cardiac muscle in patients who have inadequate coronary perfusion, by grafting in arterial connections from, say, the mammary arterial system.

Fig. 6-8.—Latex casts of the arteriovenous anastomoses of the rabbit ear. *A*, artery; *V*, vein; *arrows*, the glomus body of AVAs. Fragments of the capillary system can be seen in the two lower pictures. (From Daniel and Pritchard: Quart. J. Exper. Physiol. 41:107, 1956.)

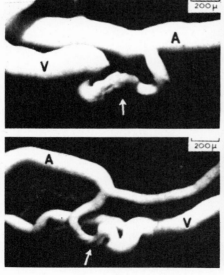
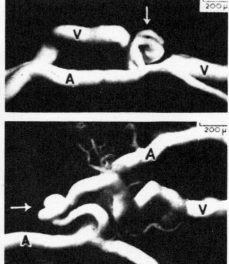

Whether or not the nutrition of the heart muscle is significantly improved, depends not merely on demonstrating an increase in total flow, but in showing that more oxygen is available to the muscle, i.e., that the new vascular bed has an adequate system of capillaries that exchange gases across their walls. One method of proof used in animals with grafts is to inject a radioactively tagged substance (e.g., radioactive iodine) into the heart muscle and show that it is "washed out" (cleared) faster by the circulation than before.

Physiologists also speak of *"physiological shunts"* where there may not be any special alternative route for blood flow in an anatomical sense, but where the function of the cells on a usual route is disturbed. An example is the use of the term "shunts" in the pulmonary vascular bed, when some of the alveoli of the lungs are poorly ventilated with air. If blood continues to perfuse these alveoli, it emerges less well oxygenated than blood from well-ventilated alveoli, with which it mixes in the pulmonary veins to the right heart. As a result, the mean oxygenation of the arterial blood is decreased by this "physiological shunt." (Special reflex controls exist which automatically tend to decrease the flow of blood through the walls of poorly ventilated alveoli.) Another example is in the complicated pattern of circulation of the kidney, where there is a variable partition of blood flow between the "cortical" and "medullary" parts of the organ. Such "shunting" can alter the amount and the reabsorption of the glomerular filtrate and so control kidney function.

"SINUSOIDS," AND OTHER VASCULAR COMPARTMENTS; INVESTIGATION BY "INDICATOR DILUTION" AND "WASHOUT" CURVES.—We tend to think of the circulation as a "closed" system of pipes, with the possibility that water and other substances in the blood stream can be exchanged with the tissues by the permeability of the vessel walls, particularly of the capillaries. In actuality, there are many special places, such as the spleen, where the direct channels of flow are in communication, through quite large openings, with other spaces where blood and its cellular elements may penetrate and remain for periods of time (analogous to the backwaters or marshes of a river system). Electronic and optical micrographs of the "sinusoids" of the spleen of animals (after the red cells are washed out) often show many sections of the walls that are "fenestrated" with holes big enough for red cells, and certainly for

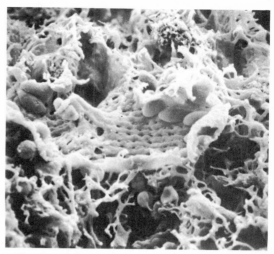

Fig. 6-9.—Scanning electron micrograph of a dog's spleen after perfusion with Ringer's solution (to wash out most of the red cells). Note the fenestrated endothelium in the central region of the picture with red cells on both sides of it. The spaces between reticular fibers were filled with red cells before perfusion began. These must have passed through the many "windows" to drain out through the large venous channel seen. From an unpublished electron micrograph by Dr. L. N. Johnson, Faculty of Dentistry, and with the kind permission of Drs. A. C. Groom and S. H. Song of the Department of Biophysics, University of Western Ontario.

platelets and white cells, to pass (Fig. 6–9). The liver is another organ with such multiple "compartments," accessible to the blood stream.

One biophysical method of learning about the several ways that blood may traverse an organ is by what is called the technique of *"compartmental analysis."* (See Chapter 19, The Measurement of Cardiac Output and of Cardiac Mechanics.) In the "indicator dilution" method, an organ is perfused with blood or solution, to which a "foreign" or "indicator" substance is added abruptly, either a "slug" of material over a short time, or continuously. The concentration of the indicator in the outflow will show a spreading out in time, indicating the existence of multiple routes with different "transit times" through the organ. The "washout" procedure is to perfuse the organ with blood and the indicator substance, then to change to perfusate without the indicator and to study the way the indicator emerges with time. If there were a single "compartment" or route of transit, the curve of concentration in the outflow would be predictably "exponential" in shape, from which the volume of that single compartment and the "half-time" associated with it could be deduced. If there are multiple compartments, the curve is described by many exponential terms, from which the volume and half-times of the several apparently separate "compartments" may be deduced. This leads to a kinetic "model" of the circulatory architecture. Great caution must be exercised in translating these "models" into a belief in separate anatomical spaces available to the blood, until identification by morphological or physiological methods has confirmed the biophysical analysis. In some cases, the results have been unequivocal. A very "slow" compartment, with a long transit time, might indicate a "backwater" of large volume and small access or alternatively that an indicator was temporarily detained on its way through (e.g., sticking to surfaces). Details of "compartmental analysis" are not appropriate here, but the student should be aware of this "black-box" or "kinetic technique," which is capable of indicating where to search for additional morphological evidence of the very many ways in which the blood halts in, or passes through, the various organs.

REFERENCES

1. Green, H. D.: Circulation: Physical Principles, in Glasser, O. (ed.): *Medical Physics*, Vol. I (Chicago: The Year Book Publishers, Inc., 1944), pp. 208–232.

2. Zweifach, B. W.: The character and distribution of the blood capillaries, Anat. Rec. 73:475, 1939.

3. Grant, R. T.: Observations on direct communications between arteries and veins in rabbits' ears, Heart 15:281–301, 1930.

4. Grant, R. T., and Bland, E. F.: Observations on arterio-venous anastomoses in human skin and in the bird's foot, Heart 15:385–407, 1931.

5. Walder, D. N.: The arteriovenous anastomoses of the human stomach, Clin. Sc. 11:59–71, 1962.

6. Zweifach, B. W.: *Functional Behavior of the Microcirculation* (American Lecture Series) (Springfield, Ill.: Charles C Thomas, Publisher, 1961).

7

Walls of the Blood Vessels
and Their Function

[*Note to the Student Reader:* If you find this chapter too difficult, read just the summary and come back to it later.]

Introduction

THE CIRCULATION PHYSIOLOGIST has a task of understanding that is much more difficult than that of the plumber or hydraulic engineer, for, instead of pipes of fixed dimensions, he deals with blood vessels that are living and constantly changing in size, not only passively with changes in the pressure of blood within them but actively because of contraction of the smooth muscles within their walls.

Variety of Sizes and Structure of Blood Vessels

Figure 7–1 is a useful summary of the range of sizes of lumen, thickness of the wall and composition of the wall in terms of the four important types of tissue—the endothelial lining, the elastin fibers, the collagen fibers and the smooth muscle. The diagram cannot be drawn accurately to scale because of the very wide range of sizes between the aorta and vena cava and the capillaries. The significant properties of the four elements mentioned and the differing proportions in which they occur in different vessels should be related to their special functions in the circulation (1).

ENDOTHELIAL LINING

A single layer of endothelial *pavement cells* is found in every category of vessel (except the glomus body of the arteriovenous anastomoses [AVAs], where modified lining cells, many layers deep, are described and called *epithelioid*, or sometimes *myoepithelioid, cells*). The role of the lining cells in the circulation is primarily to provide a smooth wall and to offer a selective permeability to water, electrolytes, sugars and other substances passing from the blood stream to the tissues. It would appear that this transport function is most developed in the endothelium of the capillaries, although transfers undoubtedly occur through the lining of the walls of other vessels. Certainly, oxygen and carbon dioxide are exchanged through the walls of all vessels. [►The differences in permeability between different blood vessels may reside, not in the endothelial cells, but in *basement membranes* behind them, and also in the very much greater surface area of the wall of the capillaries.◄]

No one now thinks that the usual endothelial lining cells are contractile, but micromanipulation studies (by R. Chambers many years ago) indicate that, once freed from the *cement substance* holding these cells to the membranes behind them, they tend to become spherical. Indeed, sections of the small blood vessels, such as arterioles (Fig. 7–2) (which were quick-frozen and sectioned under vasomotor tone so that the circular smooth muscle was contracted), show how the lining cells round up, protrude into the lumen and may eventually close the lumen altogether. The arterioles undoubtedly do close completely when their smooth muscle contracts strongly. This action of the endothelial cells helps us understand how complete closure could occur in a very thick-walled vessel. In this way, endothelial lining cells take part in the control of distribution of blood in the vascular tree.

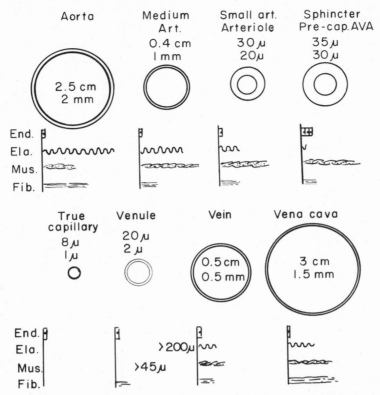

Fig. 7-1.—Variety of sizes, thickness of wall and admixture of the four basic tissues in the wall of different blood vessels. The figures directly under the name of the vessel represent the diameter of the lumen; below this, the thickness of the wall. *End.*, endothelial lining cells. *Ela.*, elastin fibers. *Mus.*, smooth muscle. *Fib.*, collagen fibers. (From Burton [1].)

Very little force is required to deform the endothelial cells, and so they play very little part in the total elasticity of the vessels. They should not be thought of as at all rigidly fixed and unchanging, for studies of developing blood vessels in tissue culture, or in a "window" in the rabbit ear or skin of the rat or mouse, show that the lining cells may migrate freely along the wall of the vessels. The vascular endothelial cells are probably being continuously renewed by mitosis.

ELASTIN FIBERS

Elastin fibers are abundant in all vessels except the capillaries and the AVAs. They form a layer, the *elastica intima*, just behind the endothelial lining, and they are also scattered through the media and adventitia. Elastin fibers are very easily stretched (about six times more easily than rubber) and are quite remarkable in that they can be extended many times their unstretched length before reaching an *elastic limit*. The function of

elastin fibers is to produce an *elastic tension* automatically, and without expenditure of biochemical energy, to resist the distending force of the blood pressure. This function they share with the collagenous fibers, in a manner described below. The elastin fibers, particularly in the elastica intima, appear in histological sections to be folded; possibly they are helical, like a coiled spring. [▶It has been suggested (1) that when the "spring" is compressed the elastica intima may resist compression, as well as resisting extension when the vessels are distended.◀]

COLLAGEN FIBERS

The collagen fibers form networks throughout the media and adventitia. Evidently collagen fibers resist stretch much more than do elastin fibers, judging from measurements on tendons, which are practically pure collagen; their modulus of elasticity is hundreds of times greater, so that a relatively small number of collagen fibers in the wall of an artery can give it a high degree of resistance to distension. However, the collagen fibers are "strung" on the wall of vessels with a degree of slackness, perhaps due to folding, so that they do not exert their tension until there has been some degree of stretching of the wall. With further stretch, more and more of these "stiffer" fibers reach their unstretched length and resist further stretch. An artery thus behaves like a garden hose, with its more stretchable rubber inside and less stretchable restricting jacket of canvas outside. This explains the shape of the curves of tension versus stretch that have been obtained for arteries.

Vascular Smooth Muscle

The function of the elastic elements (elastin and collagen fibers) in the wall is to maintain a steady tension to hold the wall in equilibrium against the *transmural pressure* exerted by the blood pressure in the vessels. In contrast, the elasticity of the smooth-muscle cells, usually arranged circumferentially or helically in the wall, probably adds little to the total elastic tension. Data on the elastic constants of vascular smooth muscle are lacking; those of other types of smooth muscle are available, and the values are much lower than

for collagen and elastin. (1) The function of the vascular smooth muscle is, rather, to produce *active tension* by contraction under physiological control and so change the diameter of the lumen of the vessel.

The greatest manifestation of the control of smooth muscle over the size of lumen is in the arterioles, where it is abundant. The arterioles, because of their small lumenal size, also can increase the total resistance to flow much more than would the constriction of larger vessels. While smooth muscle is quite apparent in the walls of the distributing arteries, even of the aorta, its physiological function is not clear in these locations. While, in pathological conditions, arteries may go into spasm, their response to physiological stimuli (e.g., to vasoactive drugs or nervous stimulation) is slight and would hardly play an important role in controlling the distribution of blood. (The next chapter is devoted to vascular smooth muscle, without which there could be no control of the distribution of blood flow to the various tissues.)

Elastic Behavior of Blood Vessels

The basic law of elastic behavior of simple homogeneous materials is that of Robert Hooke

Fig. 7-2.—Illustrating how the endothelial lining cells of arteries may round up and "crenate" the luminal cross-section, eventually closing the vessel completely under vasomotor tone. (Courtesy of R. Buck, Department of Microscopic Anatomy, University of Western Ontario.)

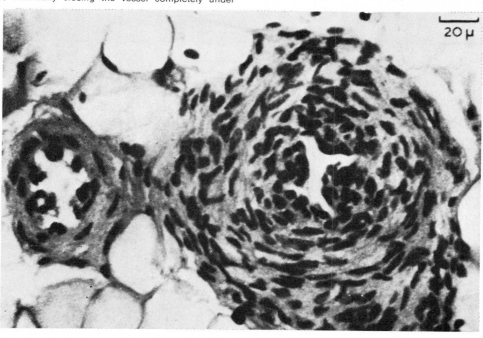

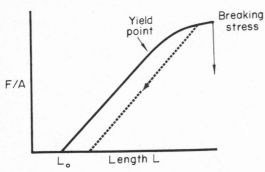

Fig. 7-3.—Illustrating Hooke's law of elasticity, that the elastic force per unit area is proportional to the stretch beyond the unstretched length, L_0—that is, to $(L—L_0)$. Eventually the line curves as the 'yield point' and 'breaking stress' are reached.

(1635–1703). *Hooke's law (ut tenso, sic vis)* is that, on stretching, an elastic tension is developed proportional to the elongation (i.e., measured by the stretched length minus the unstretched length). This is shown in Figure 7–3. The slope of the straight line on the elastic diagram is the measure of the elastic modulus, which in the case of linear stretch is *Young's modulus (Y)*. This is defined by the equation:

$$F \text{ (in dynes)} = Y \times \frac{\text{Cross-sectional}}{\text{area (in cm}^2)} \times \frac{L - L_0}{L_0}$$

where L is the stretched length and L_0 the unstretched length. In words, the Young's modulus is the force in dynes that would be developed for 100% stretch per square centimeter of cross-section of the material. (Of course, in practice the material may reach a "yield point," where it is permanently deformed, before 100% stretch is reached. The modulus is calculated from small degrees of stretch by the equation above.)

Some values of Young's modulus for different materials in comparison with that of elastin fibers (from experiments on elastic ligaments) and collagen (from tendons) are given in Table 7–1. [►The values for vascular smooth muscle are in doubt, particularly since the true cross-sectional area is hard to estimate; but probably the modulus is relatively low, even for smooth muscle in contraction.◄]

Roy, in 1905, pointed out that the tension-length, or *elastic diagram*, of arteries and veins did not obey Hooke's law but that, *universally, blood vessels resist stretch more strongly the more they are stretched* (Fig. 7–4); i.e., their effective Young's modulus increases with the degree of stretch. Roy's observations were made by cutting circumferential strips of the vessel wall and stretching them by weights. The question arises as to how much resistance to bending, as well as to stretch, is involved where the wall is not in its natural shape. Fortunately, tension-length diagrams may be obtained from pressure-volume determinations of isolated vessels (Fig. 7–4 was so obtained) by applying a simple law of mechanics—the *law of Laplace* (1821).

This law is a familiar one in connection with

TABLE 7–1.—Elastic Properties of Common Substances and Vascular Tissues

Substance	Young's Modulus, (Dynes/Cm² 100% elongation)	Tensile Strength, (Dynes/Cm²)	Maximum Extension (%)	Source of Information
Rubber	4×10^7	2×10^8	600	*Handbook of Physics and Chemistry*
Wood:				
Willow	5×10^{10}	5×10^{10}	1	"
Oak	1×10^{11}	1×10^{11}	1	"
Steel	2×10^{12}	2×10^{12}	0.1	"
Endothelium	Negligible	?	Very great	Micromanipulation studies
Smooth muscle:				
Relaxed	6×10^4?	?	300	Pecten muscle
Contracted	1×10^5?	?	300	Retractor penis muscle
Elastin fibers	3×10^6	1×10^7	>100	"Purified" aorta; distensibility of veins at low pressure; elastic ligaments
Collagenous fibers	1×10^9	Very great	50	Tendons

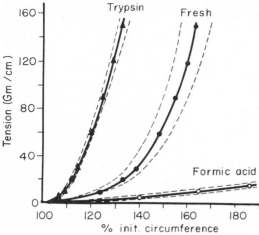

Fig. 7-4.—Tension-length diagram of human external iliac artery *(fresh curve)*, showing how the more the wall is stretched, the more it resists further stretch. The results are based on the means of nine arteries from subjects aged 20–50 years. *Trypsin curve*, after selective digestion of the elastin fibers; *formic acid curve*, after selective digestion of the collagenous fibers (see text for explanation). (From Roach and Burton [3].)

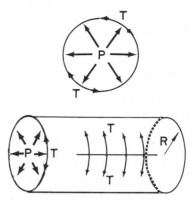

Fig. 7-5.—Illustrating the law of Laplace as it applies to a cylindrical blood vessel. *T*, the tension in dynes per centimeter length of an imaginary longitudinal slit; *P*, the transmural pressure in dynes per square centimeter; *R*, the radius in centimeters. $P = T/R$.

soap bubbles. It states that if there is a curved "membrane" (i.e., a partition separating two spaces) and the membrane has a tension in it of T dynes per cm (i.e., if we cut a slit 1 cm long in the membrane the edges of that slit would pull apart with a force of T dynes or would require that force to hold them together again) then there will be a difference of pressure of P dynes per cm² between the two sides of the membrane, given by the law:

$$P = T\left(\frac{1}{R_1} + \frac{1}{R_2}\right)$$

where R_1 and R_2 are the principal radii of curvature of the membrane at any point. This is a general law for membranes of any shape, where the two radii may not be the same. The case of a cylindrical, or nearly cylindrical, blood vessel is much simpler, for in a cylinder one radius of curvature is infinite, e.i., $\frac{1}{R_2}$ is zero while the other (R_1) is simply the radius of the cylinder. The law then becomes (for a cylindrical vessel):

$$P = \frac{T}{R_1}$$

This is illustrated in Figure 7–5.

An artery or vein is attached to an apparatus by which increments in volume of fluid may be injected, and the pressures required are recorded, giving the pressure-volume curve (see, e.g., Fig.

6–3). From the length of segment and the volume, the mean radius of the lumen may be calculated from simple geometry. The equation states that the tension in the wall is the product of the pressure and this radius, and so the elastic diagram of tension versus radius (or the circumference, which is proportional) may be constructed. Modern work on the elastic behavior of the blood vessel walls has employed this simple technique.

Reason for Shape of Elastic Diagram of Arteries

Figure 7–6 shows the elastic diagram of segments of human iliac arteries (4) obtained as just stated, with the characteristic increase in slope with stretch. The reason for this change of slope is easily postulated as the heterogeneity of the wall—that is, the presence of elastin plus collagen fibers. This has been proved conclusively by the selective digestion of these elements (Fig. 7–4) (3). Either of the elements, elastin and collagen alone, would approach Hooke's law up to a considerable degree of stretch. When they are both present, as the degree of stretch increases, more and more of the much stronger collagen fibers reach their unstretched length and add their contribution to the total tension. The curve of increasing slope results. When either element is destroyed by selective digestion, there is an approximation to Hooke's law.

On this basis, the final constant slope of the tension-length diagram represents all of the collagen fibers having been "recruited," and thus may be used as an index of the amount and state

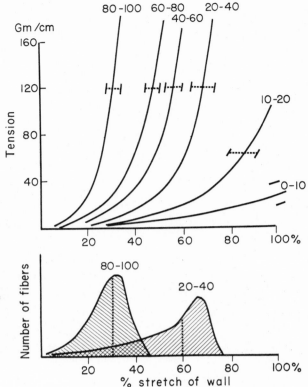

Fig. 7-6.—**Top,** effect of age on elastic diagrams of external iliac arteries of different ages (human autopsy material). The standard error of the curves is shown. The change up to 20 years of age is due mainly to increasing thickness of the arterial wall with growth but at later ages is due to a change in elasticity. **Bottom,** distribution curves of the number of collagen fibers that have reached their un-stretched length versus degree of stretch of the wall. For the young vessels, half are in action at 60% stretch; for the old vessels, half at 30% stretch. The areas under the curves represent the total amount of collagen in the wall, and this increases with age. The curves are derived from those above by differentiating twice. (From Roach and Burton [4].)

of collagen in the wall. The initial slope is more indicative of the number and state of elastin fibers (although a few tightly strung collagen fibers would greatly increase the slope). The degree of stretch before the final slope is reached is an index of how closely the collagen fibers are "strung," or the degree of "slackness" in them.

Wolinsky and Glagov (10) have made a detailed histological study of the organization of the elastic tissue in the media of arteries, fixing the tissue when the artery was under different transmural pressures, i.e., with different degrees of stretch. Figure 7–7 is from their publications. It shows how the elastin fibers become straightened as higher pressures are reached and the wall becomes progressively thinner. The collagen fibers appear to be quite randomly oriented until the higher pressures are reached, when they are all oriented circumferentially. This work gives a plausible basis for the model described, i.e., of two springs in parallel, the weaker spring (elastin) without "slack" and the stiffer spring (collagen) not stretched until there is a considerable extension. Their work has resulted in postulation of concentric, "medial unit lamellae." The number

of lamellae in the wall was found to be remarkably consistent in the aortas of many mammalian species, in which there are about 30 laminar units.

Effect of Age on Elasticity of Arteries

It has long been known that the normal aging process is accompanied by an increasing stiffness of the aorta and the distributing arteries. This shows itself in an increase in the *pulse-wave velocity,* in the shape of the *pulse curve* (Chapter 18) and in the magnitude of the *pulse pressure.* Tension-length diagrams of groups of human iliac arteries, obtained from autopsy specimens by the pressure-volume method (4), show a progressive change from birth to old age (Fig. 7–6) (the change up to age 20 is mainly due to increasing thickness of wall with growth). The observed change has two aspects, as follows:

a) The final slope is greater with increasing age. This is related to the well-known *diffuse fibrosis* of age—that is, to the increase in the total content of collagenous fibers in the arterial wall.

b) Equally important is the fact that the curves turn upward at a less degree of stretch; that is, in

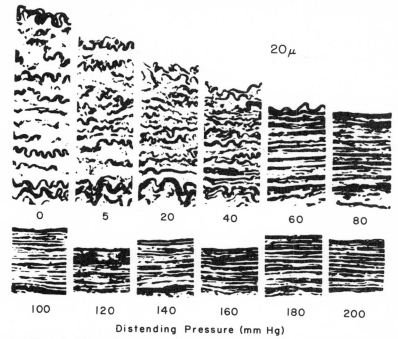

20μ

| 0 | 5 | 20 | 40 | 60 | 80 |

| 100 | 120 | 140 | 160 | 180 | 200 |

Distending Pressure (mm Hg)

Fig. 7-7.—Cross-sections of rabbit aortic walls fixed while extended to in vivo length and distended by various intraluminal pressures. Circumferential waves and folds in elastin lamellae diminish and interlamellar distances decrease uniformly throughout the wall as distending pressures increase from 5 to 80 mm Hg. At and above 80 mm Hg, all elastin lamellae are straight and interlamellar distances change little. Weigert stain. (From Wolinsky and Glagov [10].)

the older vessels, the collagenous fibers have less degree of slackness of connections to the other elements of the wall. Biophysical analysis of these curves (5) has indicated that, while in the young adult, to "recruit" half of the collagenous fibers, there must be 60% stretch of the wall, in the age group of 70–80, 25 or 30% stretch is sufficient to do this. The explanation of this "tightening-up" of the fabric of the wall is probably that the number of cross-connections (or "adhesions") between the collagen fibers increases with age.

Total Tension in the Wall of Blood Vessels

The law of Laplace gives us a way of estimating the total force, or tension, in the wall of the different categories of vessels, for we may list (see Table 7–2) the radius of the vessels and the blood pressure normally found in those types of vessels. (If the tissue pressure is negligible, as it usually is, this is equal to the transmural pressure.) The product of pressure and radius gives the total tension. Table 7–2 shows how this is of the order of 200,000 dynes per cm (200 Gm/cm) in

the wall of the aorta and only 16 dynes per cm (16 mg/cm) in the capillaries, but, in spite of the lower transmural pressures in the venous system, the total tension rises to 20,000 dynes for the vena cava. The seemingly fragile structure of the capillary can withstand the distending force of the capillary pressure of 25 mm Hg because of its very small radius (or very high curvature), which gives the tension in the wall a very great mechanical advantage over the pressure. A force of 16 dynes per cm is a very small force indeed, for experiment shows that a 1-cm strip of the thinnest paper (facial tissue) will withstand about 50 Gm, or 3,000 times as great a force, before it tears. The figures in Table 7–2 can also be used as a guide to the necessary strength of arterial suture material; for example, if a slit in the aorta were stitched with 10 sutures per cm length, the sutures or the tissues must withstand a force of at least 17 Gm (much more would, of course, be desirable).

In addition, Table 7–2 gives a clue as to the function of the different elements of the wall, already outlined. The amount of elastic tissue (elastin and collagen) is related to the *maintenance tension*. We see, also, why veins must be

TABLE 7–2.—CIRCUMFERENTIAL TENSION IN THE WALL OF
DIFFERENT CATEGORIES OF BLOOD VESSELS

TYPE OF VESSEL	MEAN PRESSURE (Mm Hg)	INTERNAL PRESSURE (Dynes/Cm²)	RADIUS (R)	TENSION (T) IN WALL (Dynes/Cm)*	AMOUNT OF ELASTIC TISSUE
Aorta and large arteries	100	1.3×10^5	1.3 cm or less	170,000	Very elastic two coats
Small distributing arteries	90	1.2×10^5	0.5 cm	60,000	Much elastic tissue but more muscular
Arterioles	60	8×10^4	0.15 mm to 62 μ	1,200–500	Thin elastica intima only
Capillaries	30	4×10^4	4 μ	16	None
Venules	20	2.6×10^4	10 μ	26	None except in largest venules
Veins	15	2×10^4	200 μ	400	Elastic fibers reappear
Vena cava	10	1.3×10^4	1.6 cm	21,000	Very elastic, fibers increasing in size

*For tension in grams, divide by 1,000 (980, to be exact).

very elastic, even though their transmural pressure is low. An increasing elastic tension is required because of the increasing size of veins.

Instability of Small Blood Vessels under Vasomotor Tone

The elastic tension in the wall, automatically increased by stretch, gives an almost complete stability to the equilibrium between the transmural pressure and the tension in the walls. Consider (see Fig. 7–8) a blood vessel in equilibrium between the transmural pressure and the tension. If the blood pressure should begin to "win" over the tension, the radius of the lumen would increase. At the greater radius, by Laplace's law, a still greater tension would be required to withstand the same pressure. However, the extra stretch may increase the elastic tension to a sufficient value. Analysis of the physics of this (1, 6, 7) shows that a minimal value of the elastic modulus is required for stability, but, in general, this is amply provided in healthy blood vessel walls. In diseased states, *particularly in syphilitic disease of large arteries*, the elastic tissue may be so weakened that, if the transmural value exceeds a critical value, equilibrium is not possible and *blowout* (e.g., aortic *aneurism*) results. From the elastic constants of normal aortas and arteries, this critical pressure would probably be over 1,000 mm Hg, instead of the maximal 200 mm Hg normally found. In disease, the critical pressure may be much less.

The situation as to stability is very different where the tension in the wall is active tension, with very little automatic adjustment to the degree of stretch by elasticity. In the extreme case of negligible elasticity, the tension would not increase at all if the transmural pressure began to win and the radius of the lumen increased. The radius would then continue to increase, for if the tension had been insufficient to withstand the pressure at the original radius, it would be still less able to do so when the radius was increased. Again, if the smooth muscle contracted more strongly, so that the active tension began to win over the pressure, the radius of the vessel would decrease. By the law of Laplace, less tension would now be required to hold the pressure than before; so we would expect the vessel to continue to get smaller in radius until it closed completely or some new factor intervened. The prediction is, then, that control by smooth muscle alone, without the participation of elastic tissue, might lead to complete instability. Blood vessels would either be widely open (a blowout might occur) or else completely closed under vasomotor tone. The prediction is verified for the case of the glomus bodies of the AVAs, which are full of contractile muscle cells but almost completely lacking in

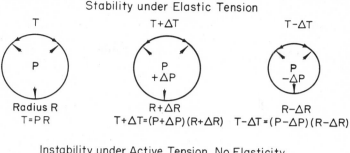

Stability under Elastic Tension

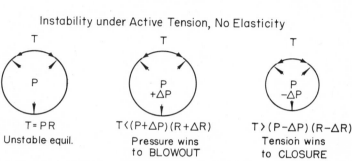

Instability under Active Tension, No Elasticity

Fig. 7-8.—Showing how, without elasticity in the wall of blood vessels (i.e., an automatic increase in tension with stretch), active tension (vasomotor tone) would lead to complete instability of the equilibrium.

elastic tissue. Such AVAs have been shown to be either widely open or else closed, never having an intermediate radius of lumen.

Analysis of the stability of the equilibrium, when both active tension (of smooth muscle) and elastic tension (of elastin and collagen fibers) are present, shows that, over a wide range of size of lumen, equilibrium is now possible. Modification of the degree of vasomotor tone of the muscle, by nervous control, can result in nicely graded vasoconstriction of arterioles. We see, then, *in addition to providing maintenance tension versus the prevailing transmural pressure (and this without energy expenditure), the elastic tissue of the blood vessel walls has a second, most important, function in the circulation. Its presence makes possible graded vasomotor control, where otherwise this would be impossible.*

There is actually more subtlety than this in the situation. Without elastic tension, there would be complete instability. While this would be unusable in general control of the circulation (although it is used in the shunts), it would provide a very great sensitivity indeed, for the smallest increase in active tension could produce a very great vasoconstriction. Elastic tissue, enough to remove the instability but not too great in amount, can still leave a great sensitivity to contraction of the smooth muscle. Those old enough to remember the days of the early triode "wireless" receivers,

where one increased the coupling between the grid and plate coils, know how very great sensitivity would be achieved by working at the point just below that of instability. (When the coupling was made too great, "howling" resulted.)

With the increase in elastic constants with age, there is a corresponding decrease in sensitivity of response to the contraction of the smooth muscle. In general, with the arteriosclerosis of age, the effectiveness of vasomotor tone in controlling the distribution of the blood flow is demonstrably reduced. Old people cannot adjust their peripheral circulation well to such factors as heat and cold.

Critical Closure of Vessels

While the cooperation of elastic tissue with the smooth muscle can stabilize the equilibrium of the wall under vasomotor tone, instability of those blood vessels which can develop large amounts of active tension (such as the arterioles) will occur when the vessel is constricted enough so that the elastic fibers are unstretched. There is no elastic tension below this point of unstretched circumference. Consequently, theory predicts, and there is ample experimental verification in peripheral vascular beds (5, 6), that vasomotor tone not only tends to decrease the lumenal diameter of the controlling vessels (e.g., the arterioles) but also creates a tendency to close altogether. This will happen for a given transmural pressure if the active tension rises above a critical value, or with a given degree of active tension if the pressure falls below a critical value. This has been called *critical closure* of blood vessels. It is of considerable physiological importance. The case of *hypotensive shock* (e.g., due to hemorrhage) illustrates this closure, for here not only is there less transmural blood pressure available to keep vessels open but there also is a violent reflex increase of the vasomotor tone of peripheral vessels. Both of the factors tending to cause closure of vascular beds are present. A patient in hypotensive shock may present limbs that seem lifeless, in which blood flow is not merely reduced but has ceased altogether. The blood vessels of the kidney are capable of very great vasomotor tone, and this may be why, in shock, kidney function seems to stop altogether when the central blood pressure is reduced below, say, 70 mm Hg instead of the normal mean of 100 mm Hg. The blood flow of the kidney is probably zero at pressures lower than a critical value.

The critical vessels, which close in these circumstances, are undoubtedly the arterioles, as their small diameter of lumen and very great amount of smooth muscle would predict. Experimental proof is provided by measurements of critical closing pressure in vascular beds of the limbs of animals, and in the blood flow in fingers and arms of men, when the effective transmural pressure is reduced by various means. The resistance to flow of the vascular bed (ratio of driving pressure to flow produced) is mainly due to the arterioles. When the vasomotor tone of these is changed (as by putting a man in the cold, which increases the vasoconstriction of peripheral vessels), the measured critical closing pressure increases. For example, in the fingers, in full vasodilation the critical closing pressure is as low as 10 mm Hg; in full vasoconstriction to cold, as high as 60 mm Hg (6). [►Critical closure of the mesenteric vessels in hypertensive shock, giving anaerobic conditions there, may be a factor in the production of *irreversible shock* through bacterial toxins from that source.◄]

Another example of the importance of recognizing the tendency of small blood vessels under tone to close completely is that of gangrene of the extremities, (e.g., the toes) where there is obstruction to the main blood supply of the limbs (e.g., embolus in the femoral artery). Dible (8) has shown, by injection of x-ray contrast material into such limbs at amputation, that where the obstruc-

tion has been chronic, there is a very good delivery of blood to the foot by long narrow collateral channels. The blood arrived at the foot in normal amount; yet none at all reached the toes (necrosis of skin denotes practically zero blood flow). The only reason that can be advanced for this is that, although blood was delivered to the foot, it was at insufficient pressure (the pressure drop down the collateral vessels would be abnormally great) to keep open the arterioles of the toes under their vasomotor tone.

Relation between Pressure and Flow in Vascular Beds

Even in vessels without vasomotor tone, we would therefore not expect linear relations between the driving pressure and the flow that results, for, if we lower the arterial pressure, we will reduce not only the *driving pressure* but also the *transmural pressure* of all of the vessels, and their geometrical factors (r^4/l) will change. With vasomotor tone, the curve will be even less like a straight line, for the effect of the active tension greatly increases as the transmural pressure is reduced.

The complete flow-pressure curves in limbs on animals, under a variety of different degrees of vasomotor tone (produced by perfusion with pressure drugs or by electrical stimulation of sympathetic nerves), have been measured. Those obtained by Girling (Fig. 7–9) for the rabbit ear are typical of the nonlinear curves that are found. Dilated vessels with very little vasomotor tone give almost straight lines, although they hit the axis of zero flow before the driving pressure is zero (the critical closing pressure is a few mm Hg). With increasing vasomotor tone, the curves are more and more nonlinear (sigmoid or concave to the pressure axis) until, with high vasomotor tone (maximal stimulation of the sympathetic nerves at 15 impulses per sec), the curves dive quite abruptly into the axis (critical closure) at as high a critical closing pressure as 60 mm Hg.

Of course, it ought to be realized that it makes no sense to speak of a single flow-pressure curve or even a single set of curves for different degrees of vasomotor tone. *The driving pressure (artery to vein) and the transmural pressures that determine the size and resistance of vessels are really quite independent.* For example, if we raised both the arterial and the venous pressures in a limb, keeping the driving pressure constant, we would get a different flow-pressure curve simply because the

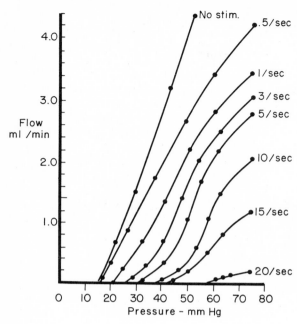

Fig. 7-9.—Flow-pressure curves of the vascular bed of the ears of rabbits, with increasing vasomotor tone produced by stimulating the sympathetic nerves (superior cervical ganglion) at the frequencies shown. Note the nonlinearity and the increasing intercept on the pressure axis (critical closing pressure). (From Girling: Am. J. Physiol. 170:131, 1952.)

Fig. 7-10.—The flow-pressure curve in the human forearm, deduced from positive-pressure plethysmography. The broken line represents data from similar experiments on the same subject when cold (i.e., with increased vasomotor tone in the peripheral blood vessels). An increase in critical closing pressure is seen. (From Burton and Yamada: J. Appl. Physiol. 4:329, 1951.)

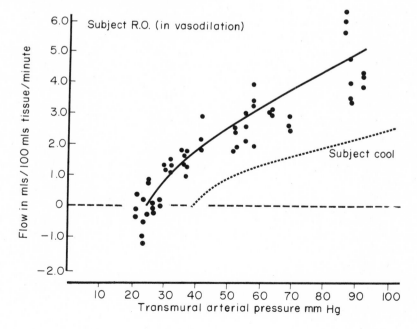

transmural pressures were everywhere increased, and the vessels would be passively dilated. This has been demonstrated for the isolated rabbit ear (9). Physiologically, this happens when the posture of a limb is altered. Lowering the limb, by the hydrostatic effect (Chapter 10), increases the transmural pressures and may thus increase the flow even though the driving pressure is not altered. Raising the limb may reduce the transmural pressures and size of the resistance vessels and so reduce the flow.

Independently changing the two factors of transmural pressures and the driving pressures has made possible the measurement of flow-pressure curves in the intact human arm without cannulation of vessels, by "positive-pressure plethysmography." The forearm (or finger) flow was measured when the tissue pressure was increased by raising the pressure in the plethysmograph. The transmural pressure was thus reduced correspondingly. Figure 7–10 shows that the flow-pressure curves so measured have the characteristics already described.

Importance of Level of Transmural Blood Pressure

The tendency of the small vessels to close when their transmural pressure is reduced, and the resulting nonlinearity of the flow-pressure curves, gives the maintenance of the level of the blood pressure a new importance. If the blood pressure is high, a given increase in vasomotor tone will reduce the flow in vascular beds—say to half the normal value. If the blood pressure is low, as in hypotensive shock, the same degree of tone (active tension) may be sufficient to reduce the flow much more drastically, even to zero if the vessels reach critical closure.

Elaborate homeostatic reflexes exist in the circulation to maintain a relatively constant level of the transmural arterial blood pressure. They are required not only to insure an adequate blood flow in vascular beds with relatively little vasomotor control but also to maintain the effectiveness of vasomotor control within normal limits.

The student may be discouraged to learn, from this chapter, of all the complications in the study of the physics of blood flow in vascular beds. Fortunately, in the case of *resistance to flow* (discussed in detail in Chapter 9), there is a convenient way to interpret physiological observations of blood pressures and blood flow, which is valid and simple despite the complexity.

Summary

For the average medical student, the arguments of this chapter may well be indigestible; hence this summary:

1. The walls of the blood vessels contain different mixtures of four basic components: the endothelial lining cells; the two elastic tissues, elastin and collagen fibers; and vascular smooth muscle. The relative proportions vary greatly in vessels of different categories.

2. The function of the elastic tissue (elastin and collagen) is to develop elastic tension in response to distension of the vessel by the transmural pressure and to hold the wall in equilibrium. The elastin fibers do this for small degrees of stretch; the collagen fibers reinforce them at higher degrees of stretch. Smooth muscle probably plays a very minor role in producing elastic tension. This function of elastic tissue does not require expenditure of energy.

3. The role of the smooth-muscle bands in the wall is to develop active tension, regardless of stretch, and so alter the size of the lumen and control the distribution of blood flow. Cooperation with the elastic tissue is necessary so that this can be done without instability. The control is greatest in the small arteries (arterioles).

4. Even with ample elastic tissue to provide stability of graded vasoconstriction by smooth-muscle action, small blood vessels tend to close completely (critical closure, or "spasm") when their smooth muscle contracts—if their transmural pressure falls below a critical value (critical closing pressure). Thus, blood flow in some vascular beds may be shut off completely (e.g., in low-blood-pressure shock). The maintenance of sufficient arterial pressure is important.

5. In spite of all these complications, we may still use a law of flow based on Poiseuille's formula if we remember that, while the flow depends on the driving pressure gradient (artery to vein), it also depends on how narrow the peripheral vessels may be. The latter depends on the degree of vasomotor tone (smooth-muscle contraction) and on the transmural pressure of each of the vessels.

REFERENCES

1. Burton, A. C.: Relation of structure to function of the tissues of the wall of blood vessels, Physiol. Rev. 34:619, 1944.
2. Burton, A. C.: The physical equilibrium of small blood vessels, Am. J. Physiol. 149:389, 1947.

3. Roach, M. R., and Burton, A. C.: The reason for the shape of the distensibility curves of arteries, Canad. J. Biochem. & Physiol. 35:681, 1957.

4. Roach, M. R., and Burton, A. C.: The effect of age on the elasticity of human arteries, Canad. J. Biochem. & Physiol. 37:557, 1959.

5. Nichol, J. T., et al.: Fundamental instability of small blood vessels and critical closing pressures in vascular beds, Am. J. Physiol. 164:330, 1961.

6. Burton, A. C.: Physical principles of circulatory Phenomena: The Physical Equilibria of Heart and Blood vessels, in Handbook of Physiology, Vol. I: Circulation (1961), pp. 85–106.

7. Burton, A. C.: Properties of smooth muscle and regulation of circulation, Physiol. Rev. 42:1, 1962.

8. J. H. Dible: Some Anatomical Observations on Peripheral Ischemia in Man, in Wolstenholme, G. E. W. (ed.): Peripheral Circulation in Man (Ciba Foundation Symposium) (London: J. & A. Churchill, Ltd., 1954), pp. 173–179.

9. Burton, A. C., and Rosenberg, E.: Effects of raised venous pressure in the circulation of the isolated perfused rabbit ear, Am. J. Physiol. 185:465, 1956.

10. Wolinsky, H., and Glagov, S.: Structural basis for the static mechanical properties of the aortic media, Circulation Res. 14:400, 1964.

8

Vascular Smooth Muscle (VSM)

"Silly and inexperienced persons wrongly attempt, by means of dialectics and far-fetched proofs, either to upset or to establish which things should be confirmed by anatomical dissection and credited through actual inspection. Whoever wishes to know . . . must either see for himself or be credited with belief in the experts."—WILLIAM HARVEY, *Second Essay to Jean Riolan* (c. 1649).

The Importance of Vascular Smooth Muscle

WILLIAM HARVEY, in his defense of his brilliant theory that the blood circulated, emphasizes in his arguments with his many critics that the activity of the heart is solely responsible for the circulation and that the arteries and veins play a largely passive role. In this main point, he was correct (except that the muscles of the limbs assist by the "muscle pump" in propelling blood through veins with valves). Active contraction of vascular smooth muscle (VSM) does not help to propel the blood stream, in fact, it impedes it by narrowing the vessels. Yet the smooth muscle is all important in governing the distribution of the total cardiac output, so that, as decreed by the Celestial Committee, each cell might receive blood "in accordance with its needs." If this function is not performed normally, serious cardiovascular disease results (e.g., hypertension, peripheral vascular diseases). In the past few years, there has been a great increase in knowledge of the morphology, contraction and response of vascular smooth muscle to physiological agents and to drugs. Many excellent and detailed reviews have resulted (1–5).

Morphogenetic Function of VSM

There is a significant amount of smooth muscle, even in such predominantly elastic arteries as the aorta and a great deal in the "muscular distributing arteries," such as the iliac, femoral and carotid. Yet reduction in the size of these large vessels by smooth muscle contraction, unless very

marked, would add little to the total resistance that governs the distribution of blood, since the resistance is dominantly in the small vessels, notably the arterioles of the terminal vascular beds. How then can we account for so much VSM in the larger vessels?

The smooth muscle cells are the *only cellular elements* in the wall of blood vessels, other than the single layer of endothelial cells lining the lumen. The network of elastin and collagen fibers in the wall is "inanimate." Thus, fibrogenesis and repair of the elastic network must be one function of the smooth muscle cells, and, in the large vessels, perhaps the contractile property of VSM is purely incidental (although in disease, it can be catastrophic, as in spasm of the distributing arteries). There has been relatively little study of the synthesis and secretion of the elastic fibers by the smooth muscle cells (6). Although the fibers are seen in the cytoplasm of the cell (Fig. 8–1), they do not seem to pass through the cell membrane to the extracellular space, and details are lacking as to how they are "secreted" to form the network outside. It is not known whether both collagen and elastin fibers are synthesized by the same cell. This should be an important field for new research. [▶It seems likely that final process in laying down of elastic networks must be some sort of "condensation" (shortening) of the "precursor fibers" when in position, for it is known that in the repair of severed tendons (collagenous) the repaired tendon tends to be too tight rather than too slack. Also, when damaged vessels have suffered dilatation by damage to the elasticity of the walls, they are capable (in vivo but not in vitro) of returning to their original smaller diameter when the cause of dilatation is removed. The newly laid down elastic fibers must contract as they "harden," like a good carpenter's glue, in pulling together the structures to which they adhere.◄]

The Smooth Muscle Cells

The media of arteries and veins is quite tightly packed with smooth muscle cells, shown diagramatically in Figure 8–1. These are fusiform, varying from 30 to 100μ in length, with a sausage-like nucleus. In the contracted state, the nuclei become serrated or wrinkled, and histologists use this as an index of the state of contraction at the time the tissue was fixed. The cells are enclosed by a "sarcolemma" outside the physiological "plasma membrane." At the ends of each cell are long processes, enclosed by the sarcolemma, which make "tight junctions" with the neighboring cells (the sarcolemma does not intervene). These junctions undoubtedly serve as electrophysiological "synapses," by which excitation spreads from cell to cell, so that the contraction of all the cells is almost simultaneous. It is to be noted that the endings of the sympathetic vasoconstrictor nerves lie at the outer layers of the media only and do not penetrate farther. This

makes electrical conduction from cell to cell a necessity. The cytoplasm is packed with contractile myofilaments arranged longitudinally in the cell. At the surface of the cell, there are so-called dense bodies, which are thought to be where attachments to the elastic network outside the cell are made. Pinocytotic vesicles may play a part in the transport of the synthesized elastic fibers to the outside. There is an absence of the highly organized systems of vesicles and the endoplasmic reticulum that is so important in the contraction of striated and possibly of cardiac muscle cells.

The smooth muscle cells are usually oriented in the vessel wall circumferentially, or helically with a very small pitch. Between the cells lies the elastic network, again oriented circumferentially, except for cross-connections to the walls of the cells (if these are made where the dense bodies are seen). This organization may give a high mechanical advantage to the VSM (see later in this chapter).

Mechanism of Contraction

The mechanism of contraction of striated, and to a less extent, of cardiac muscle has been elucidated in detail, although important problems and discrepancies in the current theories still exist. The "sliding model" of interdigitating

Fig. 8-1.—The smooth muscle cell of the media of arteries. The connections by "tight junctions" to adjacent cells serve the function of conduction of excitation, not of transmission of the contractile force, which is through the elastic network surrounding the cells and attached to the sarcolemma at many points. (Drawing kindly supplied by Prof. R. C. Buck, Department of Anatomy, University of Western Ontario.)

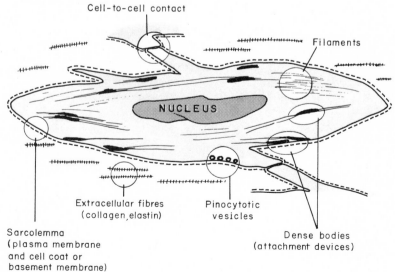

Cell-to-cell contact

Filaments

NUCLEUS

Extracellular fibres (collagen, elastin)

Pinocytotic vesicles

Sarcolemma (plasma membrane and cell coat or basement membrane)

Dense bodies (attachment devices)

"thick" (myosin) and "thin" (actin) fibers has had so many successes in explaining data (obtained, for example, by x-ray scattering) that those in this field are apt to assume their models must apply to all other contractile cells. Extraction of the contractile proteins of VSM certainly shows that they are biochemically similar to, but not identical with, the actin and myosin of striated muscle. However, the protein of the myofilaments is much more soluble than in striated muscle, and the ratio of actin-like to myosin-like protein does not fit the sliding model (the ratio actin/myosin is much higher). No third protein, like the relaxing factor "troponin" of striated muscle, has as yet been found that would regulate the interaction of actin and myosin. Also, of course, there is little seen of the regularity of spacing and organization of molecules, and of overlapping regions, that is responsible for the phenomena in voluntary muscle. It has been shown by electron micrographs of VSM that the cross-sectional area of the filaments does not increase when the muscle shortens, and it has been concluded that therefore their length has not decreased. This has been taken as evidence that the mechanism must involve some kind of "sliding" and interdigitation. [►Even here, however, there is a possibility for doubt. At the molecular level, a "hollow" helical structure (like a coiled spring) may increase, decrease or keep constant its length without changing the envelope of its cross-sectional area. It depends on the relative ease of bending vs twisting of the molecular chains in the helices.◄]

The responses of *intact* VSM to vasoactive agents and drugs are very different, in some cases opposite to those of striated muscle. It is important to realize that great differences in response exist between the smooth muscles of different blood vessels (see later, Fig. 8–5). For example, adenosine triphosphate (ATP) injected into the blood stream is one of the most potent vasodilators known, yet in striated muscle it is the basic excitor of contraction. These facts do not preclude the belief that the basic mechanism of vascular smooth muscle in contraction may be similar to that of other muscles, for peculiarities of the permeability of the cell membrane and of "active transport pumps" may be responsible for the differences. A given agent may affect the result in three ways: by altering the permeability of the membrane, the activity of the "pumps" and/or the basic contractile process. In support of this view is research on "extracted models" of VSM, in which, as with striated muscle, glycerol extraction removes the membranes. Such extracted models do show qualitative, if not quantitative, similarity to striated muscle in their response to ATP, Ca^{++}, etc.

Ions and Vascular Smooth Muscle, Electrophysiology

As in all living cells, there is a resting potential in vascular smooth muscle cells, reported as up to 60 mv (negative inside). This is considerably less than for skeletal muscle and for nerve axons. The resting potential in striated muscle is almost completely a "K^+ potential," following the equation for a "Nernst potential" between two different concentrations of K^+ on each side of a membrane, which is much more permeable to K^+ than to other ions. However, in VSM Na^+ ions play a much greater role, and the concentration of Cl^- ions inside the cell is much greater than for striated muscle (where it is very low indeed). Permeability of the membrane to Na^+ is also much greater in VSM. During the contraction of VSM, rapid and large exchanges of Na^+ from outside to inside take place. Vasodilation and vasoconstriction are accompanied by changes of Na^+ in the blood stream (7). Thus, the resting potential cannot be attributed to any single ionic species.

Bivalent ions, particularly Ca^{++}, are essential for the contraction, which is impossible in Ca^{++}-free solutions. [►The Ca^{++} ions necessary for excitation of the contraction, in the case of VSM, probably enter from outside the cell and are not, as in skeletal muscle, released from particulate stores of Ca^{++} on the inner surfaces of cellular membranes. The permeability of the membrane to Ca^{++} thus is of much more importance in VSM.◄] The concentration of Ca^{++} greatly modifies the response to other agents such as adrenaline. Mg^{++} ions are also important, but increased concentrations reduce rather than increase the strength of contraction to other agents. Removal of Mg^{++} enhances the response. These effects on reactivity of the concentrations of ions, particularly Na^+ and K^+, have been the object of much research in connection with essential hypertension, and at one time Na^+-free, high K^+ diets were a popular treatment. No simple explanations of the effect of ions is possible, because, as mentioned earlier, their effects may be multiple, on the permeability of the membrane, the activity of the "pumps" and the contractile process itself.

In both in vivo and in vitro, action potentials,

signaling the depolarization of the membrane (reduction to zero or reversal of the sign of the resting potential), can be recorded from VSM cells. The "spike potential" is of much less magnitude (5–50 mv) than in striated muscle (130 mv), and the time constant of rise and fall of potential is much longer, up to 100 msecs. [►It is most disconcerting to electrophysiologists to find that the action potentials are not always correlated with the contraction. Action potentials can occur without any contraction, and vice versa. Evidently we should apply with great caution the knowledge of the mechanism of excitation of striated muscle, with the special intervention of calcium bound to the membrane as the excitation-contraction coupling agent, when mobilized by the action potential. The recording of action potential from the wall of blood vessels remains potentially a useful tool of research on vasomotor tone but will require careful interpretation.◄]

"Myogenic" vs "Neurogenic" Tone

As with other smooth muscles of viscera, VSM often shows rhythmic, apparently spontaneous, contractions not representing a response to the impulses in the sympathetic (adrenergic) nerves that innervate the vessel wall or to vasoactive substances in the circulation. There is much controversy whether such myogenic tone represents a physiological condition. The phenomena "in vitro" are seldom consistent, so the "myogenic school" consider that when such "pacemaker" activity is seen in VSM the conditions of the experiments are ideal, whereas the opposite "neurogenic school" consider the phenomena as indicating poor, unphysiological condition of the tissue! Myogenic activity is seen more often in the veins than in arteries. Certainly in the microcirculation, rhythmic contraction of the smooth muscle of arterioles, which is independent in different neighboring terminal beds, has been routinely seen. Stimulation of sympathetic nerves, in contrast, causes simultaneous contraction of all the arterioles in the field. Zwiefach called these independent rhythmic contractions "vasomotion." [►This is an unfortunate choice of name, since the phenomena are independent of the activity of the "vasomotor nerves."◄]

The Effect of Stretch on the Response

[►Related to the controversy about "spontaneous" myogenic activity is the "myogenic theory," originally advanced by Sir William Bayliss (8). He suggested that stretch of the VMS of the wall of arteries by an increase in transmural pressure (arterial pressure) was itself a stimulus to contraction.* Ever since, there has been controversy as to the validity of this statement. Folkow and his co-workers have produced much evidence which they interpret in terms of the "myogenic reflex." Others do not find stretch of the wall, per se, produces vasoconstriction, *in isolated or denervated blood vessels.* Perhaps the argument is academic. All parties agree that for VSM the degree of initial stretch, or initial passive tension due to stretch, greatly affects the tension developed when the muscle is stimulated chemically, electrically or by the arrival of vasomotor impulses in the sympathetic vasoconstrictor nerves. Since in intact living arteries and arterioles there is probably always a stream of impulses arriving (vasomotor tone), the end result of passive stretch is the same whatever view is held, i.e., the contraction or "tone" is increased.◄]

The effect of passive stretch (Fig. 8–2) is very similar to that which is so well known for striated muscle. The tension elicited by stimuli increases from a very low value when the wall, or a circumferential strip of it, is unstretched, to a maximal value for a stretch of 50–80% over the unstretched length (for striated muscle the maximum occurs at a lower per cent stretch). Further stretch decreases the active tension. [►As with striated muscle, it is not possible to decide whether it is the passive initial tension, or the initial length of the muscle that determines the increased response, but biophysical theories for the "sliding model" of striated muscle would prefer the assumption that the initial length, i.e., "conformation," was the determinant since it governs the degree of overlap of thick and thin fibers and the number of active crossbridges between them.◄]

The effect of stretch on the response of VSM to vasomotor tone means that the level of arterial blood pressure maintained plays an important role

---

*Note, however, that Bayliss himself, 21 years later, wrote, "I fear that we must regard the question as undecided." (*The Vasomotor System* [London: Longman, Green & Co., 1923], p. 17.) The greatest tribute to the genius of Bayliss is that in the final paragraph of his 1902 paper he said that his "myogenic reflex" might lead to instability in the cardiovascular system:

"Thus, without controlling government of the latter (the sympathetic nervous system), every rise in pressure would automatically cause a further rise, and every fall, from whatever cause, a further fall of blood pressure from peripheral vascular dilatation; i.e., a vicious circle would be established in the absence of the regulating functions of the vasomotor controls." (This was written 30 years before anyone talked of "positive feedback" and "cybernetics"!)

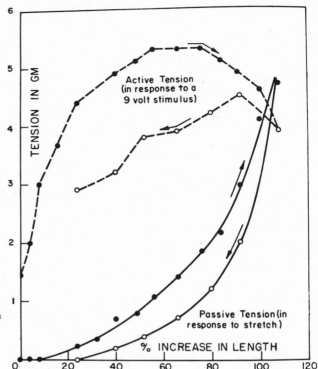

Fig. 8-2.—The effect of stretch of VSM on the *passive* (elastic) *tension* and on the *active tension* when stimulated. Note the phenomena of "hysteresis." (From Sparks, H. V., Jr., and Bohr, D. F.: Am. J. Physiol. 202:835, 1962.)

in governing the regulation of the circulation, in addition to its obvious role as the driving force for flow.

Metabolism (Oxygen Consumption) of VSM

A remarkable finding of Kosan (9, 10) is that the metabolic activity of vascular smooth muscle, as indicated by its oxygen consumption, is affected in a similar way by passive stretch (Fig. 8–3). He measured simultaneously the respiration (oxygen consumption) and the maintained tension developed by freshly isolated arteries of dogs; "passive tension" when the muscle was not stimulated; "active tension" when stimulated electrically or by adrenaline or by noradrenaline. Unfortunately, it was not possible to measure the degree of stretch of the contractile cells themselves. It was not surprising to find that the "activity oxygen consumption" increased parallel to the increased "active tension," as initial stretch altered this. It was, however, surprising to see a similar, but smaller, increase in rate of oxygen consumption in the unstimulated muscle, reaching a maximum at a certain degree of stretch. The curves of tension vs stretch compared with oxygen consumption vs

stretch are so similar, with stimulation (active) or without stimulation (passive), that a linear relation between the level of maintained tension (active or passive) and the rate of oxygen consumption is clearly indicated (Fig. 8–4). Points on such a graph can be obtained by varying the initial stretch of the muscle, by electrical stimulation or by vasoactive drugs (e.g., adrenaline and noradrenaline). No matter how the extra maintained tension is elicited, it is accompanied by a cost in increased flux of energy, indicated by the increased rate of oxygen consumption. The ratio of increased cost to the increased tension that is maintained is much less than in the case of striated muscle (although data on steady maintained tension, i.e., "tetanus" rather than isolated twitches, are not very complete). Thus, VSM is much more *efficient* in maintaining steady "tone" than is striated muscle, which in contrast is adapted to the rapid development and rapid decay of large tensions, as in the "twitch."

Our basic picture of the mechanism of contraction of VSM should thus be of a *steady-state system*. Even in the resting noncontractile state, there must be a steady flux of energy and substrate. This is carbohydrate, judging from the respiratory quotient, which is found to be very close to unity in the in vitro experiments. The magnitude of this steady flux is somehow governed by the molecular conformation, i.e., by the length of the muscle cell (the familiar curve rising to a maximum of tension and of oxygen consumption at a certain degree of stretch). If we think in the simplest terms, the heart of the matter is that even in the resting state any particular conformation of the elements of the contractile structure has a "self-decay," so that energy must be provided steadily to maintain any level of "activation" or length of the contractile unit.* Think of pouring water into a bottle with an outlet or leak at the bottom. To maintain a higher steady level of water in the bottle, the rate of pouring in water must be increased proportionately. There are two states of the molecular organization, resting and stimulated. The energy flux for a given length of the muscle cell is higher for the stimulated, but the energy flux is dependent on the length for each state (Fig. 8–4). However, whether resting or stimulated, the flux is the same for a given tension

---

*For those who want to think more deeply about essential causes, it is suggested that the crux is that myosin is an ATPase.

Fig. 8-3.—The result of simultaneous measurements of oxygen consumption, as per cent *over basal, passive* tension and *active* tension when VSM of dog arteries is stimulated by adrenaline. The symbols represent the three different experiments. (From Kosan, R.: Ph.D. Thesis, University of Western Ontario, 1967.)

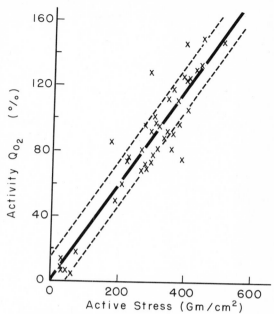

Fig. 8-4.—The relation between activity Q_{O_2}, i.e., the per cent increase in rate of oxygen consumption per unit weight of VSM, and the active stress, i.e., maintained tension in Gm/cm^2. The regression line and standard error of estimate represent points where the active tension was varied not only by different concentrations of adrenaline or noradrenaline but also by the degree of initial stretch. (From Kosan, R.: Ph.D. Thesis, University of Western Ontario, 1967.)

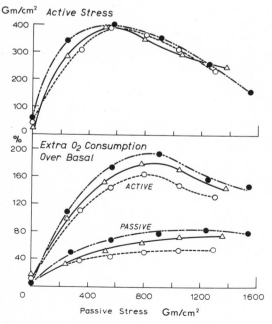

(active or passive tension). Further biophysical analysis of the model is inappropriate here. The ratio between rate of energy flux (e.g., from the oxygen consumption in L/sec × 4.8 kcal/L and the tension (dynes) would have the dimensions of energy/sec divided by force, i.e., of a *velocity*, which is related to the rate of development of tension of which the muscle is capable. The greater efficiency of VSM over voluntary striated muscle is achieved by sacrifice of the speed of response, i.e., because the VSM is much "slower" and has larger "time constants." (An extreme case of "efficiency" is the muscle of the clam that holds its two hinged shells together, where apparently a "locking mechanism" exists so that the shortening may be maintained without any extra flux of energy at all.)

Methods of Measuring the Active Tension

Our advance in knowledge of activity of vascular smooth muscle is largely dependent on development of methods of recording its response to nervous stimulation and vasoactive drugs. The classic method has been to measure the changes in resistance to flow (driving pressure/flow) of vascular beds, by cannulation of the relevant arterial supply and perfusion by a pump or by the animal's own blood pressure. If a pump, or reservoir of blood, was used, this was usually arranged to study flow under a constant perfusion pressure, which approximates the physiological conditions. With the availability of "finger pumps," which supply a constant flow, while the perfusion pressure depends on the resistance to flow of the vasculature perfused, constant flow perfusion became more popular than the method of perfusion at constant pressure. It is important to realize that the two methods, constant pressure vs constant flow perfusion, give very different dose-response curves, even though the same calculated resistance is used as an index. With constant pressure perfusion, the VSM has more and more mechanical advantage as the muscle succeeds in reducing the radius of the vessel. Equal increments of active muscle tension produce greater and greater increments of resistance, until "critical closure" (Chapter 7) may result when the tension and radius reach a critical value.

On the other hand, with constant flow perfusion, the decrease in radius of the vessel is very nearly completely compensated by a rise in the perfusion pressure (since the pump will not allow any decrease in flow) and the resulting passive distention of the vessel. The result is that the increase in calculated resistance (or in the perfusion pressure, since flow is constant) is approximately proportional to the active tension produced by the VSM (11). The relation has been proved by experiments in which an independent method of estimating the active tension was simultaneously applied. Pharmacologists like to apply their results on response vs strength of stimulus to theories of interaction of the drug with a "receptor," according to chemical kinetics (e.g., Michaelis-Menton kinetics of complex formation). It is essential that the data they use for such mathematical theories should be such that they have a reliable index of the response, linearly related to the force generated by the muscle. *The method of constant flow perfusion offers data applicable to this; the constant pressure method does not.*

An ingenious method of more direct study of the contraction of the vessel wall has been highly developed by Bohr and his associates (12). A helical strip of the wall is prepared from the artery on a jeweller's lathe and mounted so that it stretches a strain-gauge transducer when the VSM contracts (Fig. 8–5). This has been done with quite small arteries, and the responses to many stimuli are quickly and repeatedly recorded by this method. Figure 8–6 illustrates some results obtained by this method, the features of which have already been discussed. The absolute magnitudes of the force developed by the wall of course

Fig. 8-5.—The helical-strip method of preparing arterial smooth muscle for recording of tension developed. (See text.) (From Bohr *et al.* [10].)

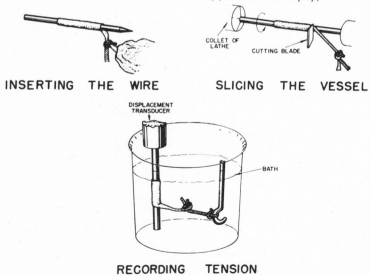

INSERTING THE WIRE   SLICING THE VESSEL

RECORDING TENSION

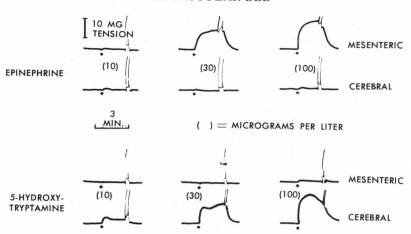

EPINEPHRINE

5-HYDROXY-
TRYPTAMINE

( ) = MICROGRAMS PER LITER

Fig. 8-6.—Results obtained from helical strips from the arteries of different organs, illustrating the difference in the responses to various stimuli. The vertical lines that intercept the tension record are artifacts when the solution in the bath was changed. (From Bohr *et al.* [10].)

may be unrepresentative of those in situ, because unless the "pitch" of the helix is correct, some VSM fibers will have been cut, and, also for small active tensions, the force required against the natural curvature of the strip will not be negligible.

Transmission of the Force to the Wall

There is nothing like the tendon of striated muscles in the case of vascular smooth muscle, by which the contractile force of the cells is transmitted to the structure of the wall. The smooth muscle cells are, it is true, connected to each other by the "tight junctions" at their ends, but it is not likely that these are mechanical linkages. The contraction of the smooth muscle cells must somehow tighten up the network of elastic fibers in which they are embedded, through the attachments of these fibers to the cell membranes.

As indicated in Figure 8–1, these attachments tend to be not at the ends of the cells but along the sides, i.e., at right angles to the circumference of the blood vessel wall. These cross fibers are connected to the circumferential fibers, which are an obvious feature of the organization of the media. This indirect transmission of the force of contraction, causing a decrease in circumference of the vessel, may well give the VSM a unique mechanical advantage in resisting the counter force, which is the circumferential tension due to the transmural pressure (by Laplace's law). If this tension were directly applied to prevent the contraction of the smooth muscle cells, it is difficult

to see how they would be able to resist being stretched, since the elastic modulus of the VSM is not great, even in the contracted state.

The paradox had been previously noted from data on the passive distention of arteries by transmural pressure when relaxed, and when contracted. As the pressure increases, the radius of the lumen increases, at first considerably, then much less and finally very little at high pressures, because of the high resistance to stretch of restricting collagen network. With the constricted artery, distensibility at any given pressure is less. The puzzling feature is that the final, almost constant, radius of the constricted vessel is so much less than that of the relaxed muscle, and it seems that increasing the transmural pressure to very high levels would still not make the vessel radius as great as in the relaxed vessel. *Apparently the active tension of the VSM can always prevent the transmural pressure, however great, from completely stretching the elastic network.*

We are so accustomed to using levers and fulcrums, or sheaves of pulleys, that the very great mechanical advantage obtainable by simple arrangements of ropes is largely forgotten (Fig. 8–7). Simple mechanics, by resolving forces in various ropes at their junctions, demonstrates that in an arrangement such as illustrated, which may well represent the actual mode of linkage of VSM to the collagen network, there is a mechanical advantage given by $\dfrac{1}{2 \cos \theta \cos \phi}$ (see Fig. 8–7). If θ and ϕ are close to 90°, i.e., the ropes are almost straight and the cosines are very close to

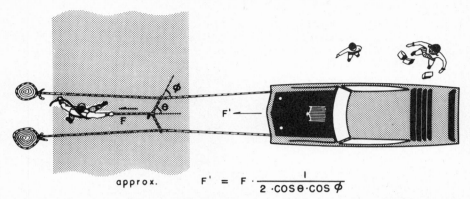

$$\text{approx.} \qquad F' = F \cdot \frac{1}{2 \cdot \cos\theta \cdot \cos\phi}$$

Fig. 8-7.—A physiologist pulls his car out of the ditch with an arrangement of ropes which he learned from the study of how VSM is linked with the elastic network of arteries. (See text.) (Kindly drawn by Alfred Jay.) The famous engraving by Gustav Doré, *The Death of Samson,* shows the blinded Hebrew hero utilizing the same kind of mechanical advantage (though he pushed on the pillars rather than pulled) in demolishing the temple of his enemies.

zero, the force applied, when the man in Figure 8–7 is pulling on his rope, effectively can exert a force hundreds of times greater on the car. Of course, he will have to move his rope many feet to move the car an inch (the "displacement ratio" is correspondingly low), but, if his wife is ready with a brick under the rear wheel and he has enough patience to readjust the ropes repeatedly, he will succeed in getting home that night. The interested reader might make a simple model of strings (13) and verify that a very small weight can prevent the stretching of the network by a much larger weight.

Note that the mechanical advantage increases, toward infinity, as the tension in the wall increases, so that the paradox that the muscle can prevent complete stretching of the wall, by whatever transmural pressure, is explained.

Summary

The important points made in this chapter are as follows:

1. The media of arteries and veins are tightly packed with vascular smooth muscle cells. Although these communicate with each other through "tight junctions," serving to conduct excitation from cell to cell, the transmission of the force of contraction to the vessel wall is by linkages with the circumferential network of elastin and collagen fibers.

2. VSM also has a morphogenetic function in synthesizing elastin and collagen fibers and somehow, in a way yet unknown, laying down the elastic network in embryonic development, growth, and repair of blood vessels.

3. The contractile mechanism is by myofibrils, which probably basically resemble the actin and myosin complex of striated muscle (the sliding model), but there are important qualitative differences in the role of specific ions. There are great differences in response between striated and VSM and between VSM of vessels of different kinds (e.g., arteries and veins) and of the same kind from different organs. A drug may alter the permeability of the membrane to other agents, the activity of metabolic pumps maintaining ionic gradients, or the contractile mechanism itself. Hence, the variety of different effects on VSM.

4. The degree of initial stretch of the arterial wall by the transmural pressure greatly affects the response to vasomotor stimulation by the vasoconstrictor nerves (vasomotor tone) and to circulating pressor substances. Thus, the level of the maintained blood pressure governs the vasomotor response of the vessel wall.

5. The VSM is a "steady-state" system, which requires a steady transformation of energy (as shown by the oxygen consumption) to maintain a steady active tension. In this function, VSM is more efficient than striated muscle. The increased efficiency is at the expense of rapidity of development of tension and of relaxation.

6. The mechanical arrangement by which the VSM transmits its force to resist the tension in the wall is such as to give it a high mechanical advantage of a special kind.

REFERENCES

1. Holman, M. E.: Electrophysiology and vascular smooth muscle, Ergebn. Physiol. 61:137, 1969.
2. Mellander, S., and Johansson, B.: Control of resistance, exchange, and capacity functions in peripheral circulation, Pharmacol. Rev. 20:117, 1968.
3. Somlyo, A. P., and Somlyo, A. V.: Vascular smooth muscle: I. Normal structure, pathology, biochemistry, and biophysics, Pharmacol. Rev. 20:197, 1968.
4. Somlyo, A. P., and Somlyo, A. V.: Vascular smooth muscle: II. Pharmacology of normal and hypertensive vessels, Pharmacol. Rev. 22:249, 1970.
5. Bohr, D. F.: Electrolytes and smooth muscle contraction, Pharmacol. Rev. 16:85, 1964.
6. Haust, M. D.; More, R. T., and Morat, H. Z.: The role of smooth muscle cells in the fibrogenesis of arteriosclerosis, Am. J. Path. 37:377, 1960.
7. Friedman, S. N.; Nakashiwaa, M., and Friedman, C. L.: Sodium, potassium, and peripheral resistance in the rat tail, Circulation Res. 13:223, 1963.
8. Bayliss, W. M.: On the local reactions of the arterial wall to changes in internal pressure, J. Physiol. 28:220, 1902.
9. Kosan, R. L.: The oxygen consumption of relaxed and active arterial smooth muscle (Ph.D. diss., University of Western Ontario, 1968).
10. Kosan, R. L., and Burton, A. C.: Oxygen consumption of arterial smooth muscle as a function of active tone and passive stretch, Circulation Res. 19:79, 1966.
11. Burton, A. C., and Stinson, R. H.: The measurement of tension in vascular smooth muscle, J. Physiol. 153:240, 1960.
12. Bohr, D. F.; Goulet, P. L., and Taquini, A. C., Jr.: Direct tension recording from smooth muscle of resistance vessels from various organs, Angiology 12:478, 1961.
13. Burton, A. C.: Relation of structure to function of the tissues of the wall of blood vessels, Physiol. Rev. 34:619, 1944.
14. Folkow, B.: Neuronal control of the blood vessels, Physiol. Rev. 15:629, 1955.

9

Transmural Pressures, Pressure Gradients and Resistance to Flow in the Vascular Bed

Fluid Pressure

THE FIRST LAW OF FLUID PRESSURE, enunciated by Pascal (1623–1662), is that at every point in a fluid system there is a *hydrostatic pressure which acts equally in all directions.* This pressure is measured by the force, in dynes, acting on each square centimeter of an imaginary plane, facing in any direction, at that point. The fundamental unit of pressure is, therefore, "dynes per square centimeter." In practice, it would be very difficult to measure the pressure in the way in which it is defined, although this could be done by making, say, a square centimeter of the wall of a containing vessel (sides or bottom) movable and measuring the thrust upon it by some device. It is much more convenient to use the second and third laws of Pascal, which state how, under gravity, the pressure changes as we move from one level to another in a fluid. The second law is that the *pressure is the same at all points,* in a continuous connected fluid, *at the same level.* The third law is that the *pressure increases with depth,* by an amount given by:

$$\Delta P = \rho\, g\, (\Delta h)$$

where ΔP is the increase in pressure (dynes per cm^2), ρ is the density of the fluid (Gm per cm^3), g is the acceleration due to gravity (about 980 cm per sec^2) and Δh is the increase in depth in centimeters.

Manometers

The familiar *U*-tube manometer measures pressure by the height of a fluid column (Fig. 9–1, *A*).

The fluid may be water ($\rho = 1$) or mercury ($\rho = 13.6$). The argument runs as follows: The pressure at the open meniscus *(a)* is atmospheric, B dynes per cm^2. By the third law, at level b, h cm below, the pressure must be $B + \rho gh$. By the second law, the pressure at b' must be the same as this, since it is at the same level in a continuous fluid. The pressure, P, to be measured must then be given by:

$$P = B + \rho gh \text{ dynes/cm}^2$$

Since this argument does not involve the relative cross-sectional area of the limbs of the U tube, it applies equally well both to the case where the two limbs are of equal area and to the type where, on one side, there is a reservoir of relatively larger area (Fig. 9–1, *B*). The difference comes merely from the relative convenience of using a fixed scale on the manometer, rather than measuring the *difference* in height, Δh, each time. In the U-tube type with a fixed scale, the two limbs must be accurately of equal cross-sectional area, and the scale is as shown, 1 mm Hg pressure being represented by 0.5 mm on the scale. With the reservoir type, the scale is 1 mm Hg pressure for each millimeter on the scale since the level in the reservoir hardly alters as the column is driven up the tube (for this to be true, its area must be at least 100 times that of the vertical tube).

Columns of mercury are so often used to measure pressure (as in the barometer) that the practical unit, "millimeters of mercury," is universally used. However, to include in the equations of hydrodynamics other forms of energy of flowing fluids (such as the kinetic energy), we should always use the fundamental unit—that is, dynes

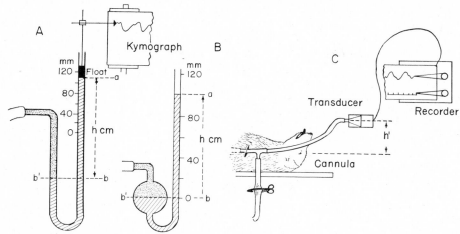

Fig. 9-1.—The types of manometer used by physiologists: **A,** the mercury manometer, U-tube type. If a fixed scale is used, it is essential that the cross-sectional area of the two limbs be equal. **B,** the reservoir type. The cross-sectional area in the reservoir must be at least 100 times that of the vertical limb. Note that the scale is twice that of **A. C,** the electromanometer. With the electromanometer, as with all manometers, unless the transducer is at the level of the cannula, the pressures recorded must be corrected by the factor $\rho gh'$.

per square centimeter. The two units are easily convertible, for by Pascal's third law we may calculate the pressure in fundamental units, equivalent to a column of mercury 1 mm in height:

$$P = \rho gh = 13.6 \times 980 \times 0.1 = 1{,}330 \text{ dynes/cm}^2$$

Therefore, *1 mm Hg pressure = 1,330 dynes per cm²*.

In experiments on anesthetized animals, the physiologist usually inserts a *cannula* into the artery, connecting this by tubes full of saline solution to the manometer (Fig. 9–1, *C*). The saline usually contains an agent, such as heparin or sodium citrate, to prevent clotting of the blood in the artery on contact with the "foreign substances" of glass and rubber. Plastic cannulas, especially if siliconized, are much better than glass cannulas in postponing clotting. If the level at which the saline solution meets the mercury in the reservoir of the "closed" limb of the manometer, or the membrane of the electromanometer, is the same as that of the cannula, no correction is necessary. If it differs, a correction ($\rho gh'$) must be applied, where ρ is the density of the saline solution (close to 1.0) and h' is the difference in levels, in order to transfer from the pressure, registered on the manometer, to that in the artery at the cannula. For measurement of relatively low pressure (as the pressures in the venous system), water or saline solution is used in the manometer rather than mercury, giving much more sensitivity, for the pressure corresponding to 1 mm of water is (ρgh), $1 \times 980 \times 0.1$, or only 98 dynes per cm² (instead of 1,330 dynes per cm² for mercury).

Modern physiologists use *electromanometers*, where the pressure deforms a membrane; this deformation changes an electrical resistance (or electrical capacity or voltage), and the pressure may be registered photographically, or by ink writing, on a recorder of some type. The device that changes the pressure into an electrical change is called a *pressure transducer*. It must never be forgotten that *the only way that the readings of an electromanometer can be calibrated is by comparison with the simple manometer using a column of fluid.* Pressure is ultimately always measured by the height of a column of fluid of known density that it will support. Electrical manometers possess no magical powers of defying the laws of hydrostatics; so the same corrections must be made if the transducer is not at the same level as the cannula.

Pulsatile and Mean Pressures

The very great, but the only, advantage of electromanometers over the liquid-column manometer (other than convenience in telemetering) is that they can be made to have very rapid response to changing pressures, such as the pressure in central arteries, which oscillates between a minimal value (diastolic pressure) and a maximal value (systolic pressure) with every heartbeat. For measurement of *mean pressure* throughout the cycle, the simple manometer is much better. By introducing, deliberately, a device that slows the response of an electrometer (either by a high resistance to flow in the connection between cannula and transducer or electrically in the electronic device beyond the transducer), the pulsations in the record may be eliminated. The level of pressure recorded is then the *true mean pressure*. By this is meant the *area mean* (Fig. 9–2). This is not, of course, equal to the arithmetic mean of the systolic and diastolic pressures. For the normal central arterial pulse curve, the true mean pressure is closer to

$$\frac{\text{Systolic} + 2 \text{ diastolic pressure}}{3}$$

than to the arithmetic mean.

Because of the great inertia of the mercury manometer, the oscillations of its column are far less (except in the case of "resonance") than the actual fluctuations of the arterial pressure, but the mean pressure is correctly recorded.

A manometer connected by cannula to an artery or other blood vessel records the pressure at the cannula tip (if the necessary corrections for levels have been made). However, this does not mean that this pressure is what would have existed at that point had the cannula not been inserted. Where the artery is cut and pushed over the cannula, the normal flow at that point ceases, and the pressure (end pressure) is greater than that which existed formerly. The use of a T cannula preserves the continuity of flow in the artery, and a side tube may be connected to the manometer; the pressure recorded (side pressure) may be very close to that which existed in the artery, and identical if the flow was not really altered at all. This difference between side and end pressures has confused medical students for generations. It is really very simple. There never existed in the blood of the artery two different pressures; *there is only one pressure at a given point in a fluid, and this acts equally in all directions*. It is simply that, in our way of measuring this single pressure, we may alter conditions so that what we measure is not what existed before. It is hoped that in the next chapter (Chapter 10) the confusion on this point may be finally resolved.

Mean Transmural Pressures in Different Categories of Blood Vessels

Physiologists long ago measured the pressures in the large vessels of animals and man by direct cannulation of arteries and veins.* The modern use of catheters of very small bore has extended the measurements from large veins to quite small ones, and from large arteries down to small ones. The general result is shown in Figure 9–3. A key measurement giving more of the whole picture was that of Landis (1), who succeeded in inserting fine glass cannulas, containing saline solution, into individual capillary loops of his own nail bed (Fig. 6–6, *C*). The level reached by the saline solution in the vertical part of the tubes measured the capillary pressure (here the stoppage of flow by the end-cannula would make an absolutely negligible change in the pressure recorded). The pressure at the arteriolar end of the capillary averaged about 35 mm Hg; that at the venular end, about 15 mm Hg; and the mean capillary pressure averaged 25 mm Hg. *These are most important levels of pressure for the student to memorize.* In the renal and portal circuits, where there are special arrangements, as of two capillary beds in series, the capillary pressures are, of course, not the standard 25 mm mean pressure. For example, the pressure in the glomerular capillaries of the kidney is probably from 70 to 80 mm Hg, while that of the tubular capillaries is 25 mm Hg. The pressure in the pulmonary capillaries is much less (about 10 mm Hg).

The transmural pressures and the gradients of pressure are much less in the pulmonary circuit, the mean pulmonary arterial pressure being only about 12 mm Hg for a resting cardiac output (systolic, 20 mm; diastolic, 8 mm). The intravascular pressure in the pulmonary capillaries is only

Fig. 9-2.—Illustrating what is meant by the "true mean" or "area mean" of a pulsatile pressure (e.g., central arterial pressure). The area of the curve above the rectangle must equal the sum of the two areas below.

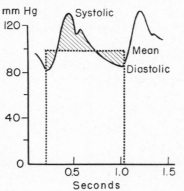

*About 1730, the Reverend Stephen Hales measured the arterial pressure of a mare.

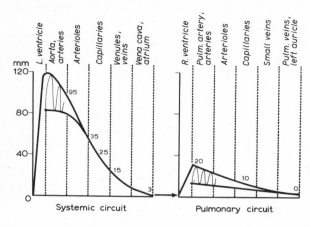

Fig. 9-3.—The distribution of intravascular pressures in the systemic and in the pulmonary circuits. The attenuation of the pulse pressure (systolic minus diastolic) is indicated. The numbers on the curves are mean pressures that are important to memorize.

about 10 mm Hg, but here there is reason to believe that the tissue pressure is below atmospheric pressure, so that transmural pressure may be greater than this (see Chapter 10).

Our knowledge of the pressures in the heart chambers and in the pulmonary circuit of man is due to the development of *cardiac catheterization* by Cournand and his colleagues, although, as Cournand (2) points out, two French physicians, Auguste Chauveau and Jules Morey, as early as 1856 had used cardiac catheters in the horse and produced records of pressures in the left atrium and right and left ventricles that agree well with modern measurements.

Cardiac catheters are now routinely pushed up (usually in the anticubital vein) in the arm, to descend the superior vena cava, thence into the right atrium to the right ventricle, in which they "curl" to pass through the pulmonary valve and record the pulmonary artery pressure. Approach to the chambers of the left heart is by a catheter in the femoral vein, pushed up the vena cava into the right atrium and piercing the septum between the left and right atria. Steering of the catheter tips is accomplished by having a curved flexible tip and utilizing the currents of flow, together with twisting of the catheter. It can now be said that the pressure in any chamber of the heart or major vessel in the human body can be measured directly with safety (3).

Knowledge of the pulmonary capillary pressure is based on what are called *pulmonary wedge pressures*. The catheter in the pulmonary artery is pushed into the vascular bed until it is wedged into a small artery (2–4 mm in diameter, according to the size of catheter tip), blocking the local flow. It then presumably records the pressure where the

column of stagnant blood joins with free-flowing streams beyond the capillary bed. Thus the pulmonary wedge pressure is likely to be between the true capillary pressure and the pressure in the left atrium, and the term "pulmonary capillary pressure" for this measured quantity has rightly been dropped. The drop of pressure (pulmonary artery pressure to wedge pressure) is used to calculate what is called the *pulmonary arteriolar resistance*, which is of great importance in the investigation of pulmonary disease (4).

Not only is the gradient of pressure greatest in the arterioles, it is also most variable here. When the arterioles are constricted (peripheral vasomotor tone), the total drop of pressure from aorta to vena cava may be the same, but the gradient will

Fig. 9-4.—Showing how the curve of **Figure 9-3** is altered when the resistance vessels (the arterioles) are constricted *(solid curve)* or dilated *(broken curve)*. The mean arterial and the mean capillary pressures tend to change very little.

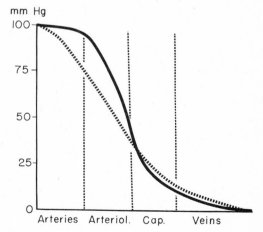

be even more dominantly in the arterioles; when the arterioles are dilated (with low vasomotor tone), the gradient is more spaced out over the whole circuit (Fig. 9–4).

Resistance to Flow: Definition

Thinking about hemodynamics is very greatly facilitated by the use of the concept of "resistance to flow." This is simply the ratio of the driving force—that is, the pressure drop from any point, A in the system to another point B,*—to the flow between A and B that results.

$$\text{Resistance to flow} = \frac{\text{Pressure drop } A \text{ to } B}{\text{Total flow from } A \text{ to } B}$$

$$_AR_B = \frac{\Delta P}{F} \qquad (a)$$

The equation has two other forms:

$$\Delta P = F \cdot R \qquad (b)$$

and

$$F = \frac{\Delta P}{R} \qquad (c)$$

Each of the three identical relations can be quickly found by using the expression ($\Delta P/F \cdot R$), by covering the quantity desired (e.g., F) and taking the remainder (e.g., $\Delta P/R$). Thus, resistance to flow is a common-sense quantitative measure of how much difficulty there is in driving the flow through a given section of the vascular bed. If the resistance is doubled, only half the flow will result for the same driving pressure difference.

The property of resistance to flow that makes it so useful is that, for flow through successive elements of a vascular bed which are effectively in series, the successive resistances are additive;

*See next chapter (Chapter 10) to realize that this is *not* the true driving force for flow.

that is, the total resistance to flow is the sum of the resistances of the elements in series (Fig. 9–5). This is true, even if the elements consist of many units in parallel and in series with each other (as in the case of the small vessels of a terminal vascular bed). For, if the elements are truly in series, the same total flow occurs through each; so we may use form (b) of the equation for each resistance in turn:

$$\Delta_A P_B = P_A - P_B = F \times {}_AR_B$$
$$\Delta_B P_C = P_B - P_C = F \times {}_BR_C$$
$$\Delta_C P_D = P_C - P_D = F \times {}_CR_D$$
$$\Delta_D P_E = P_D - P_E = F \times {}_DR_E$$

Adding, $\Delta_A P_E = P_A - P_E = F \ ({}_AR_B + {}_BR_C + {}_CR_D + {}_DR_E)$

Since, by definition of the total resistance, ${}_AR_E$ is given by:

$$\Delta_A P_E = F \times {}_AR_E$$

then

$$_AR_E = {}_AR_B + {}_BR_C + {}_CR_D + {}_DR_E$$

that is, the total resistance is the sum of the individual resistances in series. Resistances to flow obey the same laws as electrical resistances as regards the combined resistance of series and of parallel arrangements.

Relation of Drop of Pressure to Resistance

By means of form (b) of the basic equation, we can also deduce where the greatest resistance lies in the system, just by seeing where the greatest drop of pressure occurs. Therefore we conclude, from the actual measurements of pressure in the various vessels, illustrated in Figure 9–3, that the arterioles offer the major resistance in the vascular bed, the capillaries the next largest

Fig. 9-5.—Illustrating the additive property of resistances between successive points A, B, C, etc., in a vascu- lar bed where the elements are in series, that is, the total flow, F, is the same at each place.

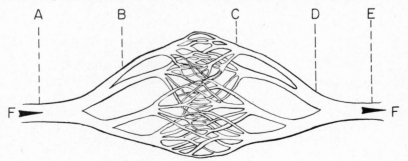

resistance, the distributing arteries much less resistance and the veins least of all.

Resistance Calculated from Poiseuille's Law

If we may use Poiseuille's law (Chapter 5), then the resistance is given by:

$$R = \frac{\Delta P}{F} = \left(\frac{8}{\pi}\right) \times (\eta) \times \left(\frac{l}{r^4}\right)$$

Since the viscosity will be the same (or approximately so) for different vessels (ignoring the Fahraeus-Lindqvist effect), we can predict the relative resistance of the different vessels by calculating their geometrical factors $\left(\frac{l}{r^4}\right)$ from data such as those in Table 6–1 (Chapter 6). If there are, for instance, N capillaries in parallel, the total resistance of the capillaries will be $\frac{1}{N}\left(\frac{l}{r^4}\right)$. Such calculation has been done, using the data of Table 6–1, with the results shown in Table 9–1.

TABLE 9–1.—Relative Resistance to Flow in the Vascular Bed: Calculated from Table 6 and Poiseuille's Law $\left(R \propto \frac{l}{r^4}\right)$

Aorta	4%	Venules	4 %
Large arteries	5%	Terminal veins	0.3%
Mean arterial branches	10%	Main venous branches	0.7%
Terminal branches	6%	Large veins	0.5%
Arterioles	41%	Vena cava	1.5%
Capillaries	27%		
Total: arterial + capillary = 93%		Total venous = 7%	

It will be seen that the relative resistances, predicted from the geometry of the vessels and from Poiseuille's law, agree with that experimentally measured by the way in which the pressure drops in the system (Fig. 9–3).

Interpretation of Resistance to Flow

In any physiological experiment where both the driving pressure (arterial minus venous pressure) and the volume flow are known, the resistance to flow may be calculated and compared with the resistance to flow in other circumstances. *Comparison tells us, without any doubt, whether the vascular bed concerned has widened or become narrower. However, the findings will not reveal the reason for this change in resistance until we examine the case carefully.*

A reduction in resistance might be purely *passive dilatation* if, between the two conditions compared, the transmural pressure of those vessels that give the major resistance had been increased and the vessels had widened because of their elastic properties. In this case, it would be wrong to conclude that an *active dilatation*, due to a decrease in vasomotor tone, had occurred unless the change in resistance was more than to be expected from the elasticity. On the other hand, in many cases the resistance will be found to change in the opposite direction to that expected from pressure change by elasticity, for example, if the resistance had increased even though the transmural pressures had risen (this is the usual case when a pressor drug is added to the perfusion fluid of a vascular bed). In such a case, the change must have been due to an active vasoconstriction (contraction of the vascular smooth muscle).

Changes in resistance to flow may be completely interpreted in terms of degree of vasomotor tone if the passive changes in resistance to flow with different pressures of perfusion are known. For example, the curves of flow or arterial pressure for the rabbit ear were obtained by Girling with different degrees of electrical stimulation (Fig. 9–6). These curves may be translated into curves of resistance to flow versus arterial pressure. They show that, in the case of no stimulation (dilated vessels), the resistance to flow rises only slightly as the arterial pressure (and thus the transmural pressures) is lowered, until finally it rises sharply at a *residual critical closing pressure* of about 10 mm Hg. For increasing degrees of vasomotor tone, the resistance is higher at all pressures and the increase of resistance with reduced pressure is more and more marked (the marked rise of resistance toward a very high value denotes approach to critical closure of the vessels). When such curves have been established for specific vascular beds, the use of resistance to flow will give accurate and unambiguous information as to the degree of vasomotor tone (5).

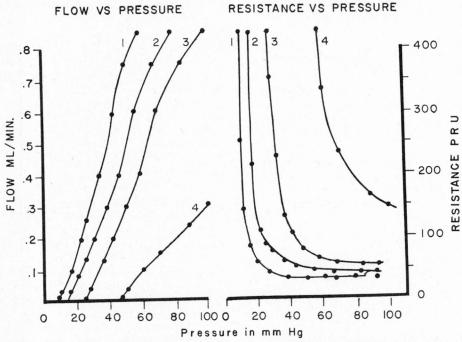

Fig. 9-6.—The almost universal shape of curves of resistance versus driving pressure in vascular beds, with increasing degrees of vascular tone *1* to *4*. *PRU*, peripheral resistance units. (From the unpublished work of Girling on the rabbit ear. Similar pressure-flow curves have been published [Girling, F.: Am. J. Physiol. 170:131, 1952].)

Examples of the Use of Resistance to Flow

The *total peripheral resistance* (TPR) is the resistance offered to the total output of the heart by all of the peripheral vascular bed. For a normal man at rest, we may take the figure of 5 L per min for the cardiac output; a mean pressure of 100 mm Hg for the aorta; and close to zero for the vena cava or atrium (say 5 mm Hg for the example). The units for these quantities may be chosen to suit physiologists. It has been agreed by many to use millimeters of mercury for the pressures, and milliliters per second, rather than liters per minute, for the flow (5 L per min equals 83 ml per sec). The unit of resistance is then in *peripheral resistance units* (PRU); and the value of TPR at rest is: $\dfrac{100 - 5}{83} = \dfrac{95}{83} = 1.1\ PRU.$ (This is why these units were chosen.)

In moderate *exercise*, the aortic blood pressure rises to values such as 180 mm Hg systolic and 100 mm Hg diastolic (with a mean pressure of, say, 140 mm Hg), while the cardiac output may have increased by as much as 3 times (i.e., to 250 ml per sec (15 L per min). Then

$$TPR = \frac{140 - 5}{250} = \frac{135}{250} = 0.54\ PRU$$

The total peripheral resistance in exercise therefore falls very greatly. Whatever the cause (both reflex and chemical actions are involved), we know that in exercise the peripheral blood vessels are dilated. The relatively small rise in mean pressure could not possibly explain this degree of dilatation on the basis of passive distention.

Another example of the usefulness of calculating resistance is that of *essential hypertension*, where the mean arterial blood pressure may be as high as 200 mm Hg instead of the normal 100 mm Hg. Research on hypertensive patients has shown, however, that their cardiac output is no greater than normal. The TPR in essential hypertension is, therefore, greatly increased above normal. *Whatever the ultimate causes of essential hypertension, we can be sure that the resistance vessels of the vascular bed are narrowed.* Moreover, since it is found that the capillary pressure in hypertension is generally normal (about 25 mm Hg), we can localize the chief narrowing to the arterioles, for the pressure drop, from arteries to capillaries (200–25 mm Hg instead of 100–25 mm

Hg), is very greatly increased, although the blood flow through them is the same.

The case of *chronic anemia,* where the hematocrit value is low, presents a different reason for an abnormal TPR. In this condition, patients have an increased cardiac output at rest, while their blood pressures tend to be normal. The TPR is thus correspondingly low. An important factor is the decreased viscosity of the blood (Fig. 5–3, Chapter 5), for even if the caliber of the vessels (i.e., their geometric factors) were normal, the reduced viscosity would lead to a lower resistance. (The change in viscosity is certainly not the whole explanation of the sustained cardiac output.)

Hemodynamic Analysis: The Example of Arteriovenous Fistula

A very good illustration of the value of thinking in simple terms of resistance to flow is provided by the case of peripheral arteriovenous "anastomoses" or "shunts." Here, illogical thinking might lead to an opposite conclusion. These shunts occur accidentally, as when a bullet traumatizes tissue in the neighborhood of, say, the adjacent femoral artery and vein. They also occur in multiple lesions of small arteries and veins in a disease called *hereditary telangiectasia* (Osler-Weber-Rendu's disease). The open ductus between aorta and pulmonary artery (patent ductus arteriosus) also would serve as a hemodynamic example. Figure 9–7 illustrates the case of a shunt between femoral artery and vein. The natural thought might be that this would result in a serious depletion of the circulation of the limb and that signs of peripheral ischemia, such as tissue necrosis or gangrene, would appear in the feet. In contrast, thinking in terms of hemodynamics leads to the conclusion that *very little diminution of flow will occur in the limb, while a serious*

overloading of the heart will result. The argument runs as follows: Before the shunt is present, the pressure in the femoral artery at *A* will be only slightly lower than in the aorta, because there is so little resistance to flow in the large arteries. The pressure drop in this segment of the tree (given by $F \times R$) will amount to perhaps only 3 mm Hg, from a mean pressure of 100 mm in the aorta to 97 mm in the femoral artery. Similarly, the venous pressure at *B* will be only slightly greater than in the atrium—say, 5 mm Hg instead of 3 mm Hg. (The exact figures assumed do not alter the outcome of the logic.) The driving pressure difference will be 97 − 5, or 92, mm Hg.

The opening of the shunt between *A* and *B* will very greatly lower the TPR of the limb. Instead of the peripheral resistance of the arterioles of the leg, there is now, in parallel with this, the very low resistance of the shunt. The total flow down the femoral artery above the shunt, and back to the heart in the femoral vein above the shunt, will in consequence increase greatly—let us say to as much as four times the original values. The pressure difference ($F \times R$) between the heart and points *A* and *B* will therefore increase proportionately. The arterial pressure at *A* will now be 100 − 12, or 88, mm Hg instead of 100 − 3, or 97, mm Hg. The pressure at *B* will be 2 + 12, or 14, mm Hg, instead of 2 + 3, or 5, mm Hg. Thus the driving force for flow through the vascular bed of the limb, which was 97 − 3, or 94, mm Hg, is now 88 − 12, or 76, mm Hg, a decrease of only about 20%, and the blood flow will decrease proportionately. We would certainly not expect any signs of ischemia in the leg from such a relatively slight decrease in blood flow.

On the other hand, the decrease in TPR will tend to increase the cardiac output very greatly, for the cardiovascular reflexes always tend to keep the arterial pressure to the standard level.

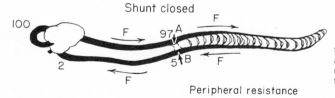

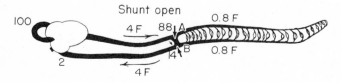

Fig. 9-7.—Schematic diagram to illustrate how the presence of a shunt (e.g., arteriovenous fistula in the thigh) will lead, not to any serious diminution of flow in the limb, but to an overload on the heart.

The patient with a shunt of this kind will have a cardiac output at rest like that of a normal person in continuous moderate exercise. Such arteriovenous fistulas therefore impose a stress on the heart, rather than leading to signs of peripheral ischemia. This conclusion, based on thinking in terms of simple hemodynamics, agrees with clinical experience. Actually, there is a close analogy in terms of electrical circuit theory (for the law of flow $F = \dfrac{\Delta P}{R}$ is analogous to Ohm's law, $C = \dfrac{\Delta V}{R}$). When there is a short circuit across the connection of the "mains" to a house on the street, say from damage by rats or by water, the lights of that house may dim a little but they do not go out. In a few seconds, however, the increased load on the generator at the substation (like the heart) may blow a fuse and the whole district will be in darkness.

Many other examples of the use of resistance to flow in the interpretation of results in circulatory physiology are given in later chapters and figures. Changes in resistance always indicate changes in caliber of the small vessels, and the other data (e.g., pressure changes) can usually help to decide whether such changes are "active" or "passive."

[►Some physiologists have held the opinion that, in view of the dependence of resistance on transmural pressures, and the dependence of viscosity on rate of flow so that the flow-pressure curve is by no means linear, the use of resistance to flow is not justified or even useful. This is as illogical as to refuse to use electrical resistance in electronics, where Ohm's law is seldom obeyed in modern circuits, or to reject thinking in terms of the price per egg because that price depends on whether they are bought by the dozen or by the gross.◄] The calculation of resistance to flow remains the first step in hemodynamic analysis. The interpretation of its value requires that we consider all the factors that may change that resistance.

REFERENCES

1. Landis, E. M.: Micro-injection studies of capillary blood pressure in human skin, Heart 15:209, 1930.
2. Cournand, A.: The Historical Development of the Concept of Pulmonary Circulation, in *Pulmonary Circulation* (New York: Grune & Stratton, Inc., 1959), pp. 1–19.
3. Zimmerman, H. A. (ed.): *Intravascular Catheterization* (Springfield, Ill.: Charles C Thomas, Publisher, 1959).
4. Fritts, H. W., Jr., and Cournand, A.: Physiological Factors Regulating Pressure, Flow and Distribution of Blood in the Pulmonary Circuit, in Cournand, A.: *Pulmonary Circulation* (New York: Grune & Stratton, Inc., 1959), pp. 62–74.
5. Burton, A. C.: Laws of Physics and Flow in Blood Vessels, in Wolstenholme, G. E. W. (ed.): *Visceral Circulation* (Ciba Foundation Symposium) (London: J. & A. Churchill, Ltd., 1952), pp. 70–83.

The Energetics of the Circulation

10

Total Fluid Energy, Gravitational Potential Energy, Effects of Posture

"The truth, the whole truth, and nothing but the truth."

Total Fluid Energy

IF THIS CHAPTER had come sooner, it would have prevented the promulgation of an error. If it came later, understanding of particular applications to the circulation would be easier. The error is widespread; *it is that fluid flows always from a point where the pressure is higher to a point where the pressure is lower, that is, it is the difference of pressure which is the driving force for flow.* With the inclusion of the word "always," this statement is not true. Even without the word, the statement is only a partial truth, applying to very restricted cases. *The true driving force for flow is a difference, not of pressure, but of "total fluid energy" between any two points.*

The total fluid energy, E, reckoned per unit volume of fluid, is the sum of three terms:

$$E = P + \rho gh + \tfrac{1}{2}\rho v^2$$

where E is the total energy, in ergs per cubic centimeter; P is the pressure, in dynes per square centimeter; ρ is the density, in grams per cubic centimeter; g is the acceleration due to gravity (about 980* cm/sec²); h is the height in centimeters above some arbitrary datum level; and v is the velocity of the fluid at that point, in centimeters per second. Instead of the centimeter-gram-second (cgs) units, ergs per cubic centimeter (identical with dynes per square centimeter), we may use millimeters of mercury for all the terms (1 mm Hg = 1,330 dynes/cm²). If the total energy, E_A, at point A in a fluid is greater than the

energy E_B at point B, flow will occur from A to B, and the rate of flow will depend on the difference in energies ($E_A - E_B$). More confusion in thinking about hemodynamics has probably resulted from lack of understanding of this complete law than from any other factor.

The three items in the total energy are:

a) The *pressure energy, P;* this is a kind of "potential energy" in a fluid.

b) The item ρgh represents the *gravitational potential energy,* that is, the capability of doing work because of differences in fluid level.

c) The item $\tfrac{1}{2}\rho v^2$ is the *kinetic energy* of the fluid per cubic centimeter (cf. $\tfrac{1}{2}mv^2$ for the kinetic energy of a mass m having velocity v).

Hydrostatics

If the fluid is everywhere at rest, the expression for E becomes simpler, since the third term, the kinetic energy, is zero; that is,

$$E = P + \rho gh$$

Also, if there is no motion, there can be no dissipation of energy, and the energy E must be the same at all points in the fluid (it is assumed that all points are freely connected by fluid, not in separate compartments). This yields at once the *laws of hydrostatics,* first enunciated by Pascal, French religious philosopher and mathematician (1623–1662) and published in 1663. These laws are:

1. The pressure in a fluid is the same at all points at the same level; that is, if h is the same for all points and E the same, then P must be the same everywhere.

---

*It should be noted that the value of g varies over the surface of the earth. The author was brought up on 981, which is the value in England.

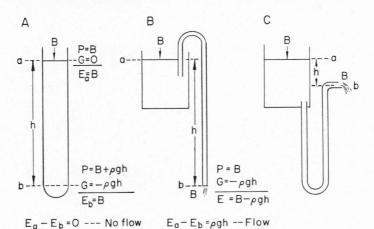

$$E_a - E_b = 0 \;---\; \text{No flow} \qquad E_a - E_b = \rho gh \;--\; \text{Flow}$$

Fig. 10-1.—Illustrating the calculation of the total fluid energy *(E)*, which determines flow. **A,** in fluid in a test tube. **B,** the syphon. **C,** the reverse syphon. *P* is the pressure energy, *G* the gravitational potential energy and *E* the total fluid energy, each calculated per unit volume.

2. The pressure in a fluid increases with the depth below the surface, by *g* dynes per cm² for each centimeter of depth. For, if *E* is a constant, then obviously $\Delta P = -\Delta(\rho gh)$.

(The minus sign is used to indicate "depth" (e.g., $-h$), since *h* is defined as the height *above* a given datum line.)

A thoughtful student, taught that flow occurs from a point of higher pressure to one of lower pressure, must have been puzzled by the fact that in a test tube of water (Fig. 10–1, *A*), where everyone knows that the pressure is higher at the bottom than at the top, there is no tendency for flow to occur from the bottom to the top. As the calculation on the diagram shows, the increased pressure (*ρgh* greater) is exactly compensated by the decreased gravitational energy (*ρgh* less); so the true driving force for flow, the total energy *E*, is the same everywhere in the fluid of the test tube.

We can extend the calculations to show the *principle of the syphon* (Fig. 10–1, *B*), although, if flow takes place, it is no longer "hydrostatics." We can imagine the velocity of flow to be so small that the kinetic energy term $^1\!/_2\rho v^2$ is negligible. If the lower end of the U tube (point *b*) is open, the *pressure here must be atmospheric.* There is, then, in this case a difference in the total energies at *a* and *b*:

$$E_a - E_b = \rho gh$$

Flow will therefore take place from *a* to *b*, driven by this force. Note that the flow depends only on the difference in levels between *a* and *b*, not at all

on the fact that in the syphon tube the flow must first proceed "uphill" to the top of the tube. Similarly, the flow in a pipe line, down to the bottom of a valley and up again (Fig. 10–1, *C*), is not in any way different from what it would be if the same length and diameter of pipe were entirely on the level.

It is only because we have so early, and so long, been taught something less than the whole truth about the law of flow that we have any difficulty answering the question: "How can the blood return from the feet uphill to the heart in venous return." It is like the question: "Why is the moon so much larger when on the horizon than when high in the sky?" It is not any larger (if measured by a physical instrument); we just think it is. It must, therefore, be repeated: *It is no harder, in the circulation, for the blood to flow uphill than downhill.* The true law of flow shows that differences in level of different parts of the vascular bed do not in any way affect the driving forces for flow and so do not *directly* affect the circulation.

Effect of Posture on Transmural Pressures

Physiological experiments on the effect of changing the posture rapidly (on a tilt table) indicate, apparently contrary to the statement above (but only apparently), that there are, indeed, marked effects on the circulation. These are due, not to a change in the driving force to flow, but to changes in the vascular bed brought about by the hydrostatic factor, together with the dis-

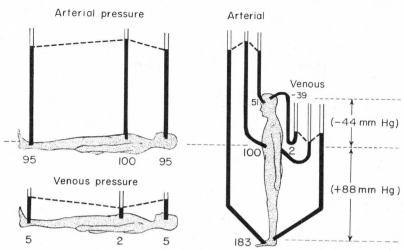

Fig. 10-2.—Effects of posture on level of arterial and venous pressures. The gradient down arteries and veins due to flow (Flow X Resistance) is included in the diagram. The figures are estimated levels of the pressures, in millimeters of mercury, referred to the level of the right atrium as datum level.

tensibility of the blood vessels, which means that their capacity for volume of blood depends on their transmural pressure.

Figure 10–2 shows that the pressures in the arterial and in the venous systems in the erect posture are very different from the corresponding pressures when the body is horizontal (in the diagram, some allowance is made for the pressure drop due to flow multiplied by resistance). In a 6 foot tall man, the feet may be about 4 feet (120 cm) below the heart level, and so the hydrostatic factor in the arteries of the foot may approach

$$\rho gh = 1 \times 980 \times 120 = 11,760 \text{ dynes/cm}^2 = 88 \text{ mm Hg}$$

and, instead of the 100 mm Hg mean pressure at heart level, the pressure will be 188 mm Hg. [►Similarly, the pressure in the arteries of the brain, say 60 cm above the heart level, will be far below 100 mm Hg—perhaps as low as 50 Hg.*◄] The arteries are not very distensible, so that these changes in transmural pressure will not produce changes in caliber and volume of blood in the arteries that are of much physiological consequence.

*This statement is debatable if by "pressure in the brain arteries" is meant the transmural pressure, for the vessels are here enclosed, or almost so, in a "box," and the "tissue pressure" in the brain box changes with posture.

Fig. 10-3—Showing how the venous pressure can be estimated by inspection of the neck veins and veins in the back of the hand. C, level at which veins collapse. B, heart level. The vertical difference. A, measures venous pressure. (Kindly drawn by R. H. Phibbs.)

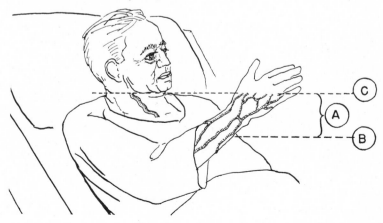

However, in the venous system, the corresponding changes (with posture) in the transmural pressures of the veins may produce profound effects in the circulation. The venous pressure in the foot could be as high as 90 mm Hg; in the veins of the brain, as low as −40 mm Hg although the fact that the brain is in some degree a closed box will prevent the transmural pressure of the cerebral veins from dropping as much as this. The peripheral veins—for example, in the neck (Fig. 10–3), well above the level of the heart—will collapse under their negative transmural pressure. Indeed, this collapse of the large neck veins at a certain level above the heart is an excellent clinical guide to the level of venous pressure, which is elevated in *congestive heart failure*. Collapsed veins, however, will offer relatively little resistance to flow, since they collapse with cylindrical "tunnels" still open at the two sides (into a dumbbell shaped cross-section, as in Figure 6–3). The level of the hand above which the superficial veins collapse is also used as a measure of venous pressure in the clinic.

The venous system is relatively very distensible (Fig. 6–3); so the very great increase in transmural pressures in the lower limbs will very greatly increase their capacity. Immediately after standing, or being tilted, much of the flow of blood emerging from the capillary bed into these veins will remain there to fill the veins to their greatly increased capacity, instead of flowing on back to the heart. Thus, immediately after standing, there is a *temporary* decrease of venous return to the heart—but only temporary, for once the "venous reservoir" is filled under the new transmural pressure, a steady state is reached and venous return will be as great as before (possibly slightly greater than before because of some decrease in resistance to flow in the veins).

Tilt-Table Experiments, Postural Hypotension, Fainting

The above conclusions from theory are entirely confirmed in the results found by physiologists (1) on the *tilt table* (Fig. 10–4), at least as to what is observed in the first 5 min after tilting. The blood pressure begins to fall, but the reflexes concerned with preserving the normal central arterial blood pressure (carotid sinus reflexes, etc.) are immediately elicited on tilting, as shown by the sudden increase in heart rate and restoration of the normal blood pressure level. However, in a few minutes of standing, or of being in the tilted

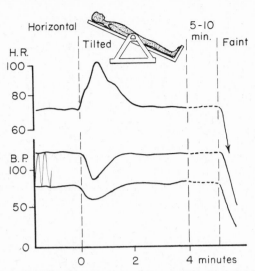

Fig. 10-4.—Typical result of an experiment on the tilt table. There is a reflex increase of heart rate *(H.R.)* on tilting (feet down), which does not, however, persist. The blood pressure *(B.P.)* is quickly restored to close to normal after a very brief fall. Fainting may occur abruptly many minutes later.

position, the heart rate subsides to the original level (as the venous return reaches the normal value once the veins are full). Undoubtedly, the reflexes include an increase in the tone of the veins of the lower limbs, for tilting an anesthetized subject will immediately cause a serious and lasting fall of blood pressure. *For this reason, drugs which tend to dilate the blood vessels acutely and drastically should never be given to patients except in the horizontal posture.*

However, continuation of the tilt-table experiment beyond the first 5 min reveals new factors not yet discussed. If the subject is cooperative in lying absolutely still, without moving the leg muscles, there will be an abrupt slowing of the heart rate and a fall of blood pressure, and usually a faint (syncope) in from 8 to 12 min. Two questions arise: (1) Why did he faint? and (2) What is the role of muscular movement?

Investigations of the signs and sequence of the faint clearly indicate that the abrupt event is associated with a discharge of the pituitary gland (2) (vasopressin [Pitressin], antidiuretic hormones, etc.), for no urine will be passed for hours after a faint. [▶This is presumably the end-result of a residual ischemia of the brain, associated with the large shift of the total blood volume into the venous reservoirs of the legs. At the time of the faint, as shown by Barcroft and Edholm, the blood vessels of the muscles widely dilate, presumably under the action of the hormone discharged, and the subject "bleeds into his own muscle vessels."◄] A plethysmograph ("fullness" or volume recorder) clearly shows the increase in volume of the limbs. In most circumstances, a faint is self-terminating, for the fainter falls to the ground and the hydrostatic factor that was the ultimate cause (plus other factors, such as emotional reaction, etc.) is no longer present. However, if the fall is prevented, death may result. Deaths have been reported of those who, presumably, fainted in the confines of a telephone booth. It is a disturbing thing to see well-meaning but ignorant persons rush to hold erect someone about to collapse to the ground from fatigue, but this is a common sight at track meets.

In *postural, or orthostatic, hypotension* there is an abrupt and considerable fall in blood pressure on standing after lying or bending down. It may be the result of several different factors:

a) Abnormally low levels of arterial blood pressure.

b) Lack of tone in the veins of the lower limbs. Even persons with healthy circulation show this after prolonged inactivity in bed.

c) An unusually large anatomical venous pool, as in *hemangioma.*

Factors *a*, *b* and *c* show a more than usually vigorous reflex increase in heart rate on standing, even though it is ineffective.

d) In contrast, in *classic orthostatic hypotension* (3) the reflex increase in vascular tone and increase in heart rate are reduced or absent. Such cases are rare and are usually due to lesions or congenital absence of brain centers controlling vasomotor reflexes.

Action of the Muscle Pump

If the leg muscles are moved from time to time, as in normal standing or walking, no faint will occur on the tilt table. This is due to the fact that activity squeezes out blood from the veins running in the proximity of the muscles. This would accomplish little but for the presence of valves in the large veins of the limbs (usually just beyond the junction of tributary veins). The valves allow blood to flow toward the heart, but not retrogradely. The venous valves were noticed by Harvey, and their action can be seen easily by any student by stroking the veins on back of the hand. When the hand is lowered below the level of the heart, the veins swell under their increased transmural pressure, but only to the point where a valve is present. Intermittent muscle activity in the legs thus serves to pump blood back to the heart and to reduce the excessive blood volume in the veins of the leg and foot. A striking demonstration of this is seen if the vein in the foot is cannulated and connected to a column of saline solution in a vertical tube. Without muscle movement, the level in the tube will stand above heart level. On contraction of the leg muscles, the level falls very greatly.

A few years ago, several British guardsmen in their heavy busby hats fainted on parade at the "Trooping of the colours." It was a particularly hot day, and some of the eager young soldiers were standing rigidly at attention in the presence of their Queen, while "old soldiers," probably ignorant of physiology but wise in experience, moved their leg muscles within the veil of their creased trousers and avoided fainting. To the Army, this disgraceful occurrence indicated that the fainters were obviously unfit, and so they were given, not as punishment but to correct this, extra duties of running around the parade square for hours. A heated correspondence to the *Times* from physiologists ensued, pointing out that soldiers should not be punished for exhibiting the normal physiology of postural effects on the circulation, particularly in hot weather, when the venous tone is reduced.

The over-all importance of the alternate contraction and relaxation of the limb muscles to the circulation is demonstrated by some data obtained by the Arbeits Physiologie (Exercise Physiology) Laboratory at Dortmund in the Ruhr. The investigators showed that for a given muscular task, such as cutting coal at the pit face by hand, there was a linear increase of heart rate with increase in the oxygen consumption. However, the increase of heart rate for a given increase in oxygen consumption depended on how "static" versus "dynamic" was the physical exercise. *For completely "static exercise" (now called "isometric muscle training"), where no motion was involved, the increase in heart rate was twice as great as for purely "dynamic exercise," such as running on a treadmill.* The increase in heart rate is a good index of the stress on the heart. It has also been shown (4) that the blood pressure, particularly the diastolic pressure, rises more in the performance of static work than in dynamic work, even if the former requires less oxygen. The importance of the muscle pump means that the cardiac patient should be warned not to exert himself in static muscular work, such as lifting pianos or trying to push his neighbor's car; but he need not necessarily be prohibited from dynamic exercise, such as walking or swinging a golf club, which puts much less stress on the heart.

Effects of Acceleration; Blackout Under G

Even in a tall man, the hydrostatic factor reduces the pressure in the brain arteries to, say, 50 mm Hg, but no less. There is still a considerable transmural pressure to keep the brain vessels from closing, even when they have vasomotor tone. However, in aerobatic maneuvers, where there is great acceleration, the effective value of g (in the term ρgh) may be many times that of gravity. A simple example is the acceleration resulting in a force toward the feet when a pilot pulls out of a dive. This may well be more than 3 times the acceleration of gravity (i.e., >3G). The term ρgh for the brain arteries becomes 3 times what it was, and the pressure in these arteries will approach zero. The systolic pressure (120 mm Hg) may fall at the level of the brain, in the example of the tall man, to $120 - (3 \times 44)$, or -12, mm Hg. The brain arteries will close, and brain ischemia will follow, resulting in loss of vision (called *blackout*) and in unconsciousness.

The tolerance to G in healthy young pilots has been measured in the "human centrifuge," where the subject is whirled in a gondola at the end of a rotating arm. Even the healthiest subject cannot stand more than about 3–4 G for more than 20 sec without experiencing blackout. This tolerance is a little greater than would be predicted from the simple calculation above; but, of course, very active vasomotor reflexes are elicited during the acceleration, which tend to elevate the blood pressure.

Blackout under high *negative G* (i.e., feetward centrifugal force) can be counteracted by use of an *anti-G suit*. In its original development, by W. Franks of Toronto, the suit, which covered the legs and lower abdomen, contained columns of water in an inextensible, close-fitting cover, so that under G the tissue pressure in the lower limbs was raised by the same factor of ρgh as the vascular pressures. As a result, the increase in intravascular pressure, particularly in the veins, did not result in a similar increase in transmural pressure and pooling of the blood volume in the lower limbs. Later it was found more convenient to use, around the limbs, rubber bags which were

automatically inflated with air pressures (graded according to the level below the heart) at the moment the pilot was submitted to the acceleration. The success of *anti-G* suits in preventing blackout proves that the decrease in transmural pressure of the brain arteries, calculated simply as ρgh, is not the sufficient cause, unless accompanied by the shift of blood volume into vessels below the heart.

[▶An ingenious use of the principle of the anti-G suit in surgical operations is to operate with the patient in a sitting position, which is often desirable (e.g., in brain surgery), but to prevent the fall in blood pressure by having the lower limbs and abdomen in an anti-G suit (air or water) or in a positive-pressure box. Increasing the tissue pressure in the lower limbs can prevent the bleeding into the veins and the fall of blood pressure in the anesthetized subject that otherwise would result. Moreover, the level of the blood pressure may be adjusted at will by raising or lowering the pressure on the limbs. Instead of using drugs to lower the blood pressure when the surgeon asks for a bloodless field, the patient can be bled into his own lower vessels and the blood volume restored in a completely controlled manner.◀]

Blackout under G can also be avoided by making arrangement so that the direction of the acceleration force in aerobatics is across the body instead of from head to feet, that is, by having the pilot prone in the cockpit. The sudden violent acceleration in the firing of men-carrying rockets is, fortunately, at right angles to the body in the normal sitting position in the nose cone. Certain maneuvers in aircraft, such as "peeling off" from horizontal flight to a power dive, expose the pilot to "positive G"; that is, the force is toward the head ("negative G" is toward the feet). Instead of blackout, the phenomenon of *redout* occurs; the vision becomes blurred and the field looks red. This is caused by the congestion of the retinal vessels with blood under the increased transmural pressures.

As might be expected, continuous accelerations under low total G (say 2 G), produced by slow rotation in a centrifuge, result in no symptoms in the subject, even when continued for hours. [▶ However, it has been found that unexpected effects of circulatory collapse may occur when the period of increased G is ended—that is, on return to the condition of 1 G. This suggests that chronic exposure to higher G than normal results in profound compensatory reflex adjustments in the circulation, which are not immediately inhibited on return to normal. The nature of these adjustments is not yet understood.◀]

Zero G (or Weightlessness) and Space Medicine

With the advent of the Space Age, some of those engaged in space medicine have expressed great anxiety about the effects of weightlessness (i.e., G = 0) on the human circulation. This anxiety seems ill-founded, since it is hard to see how the circulation can be any different in weightlessness than when a man is horizontal, or in any posture in water (such as underwater in a swimming pool). As explained, the hydrostatic factor ρgh per se does not affect the driving forces of the circulation directly. The inertial factors, represented by the term $\frac{1}{2}\rho v^2$ in our equation, are not affected at all by weightlessness (weight is affected by G; but mass, or inertia, is not). The only effects of weightlessness on the circulation to be expected would be those resulting from the disorientation of sensory function (position sense, etc.) that occurs when the limbs become effectively weightless. Since the same weightlessness of limbs is present in immersion in water, one would expect the same effects in scuba divers.

Men have now experienced zero G, or weightlessness, continuously for many days, in the "moon shots," and the above predictions that no great physiological difficulties would be encountered are verified.

Summary

To summarize the important principles of this chapter:

1. The common statement that flow occurs down a gradient of pressure is true only in the restricted case of one horizontal plane and where the kinetic energy of flow is negligible. According to the true law of flow, it takes place down a gradient of total fluid energy, which is the sum of three terms: pressure energy, gravitational potential energy and kinetic energy.

2. The hydrostatic factor, ρgh, greatly changes the level of arterial and venous pressures in the circulation, and corrections for this must be made when the vessels are not at the level of the heart, if pressures are to be compared with standard values for the horizontal body.

3. The hydrostatic factor does not in any *direct way* affect the flow of blood, since the driving force (i.e., the total fluid energy) is unaffected.

4. Considerable shifts in the volume of blood in the circulation, however, take place with change of posture, because of the change in transmural pressure in the distensible vessels (particularly the veins), when posture is changed. The shifts in blood volume may temporarily decrease the venous return to the heart and later lead to fainting as a result of cerebral ischemia. Postural hypotension occurs if compensatory reflexes are not operating, as in anesthesia.

5. The effects of the hydrostatic factor are exaggerated under high accelerations in aerobatics and reduced to zero in weightlessness. However, no drastic direct effects on the circulation are to be expected in the latter state.

REFERENCES

1. Shepherd, J. T.: Physiology of the Circulation in Human Limbs in Health and Disease, in *Fainting* (Philadelphia: W. B. Saunders Company, 1963), Chap. 34, p. 370.

2. Edholm, O. G.: Physiological Changes during Fainting, in Wolstenholme, G. E. W. (ed.): *Visceral Circulation* (Ciba Foundation Symposium) (London: J. & A. Churchill, Ltd., 1952).

3. Burton, A. C.; Jeffers, W. A., and Montgomery, H.: Types of orthostatic hypotension and their treatment, Am. J. M. Sc. 202:1, 1941.

4. Tuttle, W. W., and Horvath, S. M.: Comparison of effects of static and dynamic work on blood pressure and heart rate, J. Appl. Physiol. 10:294, 1957.

11

Kinetic Energy in the Circulation;
Streamline Flow and Turbulence;
Measurement of Arterial Pressure

The Kinetic Energy Term in the Total Fluid Energy

THE THIRD TERM in the total energy, which is the driving force for the circulation, is the kinetic energy per unit volume, $\frac{1}{2}\rho v^2$. The participation of this term in the total energy is illustrated by the *principle of Bernoulli,* which is that, where the velocity is higher, the pressure is lower; for,

Fig. 11-1.—**A,** the familiar example of Bernoulli's principle (where a tube narrows), demonstrating how flow occurs down a gradient of total fluid pressure *(E)* but not down a gradient of pressure *(P)*. **B,** illustrating the kinetic energy artifact in making measurements of pressures in blood vessels with catheters.

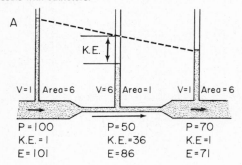

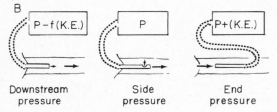

neglecting any changes in the gravitational potential energy (ρgh) (i.e., in a fluid system all at the same level), we have:

$$E = P + \tfrac{1}{2}\rho v^2$$

If the conservation of energy principle applies (i.e., the dissipation of energy is negligible), we have:

$$\Delta P = -\Delta(\tfrac{1}{2}\rho v^2)$$

A simple example is shown in Figure 11–1, *A.* Because the cross-sectional area of the tube narrows in the central portion, the velocity here must increase and the pressure decrease. Where the tube widens again, the velocity decreases once more, and part of the kinetic energy is transformed back to pressure energy. Because of the dissipation of energy in the flow, this effect is superimposed on a gradient of pressure down the tube, which would exist if the cross-sectional area were constant. The representative figures given below the diagram show that the flow is down a gradient of total energy, not of pressure.

Transformations of pressure energy into kinetic energy and back occur in the vascular bed wherever the total cross-sectional area changes. This is a most important consideration in the pulmonary circuit and for the venous filling of the heart, as explained later; much less important in the systemic arterial system.

Relative Importance of Pressure Energy and Kinetic Energy

If we assume a value for the velocity of flow in the different parts of the circulation, it is easy to

TABLE 11–1.—AMOUNT AND RELATIVE IMPORTANCE OF KINETIC ENERGY IN DIFFERENT PARTS OF THE CIRCULATION*

VESSEL	RESTING CARDIAC OUTPUT				CARDIAC OUTPUT INCREASED 3 TIMES		
	Velocity (Cm/Sec)	Kinetic Energy (Mm Hg)	Pressure (Mm Hg)	Kinetic Energy as % of Total	Kinetic Energy (Mm Hg)	Pressure (Mm Hg)	Kinetic Energy as % of Total
Aorta, systolic	100	4	120	3%	36	180	17%
Mean	30	0.4	100	0.4%	3.8	140	2.6%
Arteries, systolic	30	0.35	110	0.3%	3.8	120	3%
Mean	10	0.04	95	Neg.		100	Neg.
Capillaries	0.1	0.000004	25	Neg.	Neg.	25	Neg.
Venae cavae and atria	30	0.35	2	12%	3.2	3	52%
Pulmonary artery, systolic	90	3	20	13%	27	25	52%
Mean	25	0.23	12	2%	2.1	14	13%

*The cases where kinetic energy should not be neglected—that is, where it is more than 5% of the total fluid energy—are indicated by italic figures. When an artery is narrowed by disease processes, the kinetic energy becomes very important.
NOTE: Neg. = Negligible.

calculate the kinetic energy from $\frac{1}{2}\rho v^2$. The result will be in dynes per square centimeter. By dividing by 1,330, the figure is converted to milligrams of mercury, to be compared with the pressure, P. Table 11–1 shows how the importance of the kinetic energy is very different in different parts of the circulation. The calculations are made (*a*) for a resting cardiac output and (*b*) for an output 3 times the resting value, when all velocities will be multiplied by 3, and the kinetic energies by 9 times (3^2).

[►Physiologists might argue about the actual values assumed in Table 11–1, particularly since many of the pressures have been measured incorrectly, without proper consideration of the *kinetic energy artifact* described under the following heading, Kinetic Energy Artifact in Measuring Vascular Pressures.◄] There is, however, no room for argument about the conclusions, which are:

1. In the aorta, the kinetic energy factor is small for resting cardiac output, but it may be of considerable importance in conditions of exercise and increased cardiac output.

2. In the smaller arteries, capillaries and small veins, kinetic energy is always quite negligible.

3. In the venae cavae, kinetic energy is very important in exercise, not at rest.

4. In the atria and in the pulmonary artery, the kinetic energy factor is by no means negligible at rest and is of great importance when the cardiac output is increased.

The gradient of pressure from the left atrium to the left ventricle, during the filling of the heart, is only a few millimeters of mercury. It has been a source of wonder that in exercise, where the rate of filling of the ventricle is many times increased, so little rise of atrial pressure could be recorded. There are two reasons for the confusion. First, it is the gradient of total energy, not that of pressure, that determines the flow from atrium to ventricle, for the kinetic energy in the ventricle is much less than in the atrium during filling. Second, as explained below, the pressure in the atrium, particularly in exercise, has not been measured correctly by the usual catheterization procedure. The filling of the heart, in conditions of rest as well as in exercise, is very much a kind of "jet" or "impact" filling, utilizing the kinetic energy of flow in the atrium.

Kinetic Energy Artifact in Measuring Vascular Pressures

Pressures in many parts of the vascular system are now measured by catheters, introduced into a peripheral artery or vein and pushed centrally toward and into the chambers of the heart (Fig. 11–1, *B*). Unless the tip of the catheter has its opening at right angles to the stream (i.e., measuring what is called a "side pressure"), the pressure recorded is not accurately the pressure existing at that point in the blood. This is the familiar principle of the Pitot tube, by which the air speed is measured on aircraft.

If the catheter faces the oncoming blood stream, or if end-cannulae are tied into arteries in physiologists' animal experiments, the flow of the blood is prevented; the kinetic energy at that point is transformed into pressure energy. Consequently, the manometer at the end of the catheter or cannula records, not the pressure in the blood stream, but a pressure higher than this by the amount $1/2\rho v^2$. (This has been called "end pressure.") Conversely, if the catheter opening faces downstream, the pressure recorded is lower than the pressure in the fluid. In this case, the difference is not accurately equal to $1/2\rho v^2$ but to some fraction of this (say, 0.8 of $1/2\rho v^2$). The reason for this is that the flow is distorted in flowing around the tip by an amount depending on the streamlining of its shape. *These so-called "side pressures," "end pressures" and "downstream pressures" should not be considered to be different pressures, all existing in the blood stream at one point, for there is only one pressure at a point in a fluid, and this acts equally in all directions. The differences between the different pressures above represent artifacts which occur when we measure that single pressure by inserting a catheter or cannula.*

Since it is much more convenient to push catheters in the direction of flow, pressure readings are nearly always made with the tip pointing downstream (side-opening catheters are not so popular). Consequently, the pressure readings are too low, by amounts comparable to those given in Table 11–1. This error has probably led to serious misinterpretation of the resistance to flow in the pulmonary circuit.

Pulmonary artery pressures are usually obtained by pushing a catheter up the veins into the right atrium and right ventricle and thence through the pulmonary valve into the root of the pulmonary artery. The mean pressure for a resting cardiac output is found to be about 12 mm Hg (e.g., systolic 20 mm Hg, diastolic 8 mm Hg). To this should be added, for resting output, 1 or 2 mm for the kinetic energy artifact in systole, less for mean pressure. In exercise, the cardiac output may be 4 times as much as resting values, yet the pulmonary artery pressure, as recorded by such catheters, rises very little indeed—in fact, cases are recorded where it apparently did not change at all or apparently fell. Actually, the true pulmonary artery pressure must have increased considerably; for the kinetic energy artifact to be added, in systole, instead of, say, 1 mm Hg, should now be 16 times as great (v would be 4 times as great), that is, 16 mm. [►But even the corrected pressure in the pulmonary artery is misleading, for it should be the total energy (pressure plus kinetic energy) that is measured as the driving force for pulmonary flow. As the pulmonary bed widens, the velocity falls far below that in the pulmonary

artery, and the kinetic energy is transformed into pressure energy, so that (as in the model of Figure 11–1, *A*) the pressure before the pulmonary vascular resistance is reached may, in exercise conditions, exceed that of the pulmonary artery.◄]

The wrongly measured pulmonary arterial pressures and the wrong concept of the force causing flow had suggested that the pulmonary vascular bed was of quite remarkable distensibility, since apparently 4 times as much flow occurred in exercise with a negligible small increase in pressure (i.e., the resistance had dropped to one-fourth apparently passively, due to a rise in transmural pressures of the resistance vessels that was hardly measurable). When the correct values of pressure are measured, the pulmonary vascular distensibility is comparable to that of other vascular beds.

Kinetic Energy and Pathological Narrowing of Arteries

While the kinetic energy factor amounts to less than 1 mm Hg for distributing arteries, such as the coronary arteries of the heart, it becomes of great importance when such arteries are narrowed by internal lesions (*atherosclerotic plaques*) or external pressures (e.g., from tumors). Suppose the diameter of the lumen is narrowed at the stenosis to one-third the normal. The cross-sectional area will be one-ninth, and the velocity of flow through the narrowed orifice will be 9 times normal (assuming the resistance of the stenosis is still small compared with the total vascular resistance). The kinetic energy term, $1/2\rho v^2$, will be 81 times as great as normally. Thus, the pressure in the orifice will be reduced very greatly (Fig. 11–2). If the kinetic energy normally was equivalent to 1 mm Hg, it will now be 81 mm Hg and the mean pressure will fall from, say, $100 - 1 = 99$ mm Hg to $100 - 81 = 19$ mm Hg. In the case of an external stenosing force, the blood pressure supplies the opposing force, but this will now offer far less opposition. Bernoulli's principle thus makes constrictions of arteries tend to persist, where

Fig. 11-2.—Illustrating how the narrowing of an artery by an atherosclerotic plaque may lead to rupture of the breaks in the plaque. See text for explanation.

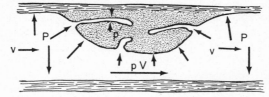

otherwise they might be compensated and recover normal size. If the kinetic energy increases enough to lower the pressure to less than atmospheric pressure (as in the filter pump), the artery will close completely. However, once the flow has been stopped by this, the pressure will rise once more and reopen the stenosis. A rhythmic closure and opening would result. This is called *flutter*, and it has long been recognized to be the principle of the functioning of such reed instruments as the oboe. Flutter of the nearly closed lips when one blows through them results in the "Bronx cheer." [▶Probably snoring is another example of flutter. The passage through the larynx is narrowed by the rise of the base of the tongue. (Look in the mirror as you make a snoring sound.) Note that it is easy to snore on inspiration, not on expiration. Why?◀]

Bernoulli's Principle, Atherosclerotic Plaques and Coronary Thrombosis

Not only does Bernoulli's principle tend to make constrictions of an artery persist, and even become narrower, but also it plays a role in the breaking up of atherosclerotic plaques protruding into the lumen (Fig. 11–2). These develop clefts or blind channels through the mass of tissue. [▶Some pathologists see these as "blind capillaries" originating from the lumen, others as faults or clefts.◀] If there is no flow in these channels, the pressure within them will be that of the vessel at their point of origin. Those that open from the narrowest position of the stenosis will have low pressure, those from the margin of the plaque will have relative high pressure. The tissue is thus submitted, with pulsatile arterial pressure and flow, to a pattern of violent pressure differences in different places. This may well lead to extension of the clefts and rupture of the plaque, pieces of which would be carried downstream to block smaller coronary vessels as "emboli." There is clinical evidence, collected by J. C. Paterson (1), that coronary thrombosis occurs more frequently when the blood pressure is elevated and flow through the stenosis is increased, at which time the pressure vibration of the plaque would be greatest.

As Edward Lear, 1812–1888 (who published 212 limericks) might have put it:

> The principle preached by Bernoulli
> Can lead to results most pecoulli,
> It may favour stenosis

> And lead to thrombosis
> If the blood flow is increased undoulli.

Streamline Flow and Turbulence

Table 11-1 is based on calculations on the assumption that the flow in the vessels is "streamline" and that the kinetic energy is entirely due to the velocity in the direction of the flow, i.e., down the streamlines. However, when the rate of flow in a system of tubes is increased above a critical limit, the character of the flow changes markedly from "streamline" to "turbulent." Elements of fluid move in all directions, and a greater proportion of the total fluid energy is kinetic energy, which is dissipated as heat and vibration. Knowledge of turbulence is essential to the understanding of the origin of sounds in the circulation such as murmurs (see Chapter 15), since undisturbed streamline flow is essentially silent. *Disturbances of the pattern of flow, as in turbulence and other hydrodynamic phenomena, can lead to transfer of energy from blood stream to the blood vessel wall, which may cause vascular pathology.*

A classic experiment was to inject into the middle of the stream in the aorta a thin lamina of dye. When seen in a glass tube interposed in the femoral artery, the dye was still unmixed and in a separate lamina along the axis of flow. This agrees with the work of the great engineer and physicist, Sir Osborne Reynolds. He used a long cylindrical tube (Fig. 11–3) and a stream of dye introduced into the axial stream to study the nature of the fluid motion. This was *laminar* (streamlined) until he increased the rate of flow to a critical value, when it became turbulent instead. In turbulence, the whole tube was filled with vortex-like eddies. The energy of flow was now being used to create the kinetic energy of these eddies. The dye now filled the tube, i.e., velocities of flow at right angles to the axis were abundant. Reynolds showed that the *critical velocity* of flow at which turbulence appeared depended on the viscosity and density of the fluid (streamline flow does not depend on density) and on the radius of the tube, by the formula,

$$V_c = R.\eta/\rho r$$

where η is the viscosity in poises, ρ is the density in grams per milliliter and r is the radius of the tube. The term R is called *Reynolds' number*, which is dimensionless and is, from the foregoing formula,

$$R = \frac{V_c \rho r}{\eta}$$

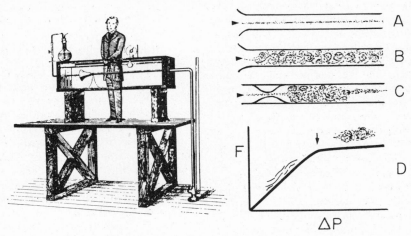

Fig. 11-3.—Left, Sir Osborne Reynolds' apparatus by which he discovered the critical velocity for turbulence (from his original paper of 1883). **Right: A,** below the critical velocity. The dye remained separate for the whole length of tube (streamline flow). **B,** above the critical velocity. The tube, from close to the entrance, filled with the eddies of turbulence. **C,** turbulence for a short distance beyond a stenosis, at much lower critical velocities. **D,** showing how the flow-pressure curve changes slope at the critical velocity. At higher flow, much more energy is dissipated in creating the kinetic energy of the eddies, in addition to overcoming viscous resistance.

For a long straight tube, Reynolds found that if R exceeded a value of about 1,000 (if v is the *mean* velocity of flow) or 2,000 (if v is the maximal velocity on the axis, which is twice the mean) the flow became turbulent. Pappenheimer, using blood in glass tubes, obtained a critical value of R of about 960. *It has not been sufficiently emphasized that the critical value of 1,000 applies only to long straight tubes.* If there is a narrowing of the tube (stenosis), the velocity through the narrowest part is, of course, greatly increased, and we would expect to have turbulence beyond the stenosis. This indeed occurs, and a vibration of the wall of the tube can be felt (palpation) and a murmur heard with a stethoscope applied to the tube at the point downstream to the constriction. However, turbulence due to a stenosis will occur at Reynolds' numbers (R) much lower than the critical value of 1,000 for straight tubes. Values as low as 150 have been found experimentally in models and in arteries, and the critical value depends very much on the particular profile of the stenosis. Further down the tube, flow becomes streamline once more (Fig. 11–3, C).

If, then, conditions in the circulation provide sufficient velocity of flow in the cylindrical vessels, or a less, but critical, velocity through narrow orifices, there will be turbulence in the blood stream; this can create vibrations, which will be shared by the elastic walls, felt as a "thrill" and heard as a "murmur."

Murmurs are therefore always associated with abnormally high velocity of flow through valves or a blood vessel. From Reynolds' criterion and the radius of the aorta (about 1 cm), we would not expect the critical velocity to be reached, except at the height of systolic ejection, for taking the viscosity of blood as 0.04 poise and the density was 1.0, we find:

$$V_C = \frac{1,000 \times 0.04}{1.0 \times 1.0} = 40 \text{ cm/sec}$$

The mean velocity for the aorta, for an output of 5L per min, is about 25 cm per sec; so we would expect the conditions for turbulence to be reached for a short period at the beginning of systole, not later. In heavy exercise, the velocity is much greater; so perfectly *"innocent"* systolic murmurs will be heard in normal individuals (especially children) in conditions of increased cardiac output during exercise.

Poststenotic Dilatation in Arteries

It has been observed for many years (first described in 1846 by Chevers in *Guy's Hospital Report*) that when an artery is narrowed by a "stenosis" from an external object, such as an extra rib or a tumour, or by internal protrusions, as in atherosclerosis, a fusiform dilatation of the artery is often found just downstream from the stenosis (Fig. 11–4). This remained an apparent hemodynamic paradox, until the work of Roach

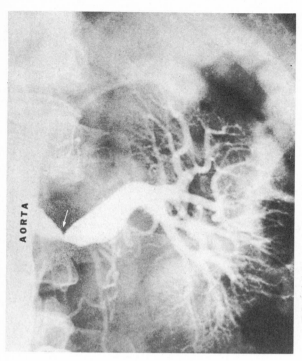

AORTA

Fig. 11-4.—Arteriogram from a patient, showing a stenosis of the renal artery *(arrow),* which had led to a marked poststenotic dilatation of the renal arterial tree. (Some retouching to eliminate irrelevant shadows has been done.) (From Roach, M. R., and MacDonald, A. C.: Invest. Radiol. 5:311, 1970.)

(2, 3). Vague explanations of the dilatation had been advanced in terms of an increased "side pressure" in the region of the dilatation, associated somehow with the disturbance of flow by the stenosis, but of course the transmural pressure here must be reduced, not increased, by the presence of the stenotic resistance.

Roach produced chronic stenosis in arteries of dogs by restricting the lumen with an external nylon band and followed changes in the artery by painting the outside wall of the artery with a radiopaque material at the time of operation, with sequential radiographic observation. The stenoses could be classified as to three degrees of severity of narrowing:

a) Minimal stenoses, where no murmur of turbulence beyond them was heard.

b) Moderate stenoses, when a bruit or a murmur was heard and could be felt as a "thrill" (vibration).

c) Severe stenoses, in which no murmur was heard.

The results were unequivocal. No poststenotic dilatation was seen in *a* and *c,* but, with moderate stenosis, *b,* a characteristic fusiform dilatation developed and increased up to 10 days. It persisted as long as observations were continued (up to 10 months in some dogs). This means that turbulence, as indicated by the presence of the murmur, is the cause of the dilatation. The extent of the dilatation is well correlated with the region of highest intensity of the murmur. The vibration of turbulence somehow weakens the arterial wall, as shown by the elastic behavior of the pre- and poststenotic portions of the arteries that had shown dilatation (Fig. 11–5). Later work by Roach and Melech (4, 5) showed that application of vibrations from an external source produced similar weakening of the wall, so that it became more distensible. The low-frequency range up to 400 Hertz (cycles/sec) seems most effective. The most damaging frequency within this range is higher with older vessels. It would appear that the damage is to the elastin fibers rather than to the collagen network of the arterial wall, perhaps to the elastin "cross-linkages" between collagen fibers. Adequate histological evidence of what has happened is not yet available, but the change in elastic behavior is very easily demonstrated.

Poststenotic dilatation can be produced by turbulence in isolated perfused segments of arteries (4), in a much shorter time than in vivo, indicating a continual repair process in vivo. It is astonishing that even after a dilatation in vivo has been

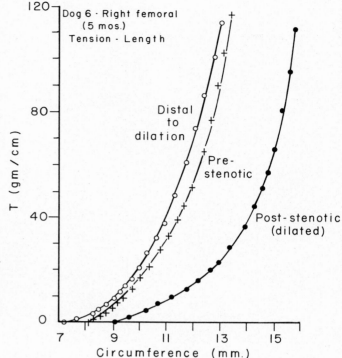

Fig. 11-5.—Tension-length curves from segments of a dog artery with an artificial moderate stenosis and associated murmur; prestenotic, the dilated area beyond the stenosis, and distal to dilation. The dilated area had a greater circumference and distended more to a given transmural pressure. In five control arteries without turbulence or murmurs, the corresponding curves all coincided. (From Roach [2].)

established for a very long time (10 months in dogs), removal of the stenosis results in a return of the poststenotic segment to the original cylindrical shape, without any dilatation, in the course of 24 hours (5). No such reversibility is seen in isolated arteries. [▶In a small number of patients, when the surgeon has been persuaded merely to remove the stenosis rather than to "resect" the dilated segment or to insert a length of prosthesis, complete recovery of original shape has occurred. Correction of the narrowing alone may "cure" poststenotic dilatation.◀] The mystery of poststenotic dilatation seems to be solved, although it is puzzling how vibration of such low frequency can be so damaging to the vessel wall. One wonders what may happen to the arteries in the hands of men who use pneumatic hammers to break up road surfaces.

The phenomena of dilatation are seen in a great variety of locations in the vessels, wherever the velocity of the flow exceeds the critical Reynolds' number that applies to their particular geometry. Stenosis is only one cause; excessive flow in the pulmonary artery due to a shunt (e.g., clinically in atrial septal defect with a left to right shunt)

causes turbulence with a murmur in that vessel, and the weakening of the elasticity of the wall is shown by unusually great pulsation ("hilar dance") in the cardiac cycle (Boughner and Roach [6]).

Another place where turbulence is generated and has an effect on the vascular wall is in human *intracranial saccular aneurysms* (7). These occur in the internal carotid arterial system, almost invariably at the "prow" of the dividing wedge of tissue at bifurcations of the arterial system (see Fig. 11-6). The cause is probably not turbulence but the impact of the high velocity pulsatile blood stream at this point. Once the aneurysm is developed, there is violent turbulence within the aneurysm,* even when the flow in the main artery and its two branches is streamline. Ferguson (7) has recorded peculiarly musical murmurs, rising in intensity at each systole, from patients at neurosurgical operation (Fig. 11-6). He also showed by models, and by measurements of the

---

*According to Ferguson, Sir Geoffrey Jefferson, on first being shown the whirlpool rapids at Niagara Falls, exclaimed, "I say—what a magnificent example of the circulation in an aneurysm!"

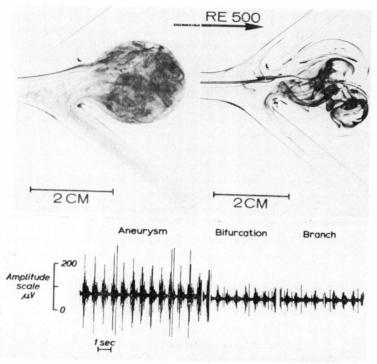

Fig. 11-6.—Turbulence in a large spherical model of an aneurysm. The Reynolds' number was 500. The streams of injected dye show that there is no turbulence in the arteries but violent turbulence within the aneurysm. **Below**, phono- catheter recording of the bruit from the aneurysm and near-by vessels (arterial pressure, 90 mm Hg) in a patient at operation. (From Ferguson [7].)

elasticity of the saccular walls, that here again the vibration of turbulent flow could weaken the wall and cause the eventual rupture of the aneurysm, usually with fatal results.

Effect of Shear Rate on the Endothelial Lining

Another case of unusually great transmission of energy from flowing blood to the wall, where it can cause pathology, is where the pattern of flow may be normal (i.e., the parabolic distribution of Poiseuille flow) but the flow so great that the "shear rate" (equal to the velocity gradient) at the wall exceeds a certain limit (Fry [8]). We should not think of the endothelial lining cells as tethered or anchored securely to the wall of vessels, for when detached from the basement membrane (as by micromanipulation) they round up and bulge into the lumen. Also, in replacement of old endothelial cells or in growth of new capillaries, the cells migrate along the wall from their point of origin. These cells have many characteristics of fluids rather than solids, and the high shear rate in the blood stream produces a shear force on the endothelium, deforming the cells and rupturing them if it is too great. By staining the elongated nuclei in sheets of endothelium lining of arteries (opened up for inspection), Fry (personal communication) has shown that there is an orientation of the cells along streamlines. The pattern can indicate the complicated nature of the streamlines near the orifice of branches of an artery and the points where the shear stress is greater. [▶These points seem to correspond with the geographic location of the initial atherosclerotic lesions found in arteries, but the matter is at the moment controversial. Some experts claim that low shear rate, or pockets of stagnation ("boundary separation"), is the source of lesions rather than regions of high shear rate. The pattern of flow may be so complicated that it is difficult to settle the matter, although high rather than low shear seems more likely to cause pathology.◀]

A remarkable demonstration of the deforming of endothelial cells by the shear at the wall was devised by Fry. Having shown that the cells were oriented in the direction of flow in a square segment of wall endothelium, he removed that section and grafted it back again, turned through an angle of 90°. In a short period of subjection to flow in the artery, the orientation of the cells of the grafted area, initially at right angles, became once more oriented parallel to the blood stream.

By partially obstructing the flow in the aorta of dogs to a cylindrical channel along part of the wall, Fry (8) was able to follow the progressive histopathological changes produced by the excessive shear rate. For example, undamaged endothelial linings are not penetrated by high molecular weight dyes, (e.g., Evans blue), but, after excessive shear, staining of injured areas indicates the first sign of damage. Resorting to the limerick:

> A proud Endothelial Cell
> Cried, "I'm all Solid, not Fluid as well."
>   But a high rate of shear
>   Soon made it quite clear
> He was mostly a Sol or a Gel.

A shear rate of 3 times the normal present in the aorta of dogs will cause endothelial damage, so evidently the safety factor in the arterial system is not very great.

The Korotkow Sounds: Indirect Measurement of Arterial Pressure

An illustration of the dictum that "streamline flow is silent" but that increased velocity of flow and turbulence can make a sound in the circulation is provided by the clinical method of measuring blood pressure by inflating a cuff on the arm (originally due to Riva-Rocci). If the stethoscope bell is placed over a peripheral artery (e.g., the brachial near the elbow or the radial at the wrist), nothing can be heard at all in normal circumstances (unless the artery is severely constricted by too much pressure of application). When, however, a wide cuff containing an inflatable bag is wrapped around the upper arm and the bag is inflated to pressures above the systolic pressure and the pressure allowed to fall slowly, characteristic sounds are heard from the brachial artery (the Korotkow sounds). Details of how the measurement should be made are best left to laboratory practice in physiology and to actual clinical experience, but it is important to understand what is happening. Otherwise mistakes will be made,

such as that made by a Committee of the American Heart Association a few years ago in choosing the best criteria for systolic and diastolic pressures.

The pressure in the bag on the arm is transmitted to the tissues of the arm lying within the cuff (the cuff must be at least as wide as the diameter of the arm for the pressure to be effectively transmitted, that is, so that the artery cannot escape being submitted to the pressure equal to that in the bag). When this is above the systolic pressure, the transmural pressure of the brachial artery is zero or negative. Consequently, even at the height of systole, the artery remains closed and no blood flows through. When, however, the bag pressure falls just below the systolic pressure, there is a brief interval (beginning of systole) in each cardiac cycle when the compressed segment of artery can open against the tissue pressure, presenting a long narrow channel through which a "jet" of blood flows. In the remainder of the cardiac cycle, the tissue pressure holds the artery closed. The velocity of the jet of blood is considerably increased above any velocity that was present when the artery was not compressed, and the criterion for turbulence is exceeded. As a result, the jet of blood reaching the uncompressed artery below the cuff generates a sound (the first Korotkow sound). It is of short duration and "sharp" and is best described as a tapping sound. The pressure in the bag at the point where the first tapping sound is heard is taken as the systolic pressure. Direct comparison of indirect and direct methods (Roberts, Smiley and Manning [9]) have shown that, in normal subjects in the standard sitting position, the two methods agree as to the systolic pressure within 5 or 10 mm Hg. There may be strong reservations as to the correctness of this systolic criterion in cases of arteriosclerosis, since the rigidity of the artery may prevent its closure by the tissue pressure unless this exceeds the arterial pressure by a considerable amount; but at any rate, the high (indirectly measured) systolic pressure in these cases serves as a clinical index of their arteriosclerosis, even if the absolute value is not correct.

As the bag pressure falls lower, the proportion of the cardiac cycle in which the artery is patent increases, and it is wider when open; yet the conditions for turbulence and instability of the stream when emerging from under the cuff are still satisfied. The sound becomes louder and extended in time; then reaches a maximal intensity and begins to diminish, eventually to "disappear" (the velocity has fallen too close to the critical value). While there has been general acceptance of the best criterion for the systolic pressure (the first tapping sound), there has been much controversy as to the criterion for diastolic pressure.

At a pressure just below that where the sound begins to diminish, there is a change in the character of the sound, known as "muffling." The sound loses its ringing, staccato quality altogether and becomes a thumping, rather than a tapping. The muffling occurs at a bag pressure very close to the diastolic pressure (as verified by direct measurements with catheters) and is undoubtedly the best criterion, both theoretically and in practice, for diastolic pressure. It tends to be a few millimeters above the true diastolic pressure.

Why should there be an association of a change in the character of the sound and the true diastolic pressure? As long as the bag pressure is above the diastolic pressure, there will be, in the cardiac cycle, a period—however brief—in which the artery is closed. The successive periods of sound are therefore interrupted by brief intervals of silence. When the bag pressure falls below diastolic pressure, the artery is never closed and the sound is not interrupted by silent periods. This can explain the change of character from staccato to muffled (e.g., from piano sound to organ sound). There is, then, a sound reason, based on theory, for the "muffling" as the best diastolic criterion. In practice (6), it proves to be more reliable than the alternative, the disappearance of the sound, in comparisons where direct measurements of pressure are made.

On the average, in a normal subject at rest, the disappearance of the sound occurs in a bag pressure about 8 mm Hg below the true diastolic pressure, and so in these circumstances it could be argued that the disappearance is about as good a criterion for diastolic pressure as the muffling. However, the complete lack of logic to suggest any reason for the correspondence must be considered. The disappearance of the sound indicates that the velocity of the blood stream has fallen below whatever the critical value may be. There is no reason why, except by chance in normal subjects, this should correlate with the diastolic pressure. Indeed, if a normal subject is compared at rest and immediately after heavy exercise, this becomes apparent. At rest, the blood pressure may be systolic, 120 mm; diastolic by muffling, 80; diastolic by disappearance, 75 mm. After exercise, these values may be systolic, 170 mm;

diastolic by muffling, 85; diastolic by disappearance, 40 mm. The pressure for disappearance has dropped to very low values (even to less than 40 mm in many cases). The reason is obvious. The increased flow through the arm after exercise means a much greater velocity, enough to be above the critical value, even when the compression by the bag is very slight. In this case, no one could claim any correspondence between this disappearance criterion and the true diastolic pressure. Another simple logical consideration ruling out this criterion as reliable is that, if the stethoscope bell is not at the point of maximal pickup above the artery (say it is 2 cm away), the disappearance will occur at a higher bag pressure; similarly, if the examiner is deaf or the stethoscopic transmission is poor.

Since there are still many professors of medicine who advocate the disappearance as the diastolic criterion (relying on the recommendation of the experts and for other reasons), the student and intern should form the habit of always recording the point of *both* the muffling and the disappearance (written $\frac{120}{80/75}$). Sometimes one or the other of the diastolic criteria may be missed, but the other will still be available. The muffling should be considered as the more reliable. If not, young men with no cardiac abnormality will continue to be referred to cardiac specialists because their diastolic blood pressure, according to the "insurance doctor," is very low (he used the criterion of disappearance), even though the muffling occurred at the normal pressures. If the diastolic pressure were, in fact, very low, this would suggest aortic incompetence, a very serious diseased state, while, in fact, it may be merely that the brachial artery is narrower than usual.

The more one inquires into the basis of the Riva-Rocci indirect method of measuring arterial pressure, the less confidence one has in its accuracy, both for systolic and diastolic pressures. Yet it remains an invaluable aid to diagnostic medicine, in no way replaced in practice by the availability of methods involving direct arterial puncture. No one has, as yet, invented any better indirect method.

The precautions to be taken in using the indirect method are important. These include: adequate width of cuff for the particular arm (standard cuffs may give falsely high pressures on a very large arm); "reactive errors" which increase the blood pressure that previously existed if the circulation is cut off too long; and the usual psychosomatic elevations of blood pressure in an anxious patient without the experience of having had his blood pressure measured.

[►It is worth noting that many patients in whom the diagnosis of mild hypertension is made are grossly overweight and have forearms so large that the standard blood pressure cuff is too narrow. This may lead to values for systolic and diastolic pressures as much as 40 mm Hg higher than the real pressures. This estimate of the error is based on comparing readings with standard cuffs with those obtained with specially constructed extra-wide cuffs. Treatment of such patients in the hypertensive clinics includes, of course, drastic weight reduction and eventually may result in an apparent lowering of the blood pressure to normal levels. One wonders if there ever was hypertension or if the lowering of the apparent hypertension actually was due to the reduction in the girth of the arm.◄]

REFERENCES

1. Paterson, J. C.: The Causal Relationship of Stress to Internal Hemorrhages and Coronary Occlusion, in Rosenbaum, F. F., and Belknap, E. L. (eds.): *Work and the Heart* (New York: Paul B. Hoeber, Inc., 1959). (Proc. of 1st Wisconsin Conference.)

2. Roach, M. R.: Changes in arterial distensibility as a cause of poststenotic dilatation, Am. J. Cardiol. 12:802, 1963.

3. Roach, M. R.: An experimental study of the production and time course of poststenotic dilatation in the femoral and carotid arteries of adult dogs, Circulation Res. 13:537, 1963.

4. Roach, M. R., and Melech, E.: The effect of sonic vibration on isolated human iliac arteries, Canad. J. Physiol. & Pharmacol. 49:288, 1971.

5. Roach, M. R.: Reversibility of poststenotic dilatation in the femoral arteries of dogs, Circulation Res. 27:985, 1970.

6. Boughner, D. R., and Roach, M. R.: Etiology of pulmonary artery dilatation and hilar dance in atrial septal defect, Circulation Res. 28:415, 1971.

7. Ferguson, G. G.: Turbulence in human intracranial saccular aneurysms, J. Neurosurg. 33:485, 1970.

8. Fry, D. L.: Certain histological and chemical responses of the vascular interface to acutely induced mechanical stress in the aorta of the dog, Circulation Res. 24:93, 1969.

9. Roberts, L. N.; Smiley, B. A., and Manning, G. W.: A comparison of direct and indirect blood pressure determinations, Circulation 8:232, 1953.

12

Dissipation of Energy in the Circulation—Work of the Heart

"Die Energie der Welt is konstant, die Entropie steigt immer."—
LUDWIG VON HELMHOLTZ (1869).

Production of Heat in the Circulation

IN THE TWO PRECEDING CHAPTERS we have used the principle of the *conservation of energy* (enunciated by Meyer, and independently by Helmholtz, about 1869) between the various kinds of fluid energy—pressure energy, gravitational potential energy and kinetic energy. Whenever there is motion of the blood, these types of fluid energy are being transformed (dissipated) into heat, which is the ultimate "degraded" form of energy. Heat energy is the random *thermal agitation* of molecules and is indicated by the temperature of the fluid. The second law of thermodynamics states that there is a tendency for all other forms of energy, in transformations from one form to another, to produce heat (which means that the *entropy tends always to increase*).

This is why the total fluid energy of the blood, when there is flow, decreases from aorta to arteries to capillaries to veins to vena cava, and must be partly restored, by the work of the right heart, to a higher value. In the pulmonary circuit, energy is once more dissipated as heat, and the total energy is restored by the work of the left heart. This dissipation of energy in the circulation is effected by the viscosity of the blood, each faster-flowing lamina speeding the slower laminae next to it, and being itself slowed. Viscosity thus tends to make the energy of all regions of the flowing blood more uniform, toward the randomness that ultimately characterizes *heat*.

Measurement of Dissipation of Energy in the Circulation

The amount of energy that is transformed into heat is therefore measured by the mechanical work of the heart in restoring the energy to the original arterial level. Mechanical work is measured, as we were taught in school, by the product of force and the distance moved by the point of application of that force. For the case of a pressure moving a fluid, this definition of work yields at once (see also Fig. 12–1, *top*):

Work = Pressure × Volume of fluid moved = PV

In the case of a ventricle ejecting blood into its artery, the bit of work done in any interval during this ejection is, then:

$$\Delta W = P_v \times \Delta V$$

where P_v is the ventricular pressure existing at that interval of time and ΔV is the volume of blood that is ejected in the interval. For ΔV we could equally well use the volume of blood ejected from a ventricle, or the diminution in volume of the ventricle in the same interval. If the ventricular pressure during the whole period of ejection were constant, at the mean ventricular systolic pressure $\overline{P}_v$, the work of the ventricle, per beat, would be:

$$W = \overline{P}_v \times SV$$

where SV is the *stroke volume*. However, to be accurate, we should integrate; that is,

$$W = \int P_v.dV$$

over the ejection period.

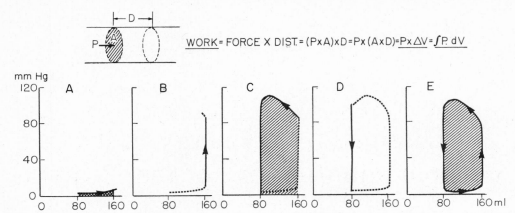

Fig. 12-1.—The work diagram of the left ventricle. **A,** filling phase. The shaded area under the curve represents work done by the blood on the ventricle. **B,** isometric (or isovolumetric) contraction phase. No work is done, but elastic energy is stored in the heart muscle. **C,** ejection phase. The shaded area represents work done by the ventricle on the blood. **D,** isovolumetric relaxation phase. No work is done, but stored elastic energy is given back. **E,** the complete cycle. The shaded area represents the net mechanical work of the ventricle in a single cycle.

Rushmer (1) has succeeded, as have others, in making measurements, in the conscious unrestrained dog, of the changes in volume and pressure of the ventricles during the heartbeat. This was done by mounting "strain gauges," measuring the increase of diameter of the ventricles, in more than one dimension of the heart. From these dimensions the volume of the ventricle was estimated. Figure 12–1 shows, schematically, the diagram of pressure versus volume so obtained, in which there is a closed loop representing the cardiac cycle. For full understanding of the shape of this loop, Chapter 15, on the events of the cardiac cycle, must be consulted. The point here is that the area under the curves of this loop represents the above integral for ventricular work. The area under the upper part of the curve represents the work done *by the heart muscle* in ejecting the blood in systole. The smaller area under the lower part of the curve represents the work done *by the blood* in filling the heart. This work is stored in the heart muscle as elastic tension (corresponding to the rise of ventricular pressure) and is later given back in helping to eject the blood. Thus the net work of the ventricle is represented by the difference in the two areas, that is, the area enclosed by the loop. The diagram for the right ventricle would be similar in shape, but the levels of pressure reached would be only about one fifth of those in the left ventricle, and the area representing work of the right ventricle would be only about one fifth of that of the left.

Physiologists have resorted to short cuts in this calculation of the work of the heart. It is more convenient, to some of them, to use the aortic pressure during the ejection phase than the ventricular pressure. This must be increased by the kinetic energy term ($\frac{1}{2}\rho v^2$) to obtain the ventricular pressure; that is,

$$\text{Work of ventricle} = \overline{P}_v \cdot (SV) = (\overline{P}_A + \frac{1}{2}\rho v^2) \cdot (SV)$$

where $\frac{1}{2}\rho v^2$ is the mean value for the kinetic energy during ejection and SV is the stroke volume. However, to confuse the student further, many textbooks omit the ($\frac{1}{2}$) from the kinetic energy term, whereupon the student cannot be blamed for giving up. The excuse apparently is that the mean value of the velocity $\overline{v}$, which is easily calculated from the stroke volume and the cross-sectional area of the aorta, is being used in these mysterious formulas. The mean value, not of v, but of v^2, is what should be used; but it is said that the way the velocity changes during the ejection is such that the true mean value of v^2 would be about twice this mean value of v. This is how the ($\frac{1}{2}$) disappeared, and the formula became "black magic," apparently unrelated to classic mechanics.

It was first pointed out by Weiss (2), in 1913, that the mechanical work of the heart is an almost trivial item of the total energy exchange of the heart; so its exact calculation, although fun for physiologists, is largely academic. This will be explained later in this chapter, when the *efficiency* of the heart is considered.

Amount of Energy Dissipated and Power of the Heart

Power is measured by the rate of working, that is, ergs of work per second. When this is calculated for the beating heart, it is found to be astonishingly small. In resting conditions, each ventricle has an output of about 5L per min, or 83 ml per sec. Using the approximate formula for estimating the power of each ventricle (i.e., Work = Mean pressure × Output/sec):

Power of left heart = (100 × 1,330) dynes/cm² × 83 ml/sec = 1.1 × 10⁷ ergs/sec

Power of right heart = (20 × 1,330) dynes/cm² × 83 ml/sec = 0.2 × 10⁷ ergs/sec

Total power of the heart = *1.3 × 10⁷ ergs/sec*

In heavy exercise, the output increases up to, say, 4 times this value and the mean pressures may increase by 50%, so that power will increase to a maximum of about 6 times this. The result may be put into more familiar units of power, for example, watts or horsepower (hp): 1 erg/sec = 1 × 10⁻⁷ watts, or 1.34 × 10⁻¹⁰ hp. Then the mechanical power of the heart (resting condition) is about *1.3 watts*, or *4 × 10⁻³ hp (0.004 hp)*. It would take about 250 resting human hearts or 50 hearts working at full power to provide a mechanical power of 1 hp (say to drive a small rotary lawn mower).

This is only the mechanical power of the heart. It takes a much higher rate of energy turnover to provide this mechanical power, since the *mechanical efficiency* of the heart is very low (less than 10%), for reasons to be explained later in this chapter. Because of this low efficiency, the rate of total energy turnover of the heart may be as much as 13 watts. The total resting metabolic rate is equivalent to about 100 watts; so the proportion used for the heart is not insignificant.

In these terms the mechanical power of the heart is not impressive. What is impressive is the ability of the heart, in a lifetime, to accomplish a very great total amount of mechanical work without cessation or breakdown. Familiar calculations are that, in a lifetime (2 × 10⁹ sec), the work of the heart (2 × 10⁹ foot pounds) would suffice to lift some 30 tons to the top of Mount Everest (30,000 feet). (But who wants to?)

Static and Dynamic Work of the Heart Muscle

The physical definition of work implies that if a force, however strong, does not move its point of application or if a pressure does not move a volume of blood, no work is done. However, in physiology we have a very different system to deal with than the examples in books on mechanics. As everybody knows, it requires a steady dissipation of energy for muscles just to maintain a force (tension). When we push with our hand against an immovable wall, our oxygen consumption increases and our muscles become tired, even though no mechanical work whatever has been done.

It has been suggested that in physiology we should amend the physicists' definition of work, but this would be a retrograde step. A simple analogy, as depicted in Figure 12–2 may make the matter clear. This figure shows (above) a crane with a hook lifting scrap iron into a truck. The work done would be calculated by multiplying the weight lifted by the height it is raised. The energy dissipated in the motor of the crane is required merely to do this external work, although far more energy will be lost, owing to the inefficiency of that motor (much of the energy will be dissipated as heat against friction of the moving parts). Modern junk yards, however, use, instead of a hook, a large electromagnet to develop the force on the scrap iron. Just to maintain this force, energy must be continuously supplied by the

Fig. 12-2.—Illustrating the analogy of an electromagnetic crane (cf. *Hook Crane*) to maintenance heat of the heart muscle. See text for explanation. (From Burton [4].)

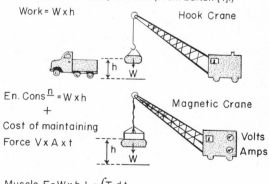

current of the electromagnet (at a rate measured by the product of volts and amperes). This extra energy consumption must be added to that required to do the external work of lifting the iron into the truck. Similarly for muscle, the total energy turnover in a given time (*t*), which might be called the *load* of the muscle, is (Fig. 12–2) the sum of two terms: the first, the mechanical work; the second, the cost of maintaining the force (tension) of the muscle. This second term is called the *tension-time integral,* expressing the fact (proved by A. V. Hill for skeletal muscle) that the extra rate of energy turnover is proportional to the tension. The total in a given time is thus proportional to the tension and to the time that it is maintained. *Muscle demands an increased rate of energy consumption proportional to the tension developed, even if no external work at all is done.* The fundamental reason for this is that the state of contraction is a steady state of "activation," which decays spontaneously unless a steady supply of activation energy is maintained. This is discussed in Chapter 8 for vascular smooth muscle.

Total Load and Efficiency of the Heart

Applying the above ideas to the heart, we find two terms in the expression for the total energy transformation (Fig. 12–2): the first is the mechanical work ($\int P.dV$); the second is the *maintenance heat,* proportional to the tension and time it is maintained ($\int T.dt$).

What are the relative magnitudes of these two terms in the *total load* on the heart? The answer has been provided by a series of research projects by many physiologists, such as M. B. Visscher, L. N. Katz, and S. J. Sarnoff and their associates (3), on the efficiency of the heart.

DEFINITION OF MECHANICAL EFFICIENCY.— There are many different types of efficiency of a machine; so the definition must be specific. By *mechanical efficiency* is meant the ratio of the external work done to the total energy transformed:

$$\text{Mechanical efficiency} = \frac{\text{Mechanical work done}}{\text{Total energy transformed}}$$

$$= \frac{\text{Mechanical work done}}{(\text{Mechanical work} + \text{Maintenance heat})}$$

$$= \frac{\int P.dV}{\int P.dV + \alpha \int T.dt}$$

The numerator of this fraction is the external work of the ventricle, from the data of the pressure-volume diagram (Fig. 12–1) or the simplified calculations for this used by physiologists. The second term of the denominator, the tension-time integral, may also be calculated from records of ventricular pressure; but the factor α by which it must be multiplied to give the maintenance heat is not well established for cardiac muscle. (It is well known for skeletal muscle, from the work of A. V. Hill and his collaborators.) However, the total energy turnover may be estimated from the rate of oxygen consumption of the heart muscle, calculated from the difference in oxygen content between coronary artery and coronary veins, and from the rate of coronary flow.

The result of all these measurements of efficiency of the heart is perhaps astonishing. The efficiency is only a few per cent, sometimes as low as 3%. It rises greatly when the external work is increased, but never reaches more than 10–15%. This means that the work of the heart is a much smaller item in its total energy exchange (i.e., the load) than is the tension-time integral (or maintenance heat). Indeed, this has been strikingly illustrated by experiments on a heart-lung preparation (by Visscher) in which, when the work was increased by a factor of 20 times, without much rise of blood pressure, the myocardial oxygen consumption increased by 5% only. In contrast, increasing the blood pressure or the heart rate, either of which increase the other term (the tension-time integral), increases the oxygen consumption almost proportionately.

The relatively small magnitude of the work of the heart in the denominator of the expression for the efficiency also explains why the efficiency increases greatly as the work is increased. For example, if the work is doubled, the numerator of the fraction is doubled while the denominator is increased by only a few per cent. As a result, the efficiency is almost doubled.

[► This knowledge of the energetics of the heart has a very great clinical importance in the management of cardiac patients (4). It is the total *load of the heart,* measured by the oxygen requirement of the heart muscle, that should be kept low, and in this the external work of pumping of the heart is a relatively small item. Increases in the arterial blood pressure (e.g., episodes of hypertension) and anything that increases the relative time that the heart muscle is in contraction (e.g., increase of heart rate) both increase the tension-time integral (see next paragraph) and, consequently, the load of the heart (proportionately). In comparison, a mild degree of exercise, particularly of the "dynamic" type, where motion of the body and muscular contraction aid in the circulation by the "muscle pump," although it increases the external work of the heart, has much less effect on the cardiac load. It may be much more dangerous for a cardiac patient to have an angry argument with his wife than to play a leisurely round of golf or take a long walk. The insistence on immobility and the prohibition of even mild exercise for cardiac patients, which has dominated the thinking of some cardiologists, is based on a fallacy as to the role of external work on the total load of the heart. ◄]

Production of Pressure in Ventricle; Shape and Size of Heart

The way in which the pressure is raised in the ventricle is by the development of "tension," or "force," in the ventricular muscle. The same mechanical principle applies as was used (in a special simplified form) to give the relation between pressure and tension on the wall of the cylindrical blood vessels. This is the law of Laplace, in its general form; that is,

$$P = T\left(\frac{1}{R_1} + \frac{1}{R_2}\right)$$

where (Fig. 12–3) R_1 and R_2 are the principal radii of curvature of the ventricular wall at any point, P is the pressure in dynes per square centimeter and T is the tension per unit length (of an imaginary slit in the wall) in dynes per centimeter.

Fig. 12-3.—Illustrating the two principal curvatures at each point on the ventricular wall. *NPOO'*, the normal to the surface. *AB* and *CD*, principal arcs of the curvatures. *O* and *O'*, the principal centers of curvature. *OP* and *O'P*, the principal radii of curvature. (From Burton [4].)

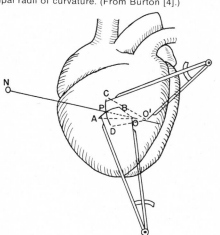

TABLE 12-1.—RADII OF CURVATURE (R_1 AND R_2) AND THICKNESS OF VENTRICULAR WALL (t) IN AN ADULT HEART*

LABEL OF POINT CHOSEN	R_1 (Mm)	R_2 (Mm)	t (Mm)	$t\left(\frac{1}{R_1} + \frac{1}{R_2}\right)$
RIGHT VENTRICLE				
z_1	60	60	1.5	0.050
c_2	65	80	2.0	0.055
d_2	32	75	1.25	0.055
a_2	75	90	2.2	0.054
e_2	30	45	1.0	0.055
f_2	55	90	2.0	0.058
Av.				0.055 ± 0.013 S.D.
LEFT VENTRICLE				
p_1	36	60	8.0	0.35
z	32	80	8.5	0.37
x_1	70	36	9.5	0.39
r_1	30	80	8.5	0.38
o_1	28	60	7.0	0.36
s_1	70	40	8.5	0.38
m_1	80	40	10.0	0.37
w_1	32	80	8.5	0.34
f_1	55	16	5.0	0.40
t_1	70	24	6.0	0.33
v_1	24	70	6.5	0.36
n_1	60	24	6.0	0.35
Av.				0.36 ± 0.023 S.D.

*From Woods (5) with statistics added.

As early as 1892, Woods (5) showed that this law applied to the heart, by measuring the curvatures at each point, in autopsy specimens of children's hearts, and calculating $\left(\frac{1}{R_1} + \frac{1}{R_2}\right)$ for a series of points (Table 12–1). The total curvature $\left(\frac{1}{R_1} + \frac{1}{R_2}\right)$ is much greater for the apex of the heart than for the relatively flat portion of the wall halfway between apex and base, but the wall is correspondingly thicker in the "flat" regions. Woods also measured the thickness of the wall at each place where he estimated the curvatures. We would expect the tension at each point to be proportional to that thickness, that is, to the cross-sectional area of the contractile muscle per unit length of our imaginary slit. Table 12–1 shows how well this relation holds for each ventricle. For the left ventricle, the product of thickness and

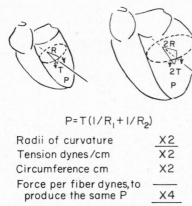

$$P = T(1/R_1 + 1/R_2)$$

Radii of curvature	X2
Tension dynes/cm	X2
Circumference cm	X2
Force per fiber dynes, to produce the same P	X4

Fig. 12-4.—The consequences of dilatation of the heart, as predicted by the law of Laplace. (From Burton [4].)

curvature is about 5 times the product for the left ventricle, which would correspond to the ventricular pressure produced being 5 times as great.

If, now, the dimensions of a heart are, say, twice as great (i.e., the heart is dilated), the law of Laplace indicates that more tension must be produced by the ventricular muscle to produce the same pressure of blood in that ventricle (Fig. 12–4). The "mechanical advantage" of the heart muscle is reduced because the curvatures are less. (In the extreme case, if the ventricular wall were truly flat [with zero total curvature], the pressure would not rise however much tension was produced in the wall.) For twice the size of the heart, the tension required for a given pressure will be at least 4 times as great. From simple physical principles, therefore, any increase in the size of the heart imposes a greatly increased load on the heart. (The tension-time integral increases proportionately.) Here, then, is an additional factor to be considered in the management of cardiac patients. *Cardiac dilation is very dangerous, for it increases the load on the heart and decreases cardiac efficiency.*

There are complications to be considered, when Starling's law of the heart and heart failure are later discussed, for stretching of the ventricular wall can increase the tension produced by contraction of the muscle and, as the heart contracts, its curvatures change (the heart becomes more spherical). The fundamental mechanical disadvantage and decrease in efficiency with increased size remains the important factor. An interesting example of this principle is the heart of a giraffe, which is very large indeed and must produce a very high systolic pressure (measured as more than 300 mm Hg) in order that the hydrostatic factor in the arteries to the brain (10–12 feet above the heart level) does not reduce the transmural pressure in the brain arteries to zero. Goetz and Keen (6) have shown how remarkably thick is the ventricular muscle of this enormous heart. In their specimen, weighing 11 pounds, the wall of the left ventricle was 7.5 cm thick, that of the right ventricle, 2.5 cm thick.

Summary

1. The production of mechanical energy is required in the heart to compensate for the dissipation of energy as heat in the circulation.

2. The amount of energy supplied to the circulation by the heart is measured by the mechanical work of the heart, which is calculated from the product (or, better, the integral) of the ventricular pressure and the ventricular output.

3. The production of this work by the heart muscle involves the maintenance of tension, and this demands an increased steady supply of energy even if no physical work is done.

4. The total load of the heart, measured by the cardiac oxygen consumption, therefore depends on the sum of two terms: the mechanical work of the heart and the maintenance heat (tension-time integral).

5. Of these two terms, the maintenance heat is much greater than the external work. As a consequence, the mechanical efficiency of the heart is always very low, even though it increases markedly as the work of pumping is increased.

6. These principles have important clinical application to cardiac patients. Mild exercise, which increases the work but does not increase the load greatly, is not so dangerous as increases in blood pressure, heart rate and size of the heart (cardiac dilation). This last factor depends on the law of Laplace, according to which the larger the heart, the greater is the muscular tension required to produce a given systolic pressure.

REFERENCES

1. Rushmer, R. F.: Continuous measurement of left ventricular dimensions in intact unanesthetized dogs, Circulation Res. 2:14, 1954.

2. Weiss, G.: Le travail du coeur, J. Physiol. et Path. gén. 15:999, 1913.

3. Sarnoff, S. J.; Braunwald, E.; Welch, G. H.; Stainsby, W. N.; Case, W. B., and Macruz, E.: Hemodynamic

Determinants of the Oxygen Consumption of the Heart with Special Reference to the Tension-Time Index, in Rosenbaum and Belknap (eds.): *Work and the Heart* (New York: Paul B. Hoeber, Inc., 1959).

4. Burton, A. C.: The importance of the shape and size of the heart, Am. Heart J. 54:801, 1957.

5. Woods, R. H.: A few applications of a physical theorum to membranes in the human body in a state of tension, J. Anat. & Physiol. 26:302, 1892.

6. Goetz, R. H., and Keen, E. H.: Some aspects of the cardiovascular system in the giraffe, Angiology 8:542, 1957.

SECTION 4

The Heart and Its Action

13

Origin and Propagation
of the Heartbeat;
Electrophysiology of the Heart

"... For it is the heart by whose virtue and pulse
the blood is moved, perfected, made apt to nourish and is
preserved from corruption and coagulation.... It is indeed the
fountain of life, the source of all action."—WILLIAM HARVEY,
Exercitatio de Motu Cordis et Sanguinis (1628).

Intrinsic Rhythmicity of Cardiac Tissues

THE BEATING of the heart is intrinsic, independent of all nervous control, which merely modifies the rhythm; it does not initiate it. If kept supplied with oxygen and nutrients, a completely isolated mammalian heart will continue to beat just as does the isolated frog or turtle heart. The difficulty in demonstrating this lies only in the greater difficulty in supplying continuously the necessary physiological conditions for the mammalian heart.

All of the nervous and muscular tissues of the heart are capable of independent rhythmic activity, not merely the cells of the *cardiac pacemaker* (located in the wall of the right atrium), which normally dominate cardiac activity. If conduction from the pacemaker area is cut off, as in the classic experiment of tying a *Stannius ligature* between the atrium and the ventricles of the frog heart, the heartbeat does not cease, but a new, slower rhythm results from a new "pacemaker" (in the region of the sinoatrial node), which takes up the role of the original pacemaker. If conduction is blocked lower in the system, for example, at the atrioventricular junction (the *second Stannius ligature*), the ventricle itself will take up its own ventricular rhythm, at an even slower rate.

New insight into the relative dominance of the rhythm of different parts of the system has been provided by studies of cardiac cells in tissue culture by Harary and his co-workers (1, 2, 3). It used to be taught that the heart represented a true "syncytium," since membranes dividing the tissue into single nucleated cells were not visible by the light microscope. Electron microscopic studies now show that the heart tissue is, rather, a collection of individual muscle or nerve cells in intimate contact with one another, each cell having its cytoplasm separated from that of its neighbors by true cellular membranes. By incubation of minced-up heart tissue of young rats with the enzyme trypsin, which breaks down the substance binding the cells together but leaves the individual cells intact, suspensions of separate cardiac cells can be prepared and cultured in nutrient material. In dilute suspension, the cells are spherical and not in contact; but, in a few days of culture on a glass plate, they assume a lenticular shape with elongated filamentous processes. Some of these isolated cells (a few per cent) begin "beating" with rhythmic contractions but with independent rhythms. As the cells multiply and grow, they establish contact with one another. At this time, it is seen that areas of many cells in contact beat in unison, evidently paced by an individual cell. Finally, all the cells of a culture beat together. In addition, fiber-like aggregations of cells appear, similar to the specialized conducting system of the heart (Purkinje fibers).

The conclusion is that two embryologically distinct types of cardiac cells exist: (*a*) the *leadcells*, which beat spontaneously in the dilute cultures and which correspond to the cells of the Purkinje and nodal systems and (*b*) *following cells*, which constitute the majority of the heart muscle and which beat synchronously when in contact with the leading cells.

What determines the dominance of certain leading cells over other leading cells, so that the whole system beats in a coordinated way? Simple, but ingenious, experiments leave little doubt that the cells that can beat with the *fastest* spontaneous rhythm dominate over the others. If a culture is divided by a knife cut, the two halves beat at different rhythms, proving that transmission is not by a humoral agent but by direct cellular contact. If one half of an undivided culture is heated or cooled, the rhythm can be speeded or slowed, but it is always that characteristic of the faster, heated region which is driving the cooler tissue.

The rate of beating of such isolated heart cell preparations is sensitive to agents that block metabolic processes (dinitrophenol [DNP], which blocks synthesis of adenosine triphosphate [ATP] and inhibits the beating of single cells) and the neurohumors and drugs (such as acetylcholine) that are known to affect the rate of the intact heart.

Factors Determining Rhythm of the Pacemaker

The rate of the pacemaker rhythm depends on the metabolism of the "leading" cells and therefore on their temperature and on the hormones, neurohumors and drugs that affect cellular metabolism. The increase in the rate of beating in isolated hearts follows the usual rule, of a 2–3 fold increase for each $10°$ C rise of temperature (Q_{10} = 2–3). In health, the temperature of the heart is kept within remarkably close limits, at about $37°$ C ($98.6°$ F); so temperature is not normally a factor governing the heart rate. However, the Q_{10} of the metabolism of the pacemaker is undoubtedly responsible for the increase in heart rate in fever, although many other factors, such as reflexes, initiated because of the increased metabolic rate of all the tissues, may play a part. In *hypothermia*, now deliberately practiced by cardiac surgeons, the pacemaker rhythm is very greatly slowed.

The substances of greatest physiological importance that affect the pacemaker are: (*a*) *Acetylcholine*, which is released at the endings of the cardiac parasympathetic nerves, that is, when impulses arrive via the vagus nerves. This decreases the rate of the pacemaker cells. (*b*) *Adrenaline* arriving via the blood stream from the internal secretion of the adrenal medulla in excitement, heavy exercise, etc. This greatly accelerates the rhythm of the pacemaker. (*c*) *Noradrenaline*, released by cardiac sympathetic nerve endings. Noradrenaline has far less effect in accelerating the pacemaker than does adrenaline. (*d*) The concentration of K^+. An increase of K^+ depresses the pacemaker activity, as one would expect from the general knowledge that the resting potential and excitability of nerve and muscle is correlated with the K^+ concentration gradient (more K^+ inside the membrane than outside). (*e*) Na^+. Increase of Na^+ increases the activity of the pacemaker up to a point.

The effects of changes in K^+ and Na^+ concentrations are very great also on the cardiac muscle, as well as on the pacemaker cells; so the effect on the intact heart (*diastolic arrest* with high K^+; *systolic arrest* with high Na^+) are not to be interpreted purely as effects on the pacemaker cells. Clinically, changes in the electrocardiogram are a sensitive index of disturbances in K^+ concentration in the blood. [► Effects on the pacemaker cells, due to changes in concentration of Na^+ and Ca^{++}, although demonstrable on dog hearts, probably play little role in health or disease and seldom threaten normal cardiac activity, since wide fluctuations are tolerated by the heart, while physiologically the concentration of these ions is controlled within narrow limits.◄]

Electrical Activity of Pacemaker Cells

West (5) has succeeded in recording the electrical potentials in pacemaker cells of the rabbit atrium by microelectrodes penetrating pacemaker cells (Fig. 13–1). The "resting potential" (negative inside) is about −50 millivolts (mv), but this spontaneously decreases (depolarization) until a critical "prepotential" level is reached, when the cell "fires" and repolarizes rapidly, only to begin the steady depolarization again. Evidently the cells act as a "relaxation oscillator," with something piling up to a critical level, at which instability occurs. The way in which the rhythm is modi-

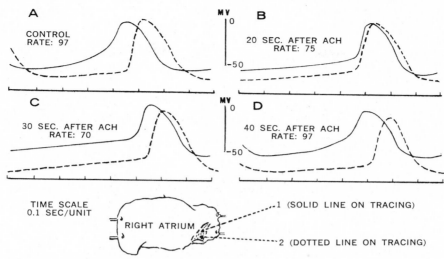

Fig. 13-1.—Records of the intracellular potentials of pacemaker cells in the isolated, but beating, rabbit atrium, showing the rate of the rise of the prepotential that precedes the discharge and how it is reduced by acetylcholine. (From West [5].)

fied (e.g., by acetylcholine) is to change (decrease) the rate of rise of the prepotential, so that the time taken to reach the critical level is altered (longer). The time course of the prepotentials of neighboring pacemaker cells is independent, although they are "discharged" by conduction from the true "leader" cell before they reach their own critical level.

The Conducting System

Figure 13–2 shows schematically the system down which the impulse from the pacemaker is conducted from cell to cell by contact. It used to be thought that there was no specialized pathway from the sinoatrial node (pacemaker) to the atrioventricular node and that the impulse spread uniformly over the atrium to converge on the atrioventricular node. This is reviewed by James (4). Now, however, there is evidence of specialized pathways of conduction over the atrium by three alternative routes, called, in order of importance, the anterior, posterior and middle internodal pathways. The multiplicity of pathways provides a safety factor, if there is focal disease (atrial infarction). From the sinoatrial node, the conduction is in the specialized *Purkinje fibers*, down the ventricular system by the common bundle, then by the two main branches (the left and right bundle branches) of the *bundle of His*, to be distributed to all of the muscle of the two ventricles. The wave of depolarization of the ventricles thus starts at the apex and moves up toward the base of the heart. It also proceeds from the inside toward the outside of the ventricular walls.

The velocity of conduction varies very greatly in different parts of the system. The velocity over the atrium from the pacemaker is about 1 meter (m) per sec, and about 0.1 sec is required for the excitation to reach the atrioventricular node. Close to, or at, the atrioventricular node, there is a major delay in conduction, which at one time was thought to be an indication of a "synaptic delay," possibly involving diffusion of a neurohumoral substance across a "gap." This assumption is no longer tenable, since conduction is known to occur by cellular contact. [▶The explanation suggested by electron microscopic studies is that probably the fibers arborize into bundles of very fine threads at this point, and, since velocity of conduction is proportional to their diameter, it is very much decreased in this region.◀] Beyond the atrioventricular node, conduction is more rapid, at 4–5 m per sec. The total interval from the pacemaker to the excitation (depolarization) of the ventricular muscle is normally 0.16–0.20 sec (estimated from the P–R interval of the electrocardiogram). A major part of this interval is spent at the atrioventricular node.

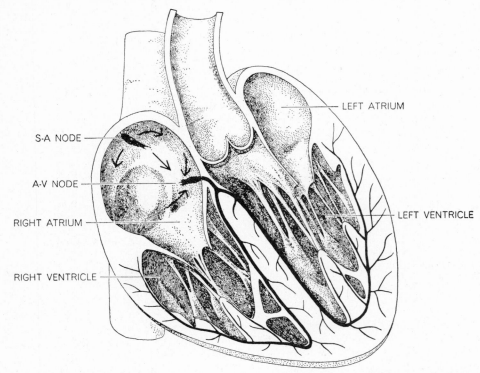

Fig. 13-2.—The conduction system of the cardiac impulse. (Modified from Harary, I.: Heart cells in vitro, Scient. Am. 206:141, 1962. Reprinted with permission. Copyright © 1962 by Scientific American, Inc. All rights reserved.)

Electrical Activity of the Cardiac Muscle Fibers

As the impulses travel over the atrial muscle, this muscle contracts (atrial systole). When the cardiac impulse arrives via the conduction system at the ventricular muscle, these muscle fibers are depolarized, and a "wave of negativity" spreads over the ventricles, accompanied by the contraction of the sarcoplasm beneath the cell membranes. The action potential of cardiac muscle has the same features as that of skeletal muscle (i.e., a spike and after-potentials), but the time course is lengthened and the shape of the action potentials is different (Weidmann [6]). Figure 13–3 shows the result of recording, by intracellular electrodes, the monophasic action potential of various cardiac tissues. The resting potential is about 90 mv (negative inside). There is a very rapid depolarization (the spike) with an overshoot to about 30 mv (positive inside), followed by a rapid disappearance of the overshoot, then a long "shoulder" of slow repolarization, complete in about 200 milliseconds (msec). The connection of this curve of action potential of a single muscle fiber with the

Fig. 13-3.—Action potentials from intracellular electrode recorded from various cardiac tissues. **A,** frog heart. **B,** dog ventricle. **C,** rat ventricle. **D,** dog auricle. **E,** sheep Purkinje tissue. **F,** rat skeletal muscle for comparison. Voltage calibration, 30 mv (inside positive), 0 mv, 100 mv (inside negative). (From Weidmann [6].)

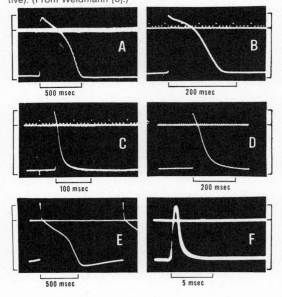

apparently unrelated shape of the electrocardiogram will be explained later (see Chapter 14). [►The ionic currents (Na⁺ in, K⁺ out) that correspond to these potential changes have been shown, although less completely, to be similar to those that have been so much studied in skeletal muscle.◄]

Spread of Depolarization over the Ventricles

A great deal of research has been concerned with the pattern of spread of the excitation over the ventricles (Scher and Young [7]). Details are obviously inappropriate here, but the two general features worth noting are:

1. The excitation usually reaches the apical region of the right ventricle slightly earlier than that of the left ventricle. However, a greater mass of muscle of the left ventricle is depolarized at a slightly later time.

2. Polarization proceeds from the inner surface of the ventricular walls toward the outer surface, as well as from the apex to the base of ventricles. As a consequence, the map of the location of negative changes on the outside of Purkinje and muscle fibers that have depolarized is changing from moment to moment, especially at the beginning of the period of activity (depolarization) and at the end of the active period (repolarization). If the whole system depolarized and repolarized simultaneously, the electrical activity could be detected by intracellular or local surface electrodes, but there would be no way of detecting the activity electrically from *distant* points, as in the electrocardiogram. As it is, owing to the asynchrony of depolarization of different parts of the heart, there is a transient distant effect, but the *voltages recorded are only a small fraction of the voltage of the action potentials.*

In order to simplify the consideration of the effect of all the positive and negative charges in the changing pattern of polarization and depolarization, we may use the concept of the *equivalent electrical dipole of the heart.*

Concept of Equivalent Dipole

Because the force between two electrical charges follows the inverse square law (such as gravitational attraction), the electrical potential due to any charge *e* at a distance *d* depends on the charge divided by the distance; that is, potential equals *e/d*. It was one of the greatest achievements of Sir Isaac Newton that he proved that, where potentials (gravitational or electrical) follow such a law, *the total effect of a number of charges at different points is the same as if all the charges were imagined to be concentrated at their center of charge* (analogous to center of gravity). Thus, Newton could consider the attraction of the earth on an apple (or on the moon) the same as if all the mass of the earth were concentrated at its center of gravity and all the mass of the apple (or the moon) at its center of gravity. (This law is hard enough for a student to prove with the modern methods of calculus; to prove it with the methods available to Newton was a fantastic intellectual achievement. Indeed, Newton first assumed this law in discovering his law of gravitation, and he proved it only later.) For this reason, we can, at any instant, replace all the positive charges in the heart by a single positive charge (equal to their total charge) at one point within the heart, and all the negative charges (mostly inside membranes that are polarized, outside as well in those that are depolarized) by a single total negative charge at another point. The center of charge of all the positive charges will not, during the process of polarization and repolarization, coincide with the center of charge of all the negative charges. When the heart is at rest, the two centers of charge will coincide. This constitutes an *electrical dipole,* characterized by three quantitative measures: (1) the magnitude of the charges; (2) their distance apart (i.e., the length of the dipole); and (3) the orientation of the line joining the two charges. It turns out that the electrical potential at a distant point (very far away compared with the length of the dipole) is given, approximately, by:

$$E = \frac{\mu \cos \theta}{d^2}$$

where *d* is the distance from the point to the center of the dipole, μ is the *dipole moment,* equal to the product of the charge and the length of the dipole, and θ is the angle between the *dipole axis* and the line to that distant point (Fig. 13–4). It therefore becomes perfectly legitimate, and very convenient, to study the changing pattern of distribution of charges during cardiac excitation in terms of a changing equivalent dipole, whose dipole moment and the orientation of its axis vary from moment to moment. The axis of the equivalent dipole is called the *instantaneous electrical axis of the heart.*

[►Since the dipole has magnitude (its dipole moment) and direction also (the dipole axis), it is a

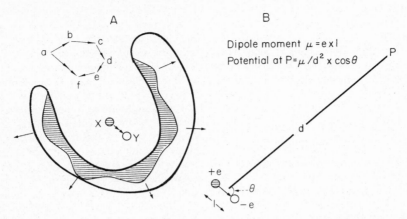

Fig. 13-4.—A, illustrating schematically the spread of depolarization over a ventricle. The shaded areas are already depolarized and are relatively positively charged. The equivalent dipoles for each region are represented by the arrows, and their resultant (shown by the vector polygon) is the instantaneous electrical axis of the heart at that moment *(XY)*. **B,** illustrating the law for the voltage at a distant point, *P,* induced by a dipole moment.

vector quantity; whereas the potential at any point, picked up at the distant point, is a *scalar* quantity, having only magnitude, without any directional quality. The fact that the magnitude of the voltage induced at a distant point depends on the cosine of the vector dipole angle does *not* make that voltage a vector. Failure to understand the distinction has led, in classic physiology texts, to appalling "howlers" in physics, as in the explanation of the classic *Einthoven's equilateral triangle* and the interpretation of *Einthoven's law* (see Chapter 14).◀]

REFERENCES

1. Editorial, Canad. M. A. J. 88:270, 1963.
2. Harary, I., and Farley, B.: In vitro studies of single isolated beating heart cells, Science 131:1674, 1960.
3. Harary, I.: Heart cells in vitro, Scient. Am. 206:141, 1962.
4. James, T. N.: Pathogenesis of arrhythmias in acute myocardial infarction, Am. J. Cardiology 24:791, 1969.
5. West, T. C.: Ultra-microelectrode recording from the cardiac pacemaker, J. Pharmacol. & Exper. Therap. 115:283, 1955.
6. Weidmann, S.: Resting and action potentials of cardiac muscle, Ann. New York Acad. Sc. 65:663, 1956.
7. Scher, A. M., and Young, A. C.: Ventricular depolarization and spread of QRS, Ann. New York Acad. Sc. 65:768, 1956.
    This is one paper of an excellent symposium on "The electrophysiology of the heart" in the same volume of this journal.

14

The Electrocardiogram and Cardiac Arrhythmias

"If it has an orange stripe just above big black beady eyes, . . .
it is a Wilson's warbler."—PETERSON, *A Field Guide to the Birds.*

The Standard Electrocardiographic Leads

TO RECORD the total electrical activity of the heart as it induces voltages at distant points, the use of three *standard leads* has long been routine. Electrodes are placed on the right arm, left arm and left leg, and the instantaneous differences of potential between the three possible pairs of these constitute the three standard leads (see Fig. 14–1).

> *Lead I* (RL): Right arm (R) to left arm (L)
> *Lead II* (RF): Right arm to left leg (F)
> *Lead III* (LF): Left arm to left leg

These three leads give electrocardiograms that show the same component waves; but the shape, amplitude and direction of the waves are different, so that the over-all patterns look quite different. The student may wonder why the left leg was chosen over the right leg. The heart is on the left side, and so this might be thought to be logical; but actually, if recordings are made from left leg to right leg, the voltage differences are very small, and so the leg lead may be thought to represent both legs or to represent an electrode in the crotch area.

To this simple convention of the three standard leads of the electrocardiograph has been added, through the years, a bewildering collection of other leads, each system with its group of devotees. F. N. Wilson and his colleagues (1) introduced the so-called zero, or central, terminal, by the use of which so-called *unipolar leads* are obtained. What was more important, he persuaded a large number of his colleagues to adopt a standard set of such leads. [►The "central terminal" is not on the body at all, but in the electronic apparatus connected to the leads, and it is connected to each of the three standard leads by a network of resistors (usually of 5,000 ohms resistance) such that a theory (of sorts) would indicate that its potential remained unchanging despite the changing cardiac potentials.◄] An "exploring electrode" connected to this central terminal is moved to a number of precordial positions over the thorax, giving *precordial leads*, designated V_1 to V_6, when one of these is used with one of the standard leads (e.g., V_1 R, V_1 L, V_1 F). [►No really sound theory exists, or probably can exist, for ascribing unique basic advantages to this system, but in practice it appears most useful. Many rival systems have been proposed and have their adherents.◄]

Actually, all the information that can be obtained about the cardiac activity from *distant* electrodes would be obtained if activity in *two* of the standard·leads were recorded simultaneously (although a third lead in the third dimension would add information). Since voltage differences are being recorded and voltage is a scalar quantity, then the potential difference between any points A and B must equal the sum of the simultaneous potential differences from A to C (any other point) and C to B; that is, *the sum of the simultaneous voltages in the three leads must be zero* (this is one of Kirchhoff's laws of electricity). If this proves not to be true on the body, then the apparatus is not measuring voltage correctly. [►The above relation, which has been called *Einthoven's law* (the name is not his fault), was thought to prove somehow that the voltages were identical with those that would exist between the corners of an equilateral triangle (Einthoven's triangle) with the equivalent electrical dipole of the heart at its center. *Obviously, the above relation has no bearing whatever on Einthoven's triangle* (which actually has little validity anyway). Since Kirchhoff's law is true, we could predict, exactly, the record from lead III, say, from the simultaneous records of leads I and II, and the recording of any more "distant" leads cannot provide any new information.◄] Recordings involving *local* leads on the heart or on the chest over the heart (precordial leads) may, of course, give new information, as would intracellular or surface electrodes directly in contact with the heart muscle.

[►On the other hand, it may be said that the usefulness of interpretations in electrocardiography depends, not on basic theory and understanding of what is happening, so much as on years of correlation of the shape of the electrocardiograms, recorded with different leads, with disturbances of normal conduction in the heart.◄] By experience with different systems of leads it is found that one particular lead shows up *infarcts* in a particular region of the heart muscle better than another. For example, inverted T waves, by clini-

cal experience, suggest this or that clinical abnormality. The student is referred to the many excellent treatises on electrocardiography (1, 2) and probably will have a detailed course in medicine from a member of one of the particular electrocardiographic parties. In this chapter, the correlation of the different parts of the normal electrocardiogram (lead II only) with different phases of activity of conduction in the heart is all that is given.

The Normal Electrocardiogram

Figure 14–1 gives the idealized normal electrocardiogram (e.g., recorded in lead II). Its features are:

THE P WAVE.—The P wave is associated with the spread of excitation and the contraction of the atrial tissue of both atria. It is normally upright, of amplitude about 0.2 mv and lasting about 0.1 sec. Atrial repolarization probably takes place in the period when ventricular depolarization is occurring; that is, the "T wave for the atria" would fall within the QRS complex of the ventricles and so is obscured in the record.

THE QRS COMPLEX.—This complex signals the depolarization of the Purkinje system (Q) and of the ventricular muscle. Q is an initial downward

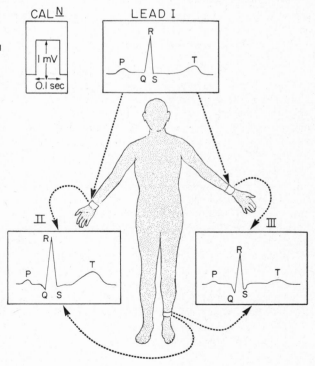

Fig. 14-1.—The standard limb leads of the electrocardiogram and the usual normal records from these leads.

deflection; R, a large upward deflection; S, a downward deflection that follows, sometimes, to below the base line, when the small upward deflection that follows is called R[1].

THE S–T SEGMENT.—The S–T segment represents the depolarized state, when all of the ventricular muscle is depolarized, and consequently there is no large resultant equivalent dipole moment of the heart. Its level is normally very close to the base line.

THE T WAVE.—The T wave represents the final difference in rate of repolarization of the different parts of the ventricular muscle. Its amplitude and form is the most variable of all the waves in the electrocardiogram, and it is the most sensitive index of disturbances in normal conduction. This is illustrated by the range given for normal amplitude in lead I: from 0.05 to +0.55 mv. A minus sign would mean that the T wave in lead I was inverted, that is, downward.

The time intervals between the different waves give valuable physiological information. The two important intervals that are routinely used are the P–R and Q–T intervals.

The *P–R interval* is measured from the beginning of the P wave to the beginning of the R wave. It represents the time taken from the start of the excitation at the pacemaker to the beginning of ventricular depolarization, i.e., depolarization of the atrium, conduction through the atrioventricular node, and through the Purkinje conduction system to reach the ventricular muscle. This is normally 0.16–0.20 sec. An increase in the P–R interval indicates a slowing of the conduction system, usually in the atrioventricular node.

The *Q–T interval* represents the total time for the ventricular muscle to depolarize and repolarize. This interval is longer for men and children than for women, and it is usually reduced as the heart rate increases (but not proportionally to the decrease in total period of the heartbeat). Table 14–1, modified from Burch, shows that, as the heart rate increases, the proportion of the total cycle which is occupied by electrical activity of the ventricle (as indicated by the Q–T interval) decreases. Speeding of the heart is thus accomplished more by shortening the electrical rest period of the heart muscle than by shortening the period of electrical activity.

Explanation of Shape of QRST Complex

The shape of the electrocardiogram from distant leads bears so little resemblance to the action potential of cardiac muscle that it is difficult for the student to see how the one can represent the sum total of the others. [►It is helpful to consider that the heart at any instant might be thought of as in two "halves," more or less, but not exactly corresponding to the two ventricles, the depolarization of which will produce opposite voltage effects in the standard distant leads. This depends on the fact that the excitation travels down the two bundles of His together, producing very small distant voltages, but at the apex the wave of excitation turns upward in the two ventricles and depolarization occurs from the inside of the walls of the ventricles to the outside of these walls. The effective dipoles of the right ventricular wall are therefore directed from left to right, those of the right ventricle, from right to left (Fig. 13–4). The effects on the voltage difference in lead I will, thus, tend to be opposite. If, now, we are permitted to take a few slight liberties with the published curves of the action potential of ventricular muscle, a plausible (but rather phony) QRST complex can be deduced (Fig. 14–2). The essence of the trick is to plot the action potential curve for the left side of the heart as upright, and invert the curve (plotted below) but with a "lead" of a very short interval of time (the curve for the right ventricle ahead of that for the left). Taking the algebraic sum of the two sets of ordinates gives a resultant with the salient features of the electrocardiogram.◄] The actual summation is, of course, much more complex than this analysis in terms of just two opposite factors, but the concept has two important features for teaching:

1. It is apparent that the "isoelectric" S–T

TABLE 14–1.—MEAN Q–T INTERVALS AND PER CENT OF CYCLE THAT IS ELECTRICAL VENTRICULAR SYSTOLE AT DIFFERENT HEART RATES (FOR MEN AND CHILDREN)*

HEART RATE (Beats/ Min.)	TOTAL CARDIAC INTERVAL (Sec.)	Q–T INTERVAL (Sec.)	% VENTRICULAR ACTIVITY	% VENTRICULAR DIASTOLE
40	1.50	0.45	30	70
60	1.00	0.39	39	61
80	0.75	0.35	45	55
100	0.60	0.31	52	48
120	0.50	0.28	56	44
150	0.40	0.25	62	38
180	0.33	0.23	70	30

*Modified from Burch and Winsor (2).

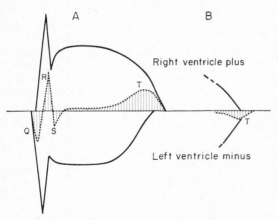

Fig. 14-2.—Illustrating how the complicated waves of the electrocardiogram can result from the subtraction of curves (similar to the action potential of cardiac muscle) of one side of the heart from those of the other side, if there is a slight lag in conduction on one side. **A**, complete curves for the muscle of the two ventricles. **B**, the detail of the termination of the curves if conduction and repolarization in the left ventricle were slowed, resulting in an inverted T wave.

segment results from the flatness of the after-potential of the action potential before the final more rapid repolarization.

2. It is obvious that the T wave results from the fact that the left ventricle has completely repolarized at a moment when the right ventricular muscle has not yet reached this state.

[►Figure 14–2 must not be interpreted as anything but a device for showing how the opposite effects on the distant electrodes of action potentials of various parts of the heart can, by partial mutual cancellation, produce unexpectedly complicated waves in the electrocardiogram. It must be pointed out that, at the time of the Q wave, depolarization has not yet reached the ventricles, and that the Q wave represents events in the septal region at the apex. Again, although the electrical activity reaches the *inside* of the left ventricle a fraction of a millisecond ahead of the first activity in the right ventricle, the spread of depolarization over the whole ventricle, toward the base and outwardly through the muscle, is completed earlier in the right than in the left ventricle, probably because there is so much less muscle to depolarize.◄]

Relative weakness of the left or right heart can be imitated in Figure 14–2 by altering the relative amplitudes of the two curves, that is, the left or right heart predominance. A very slight change in the relative conduction velocities or in the rate of depolarization of the two sides will greatly alter

the T wave; for example, if the left ventricle depolarized a little later than the right, because conduction was slowed on that side, the T wave will be inverted. The *differential* nature of the resultant electrocardiogram at once explains how relatively slight changes in conduction, and in times of polarization or repolarization in different parts of the heart, will result in marked changes in the electrocardiogram. While the action potential of cardiac muscle is more than 100 mv, the electrocardiogram voltages seldom exceed 1 mv, because most of the potentials cancel one another.

The Mean Electrical Axis

[►Simply because it has been almost universally adopted, allowing a great deal of correlation with clinical experience, it is useful to calculate from the electrocardiogram, using two of the standard leads, what is called the *mean electrical axis.* There is no sound theoretical justification of the method used, although it might be consistent, in a very approximate way only, with the dipole theory. Since the usefulness of the method thus depends completely on making the calculation in the exact standard, but arbitrary, way described in textbooks of electrocardiography, no basic principles are really involved, and the student is referred to these textbooks. The result of the calculation gives an angle for a supposed mean dipole vector, which, by clinical experience, lies normally within certain limits and, if outside these limits, can indicate roughly the type of disturbance in cardiac excitation and conduction, for example, left or right heart "preponderance," or *axis deviation.*◄]

The mean electrical axis, in spite of its pretentious name, is merely an attempt to characterize the differences in shape of the QRS complexes in the different classic leads by one number. Although it would seem unlikely that such an attempt would succeed, it has proved most useful. To attempt to popularize any one of the large number of other single-number descriptions of the curves that could be suggested would be futile.

The Vectorcardiograph

A device for visualizing, in a more unitary way, the information contained in electrocardiograms from any two distant leads is the vectorcardiogram. This device, however, has the advantage over the arbitrary calculation of the electrical axis

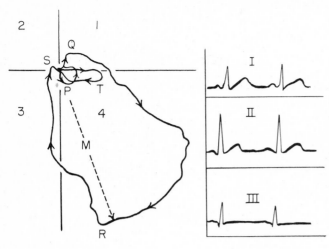

Fig. 14-3.—**Left,** tracing from a planar vectorcardiogram. This can be regarded as normal. Note the P, QRS and T loops, also that the QRS loop is mainly in the fourth quadrant. The major axis, *M,* of this loop corresponds roughly with the calculated electrical axis. (From Hession, L. B.: M.Sc. Thesis, University of Western Ontario, 1949.) **Right,** tracings of the electrocardiograms of the three standard leads for the same person.

that all of the information available in any two leads is retained. The device is very simple. The voltage in lead I is made to govern the horizontal deflection of the spot on a cathode-ray oscillograph (the horizontal axis otherwise is used as a time base), while the vertical deflection is governed by the voltage that is present at the same instant in lead III (i.e., the cathode-ray oscillograph is used as an *X–Y* recorder). The spot therefore traces a loop, or rather three loops—one for the P wave, one for the QRS complex and one for the T wave—with the spot pausing at the "origin" between these loops on the isoelectric portions of the electrocardiograms (zero voltage in both leads) (Fig. 14-3). The time variable is retained by modulating the intensity of the beam, and so the trace is interrupted by signals at equal intervals of time.

The outstanding advantages of the vectorcardiogram over the classic leads are:

1. Changes in the classic leads, such as during normal respiration, may reflect merely a geometrical change in the orientation of the heart with respect to the geographical frame of reference of the body; that is, the movement of the diaphragm shifts the geometrical, and thus the electrical, axis of the heart with respect to the leads. Changes during respiration and with posture in the classic electrocardiogram due to this shift might be wrongly interpreted as indicating changes in the pattern of conduction. The vectorcardiograph clearly shows this, for during the respiration and with changes of posture, the loop is seen to "swing" on the face of the cathode-ray oscillograph without significant changes in the shape of the loops (which would indicate changes in conduction pathways). Violent respiratory movements will, however, change the shape of the loops, indicating actual changes in conduction (these are reflex in origin). The orientation of the major axis of the QRS loop serves as an indication of the mean electrical axis, as well as, or better

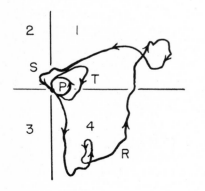

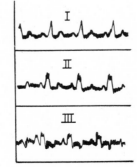

Fig. 14-4.—**Left,** vectorcardiogram (compare with **Fig. 14–3**) indicating grossly abnormal conduction in the heart (probably bundle-branch block in a patient with atrial septal defect). The accessory loops and deviations in the QRS loop correspond to the prolonged duration and splitting of the R waves, which are obvious in the standard leads. The vectorcardiogram shows abnormal conduction pathways much more dramatically than the standard electrocardiogram **(right).** (From Hession, L. B.: M.Sc. Thesis, University of Western Ontario, 1949.)

than, the arbitrary calculation from the leads and has the advantage that the voltages in the two leads were truly simultaneous. (The calculation of mean electrical axis is seldom made on records that were taken simultaneously, and there is a fluctuation from beat to beat with the respiration and other factors.) Figure 14–4 shows how different the vectorcardiograms of abnormal hearts may be.

What has been described is the "frontal plane" vectorcardiograph. The voltage at right angles, across the heart, can also be recorded by leads using electrodes on the front and back of the thorax. Ingenious vectorcardiographic enthusiasts have developed "three-dimensional" vectorcardiographs that indicate the movements of the cardiac vector in space, viewed by stereoscopic devices, or by representation in a plane, but with perspective added by altering the width of the trace. Elaborate computers have been devised to report the position of the "equivalent cardiac dipole" in space at every instant.

2. Infarcts in the heart muscle cause deviations of the conduction pathway and delays in time, which show up on the classic leads as "notchings" in the waves (usually in the R or S waves), but only if the recording apparatus has a sufficient speed of response. Perhaps simply because the vectorcardiograph uses a cathode-ray oscillograph, with its extremely rapid speed of response, the presence of such infarcted areas is more dramatically shown by a halting of the spot or reversal of its direction (called "beading") as it describes the QRS loop. Indeed, there have been cases where the records from classic leads would not be diagnosed as abnormal, yet the vectorcardiographic pattern was remarkably abnormal.

Varieties of Heart Block

Since the primary information from the electrocardiogram concerns the conduction pathways, it is most useful in the diagnosis of cases of interruption of normal pathways. *Bundle-branch block* means that the impulses have come from the atrial pacemaker, reached and passed the atrioventricular node, but travel down only one of the two main branches of the Purkinje system (left or right bundle-branch block). Excitation of the "blocked" ventricle still occurs, but by spread from the normal ventricle. The QRS complex of the electrocardiogram is greatly prolonged from the normal 0.06–0.10 sec to more than 0.12 sec. This is because conduction takes a longer route to the

blocked ventricle and because the velocity is less in the muscle than in the Purkinje system. In total *sinoatrial block,* the ventricles may continue to beat in a new rhythm, called a "nodal, or ideoventricular, rhythm," according to whether the initiation of the impulse is taken up by the sinoatrial node itself or an *ectopic* focus in the ventricular muscle becomes the pacemaker. Such varieties of block are diagnosed from the electrocardiogram by noting a dissociation of the P waves (atrial activity) from the QRST waves (ventricular activity). The P wave may be absent (atrial standstill) or present from an abnormal origin in the atrium. In cases where the atrioventricular node is partly blocked, the atrial rhythm may be conducted to the ventricles only every second beat, or in groups of two or three beats (*bigeminal* and *trigeminal* rhythms). For details, consult the books by electrocardiographers.

Flutter and Fibrillation—Arrhythmias

The normal rhythms dominated by the atrial pacemaker are known as "sinus rhythms." Nodal and ventricular rhythms, already mentioned under heart block, are examples of escape from the dominance of the normal pacemaker. In a different category of arrhythmias are *atrial flutter and fibrillation* and *ventricular fibrillation.* The very practical book by Phibbs (4) on cardiac arrhythmias is highly recommended to the medical student.

In atrial flutter, a regular succession of P waves is seen in the electrocardiogram at a rate many times the normal sinus rhythm. Only every second, third, fourth or fifth of these waves may be followed by the ventricular complex. [▶One explanation for flutter is that the wave of depolarization is following some unusual path in the atrial tissue and is returning to re-excite repetitively the pacemaker tissue, which is capable of responding to stimuli at intervals much shorter than those of its own normal spontaneous rhythm. If the wave of depolarization spreads normally from the node in all directions, it could obviously not so return (because of the refractory period); but if conduction were blocked in certain areas, one could conceive of such a "circus" route.◀]

In fibrillation, which often develops from flutter, the whole atrium beats in an uncoordinated manner with multiple apparent foci of the impulses (it quivers like jelly). The atrioventricular node is thus bombarded with hundreds of impulses every minute, and only now and then does an impulse find the atrioventricular node out of its refractory state. The ventricular rhythm that results is very irregular. The whole base line of the electrocardiogram shows tiny irregular waves, less regular and more frequent than those of flutter. [►The atria no longer achieve a significant pumping of blood; but it turns out that this does not, per se, reduce the output of the heart greatly, although the accompanying irregularity of the ventricular contractions does significantly reduce the output.◄] Ventricular fibrillation is a similar quivering of the ventricles (the ventricle feels to the hand like a sack of worms). In this case the cardiac output ceases, and this is an emergency with fatal outcome unless *cardiac massage* and a means of *defibrillation* is at once employed. Defibrillation is accomplished by administering a severe electrical shock to the heart, which arrests all excitation and conduction. On recovery from the refractoriness produced by the shock, a normal rhythm may be taken up. It is not surprising that electrocardiographic records of human ventricular fibrillation are not readily available for illustration.

Physiological Mechanism of Fibrillation: Circus Theory

[►Sir Thomas Lewis suggested an explanation for fibrillation in terms of "circus movements," which has been most useful in supplying a rationale for treatment, even if many have challenged this explanation. In essence, the idea is that a wave of depolarization from a single focus or from many foci may travel in a closed loop, returning to the point of origin. If, on arrival back at its point of origin, it finds the tissue emerging from its refractory state, it may trigger another discharge, and so on.◄] Obviously, factors that will favor fibrillation are (1) areas of poor conduction (local blocks) in the sheet of tissue, which will lead to the propagation of waves of depolarization in such loops, rather than uniform spread of excitation; (2) sufficient time, before the excitation returns to its origin, for refractoriness to have worn off at the original point (a shortened refractory period will favor fibrillation); and (3) a decreased velocity of propagation and a long pathway in the loop, which will favor fibrillation by allowing more time for refractoriness to wear off.

The drug *quinidine* is administered to convert atrial fibrillation into normal rhythms, and *digitalis,* to slow the ventricular rhythm and so improve the coronary perfusion. [►The action of quinidine has been attributed to its effects on refractory period and on velocity of conduction; that is, it lengthens the refractory period and slows the rate of conduction. Evidently, the first of these is effective in spite of the second factor. Quinidine does not always work.◄]

[►Other hypotheses are based on multiple ectopic foci in the tissue and largely reject the idea of circus movements of the excitation. There remains considerable suggestive evidence that the original theory of Lewis, or at least some modification of it, is applicable. One interesting point is that it has been shown that the ease of production of fibrillation tends to decrease with the size of the heart from species to species (e.g., it is most difficult to produce fibrillation in the frog heart). This would favor the circus theory, for, if the circuitous route is too short, the impulse will come back too soon, arriving in the refractory period. The concept of circus movement is valuable in any case, for it is similar to that of "reverberating circuits" as an explanation of rhythmic activity of the brain cells, except that in the brain the circuits are defined by specific neuronal connections and are not due to pathology.◄]

What the Electrocardiogram Cannot Tell Us

The electrical activity of the heart is due to the depolarization and repolarization of the physiological membranes of the neuromuscular and muscular tissues of the heart. Depolarization normally is accompanied by contraction of the muscle (the sarcoplasm) beneath these membranes. The magnitude of the voltages recorded by local or distant electrodes depends on the amount of the resting and action potentials. In contrast, the strength of the contraction depends on the amount and state of the muscle contractile substance. Thus, it is a mistake to expect that the amplitude of the electrocardiogram can tell us, except in extreme cases, anything about the strength of contraction or the force of the heart beat (e.g., level of arterial pressure pulse produced). This is dramatically illustrated by the existence, in rare cases, of *pulsus alternans.* In "electrical alternans" the QRS complexes alternate in magnitude and form, yet the arterial pulse may not change from beat to beat. Conversely, cases exist where the pressure pulse alternates in magnitude but the electrocardiogram shows no alteration.

Where changes in the ionic environment (e.g., abnormal K^+) or in the metabolic state of the tissue have altered the resting and action potentials of the muscle, there will, of course, be some correlation of the amplitude of the electrocardiogram with the strength of the beat. The amplitude of the electrocardiographic waves is also affected by the electrical resistance of the pathways to the distant electrodes; in addition, as has been already pointed out, the recorded voltages represent only the difference between the influences of simultaneous and opposite electrical dipoles in a complicated pattern. The resultant depends as much on the synchrony or asynchrony of the component dipoles as on the magnitude of the original potentials.

Science or Bird Watching?

[►The science of electrocardiography is not purely empirical but is based on fundamental experiments and physical laws. However, its enormous usefulness in clinical diagnosis has a basis that is almost entirely empirical. Electrocardiography is like bird watching, which depends, not on theory, but on rules like that given as a quotation at the head of this chapter.

The complete omission from this chapter of the famous equilateral triangle of Einthoven is deliberate. With the greatest respect for the very great contributions to cardiac electrophysiology made by Einthoven, the author believes that the time has come to forget this particular contribution or, at least, not to ask the student to remember it. If he has to do so, there are other textbooks.◄]

REFERENCES

1. Wilson, F. N.; Johnston, F. D.; Rosenbaum, F. F.; Erlanger, H.; Kossmann, C. E.; Hecht, H.; Cotrim, N.; Menzes de Olivera, R.; Scarsi, R., and Barker, P. S.: The precordial electrocardiogram, Am. Heart J. 27:19, 1944.
2. Burch, G. E., and Winsor, T.: *A Primer of Electrocardiography* (4th ed.; Philadelphia: Lea & Febiger, 1960).
3. Schaefer, H., and Haas, H. G.: Electrocardiography, in Dow, P. (ed.): *Handbook of Physiology*, Sec. 2, Vol. I: *Circulation* (American Physiological Society) (Baltimore: Williams & Wilkins Company, 1962), pp. 323–415.
4. Phibbs, B.: *The Cardiac Arrhythmias* (St. Louis: C. V. Mosby Company, 1961).

    This is a very practical guide on reading electrocardiograms, written for the general practitioner.

15

Events of the Cardiac Cycle, Heart Sounds and Murmurs

(Much of this chapter was kindly written by J. J. FABER.)

Streamline flow is silent
Remember that my boys!
But when the flow is turb-u-lent
There's bound to be a noise.

So when your stethoscope picks up
A bruit, murmur, sigh,
Remember that it's turbulence
And you must figure why.

Sung by a barber-shop quartet of graduate
students in the author's department (1949).

General Characteristics of the Cardiac Pump

THE HEART is a very simple kind of pump (or, rather, pair of pumps) of the two-stroke, automatic valve variety, analogous in its action to the common kitchen pump. The two "strokes" are the filling phase and the emptying, or power, phase. Two of the four cardiac valves (the inlet valves) are equipped with elaborate "strings," the chordae tendineae, which are connected to contractile muscles (the papillary muscles), but these serve merely to guide the valve leaflets into place and do not initiate the closure or opening of the valves. As in the kitchen pump, the valve action is purely passive; that is, whenever the pressure on one side of a valve exceeds that on the other, the valve moves either to open or to close.

The two sides of the heart, left and right, act mechanically quite independently, and the cardiac efficiency does not depend at all on synchrony of the two sides. The heart might pump efficiently even if the two sides had a different rhythm (although the movements of the interventricular septum would be peculiar). The beginning of contraction of the two atria, and of the two ventricles, is approximately simultaneous only because the two hearts share a common pacemaker and parallel Purkinje systems. Later events are completely independent in the two ventricles, although they may almost coincide in time.

[►The contraction of the atria plays only a very minor role in the pumping, although it may assist in the final filling of the ventricles. For the atria to pump to any significant degree, there would have to be valves upstream from the atria (i.e., in the entrance to the atrium and in the pulmonary vein). There is such a valve in the single-chambered heart of fish. In patients with atrial fibrillation, in whom, obviously, the blood cannot be pumped from atrium to ventricle, it is true that the cardiac output is reduced; but this is due, rather, to irregularity of the ventricular rhythm in this condition.◄] In outlining the events of pumping, then, we need consider only what happens in the ventricles.

The sequence of contraction of the ventricles from apex to base (determined by the way the Purkinje system is arranged) has been described as a "milking" action, which is thought to be superior, in emptying the ventricle, to other patterns of spread of contraction. [►It is doubtful whether this argument is sound hydrodynamically; ectopic ventricular beats, arising often from parts of the ventricle other than the apex, do not appear to be markedly less efficient in producing the normal stroke volume.◄]

Many years ago, a public lecture was given in which the trabeculae of the ventricular walls (ridges on the inner surface) were praised as making possible the complete emptying of the ventricle in each beat and so increasing the "efficiency of the pump." Long since, it has been possible to measure how much blood is ejected from a ventricle and how much is left behind (the "endsystolic" volume). About as much is left (e.g., 70 ml) as is ejected (80 ml); so the basic assumption of the lecturer was completely wrong. In addition, *the efficiency of the heart has nothing whatever to do with whether or not it empties completely.* In fact, the ventricular volume provides a valuable variable reservoir of the blood volume and plays an important role in the regulation of the cardiac output (Starling's law Chapter 16).

The Four Phases of the Cardiac Cycle

Physiologists have delighted in subdividing the cardiac cycle into a great number of phases, each with a name invented by its initial proponent and often bearing an alternative name preferred by some other author. Only four phases are worth

remembering (Fig. 15–1). They are based on the combinations of inlet valve open or closed, and of outlet valve open or closed. The combination of inlet and outlet valves both open does not occur in the normal heart with competent valves.

FILLING (INLET VALVE OPEN, OUTLET VALVE CLOSED)

Because of the relaxation of the ventricular muscle after its last beat, the pressure in the ventricle has fallen to only a few millimeters of mercury. The moment it falls below the pressure existing in the atrium, the atrioventricular valve opens and blood flows into the ventricle. The ventricular muscle relaxes still more; so the ventricular pressure continues to fall for a short time and the filling becomes rapid. The phase of "rapid inflow" is, rather arbitrarily, said to last about 0.1 sec, followed by what is called the "period of diastasis" (Heaven knows why, since the word diastasis means "standing apart or asunder"). Now the inflow is less rapid because the ventricular pressure is rising (due to ventricular elasticity), and the gradient of energy that is filling it is reduced. At the end of this period of slower filling, the atrial contraction "tops up" the filling of the ventricle. During the whole of this filling phase, the inlet valve (the mitral or the tricuspid valve) of the ventricle is open. The outlet valves

Fig. 15-1.—The four distinct phases of the ventricular cycle, based on whether inlet and outlet valves are open or closed. The broken line indicates the aortic pressure. The atrial pressure is not shown here since on this scale it would practically coincide, in the filling phase, with the ventricular pressure, except for small waves, which are shown in **Figure 15–4** and discussed in the chapter on the venous pulse (Chapter 18).

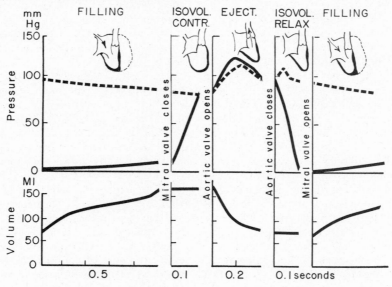

(aortic or pulmonary) are closed because the pressure on the other side of these (in the aorta or the pulmonary artery) is far above that in the ventricles.

The filling phase ends abruptly when the initial contraction of the ventricular muscle raises the ventricular pressure, by the fraction of a millimeter of mercury required, above the atrial pressure, at which time the atrioventricular valves close (creating the first heart sound). The total period of filling lasts more than half of the cardiac cycle at normal heart rates, less when the rate is increased.

ISOVOLUMETRIC CONTRACTION (INLET VALVE CLOSED, OUTLET VALVE CLOSED)

The ventricle is now a closed space, both valves being shut. As long as they remain closed, there can be no change of ventricular volume, although the ventricle changes shape as the ventricular wall develops tension. The ventricle becomes more spherical, the distance from apex to base shortening. As the contraction develops more and more tension in the wall, the pressure of blood in the ventricle rises rapidly. The moment it rises above the pressure remaining in the aorta, which has been declining by "runoff" from the high systolic value in the last beat, the outlet valves (aortic or pulmonary valve) open and this phase is over.

EJECTION (INLET VALVE CLOSED, OUTLET VALVE OPEN)

The blood in the ventricle is now ejected very rapidly into the aorta, faster than it can run out through the total peripheral resistance. The pressure in the aorta rises to keep pace with that in the ventricle, which continues to rise as contraction continues to increase. The resistance offered by the open valve is very small; so aortic pressure is only slightly below the ventricular. However, it must not be forgotten that in the aorta there has been created kinetic energy, not present in the ventricle, and so there will be 2 or 3 mm Hg difference on this score.

About halfway or two thirds through the ejection phase the contraction of the ventricle (no longer isovolumetric) ceases and is succeeded by very rapid relaxation. At first the ventricular pressure falls (because of relaxation) not quite so fast as the aortic pressure can fall by runoff; so ejection continues (the period of reduced ejection). However, ventricular relaxation increases in rate, while aortic runoff decreases; so the ventricular pressure soon falls below aortic pressure and the aortic valve closes (producing the second heart sound). The ejection phase is over. It lasts about 0.2 sec at normal heart rates. Its end is marked by a notch on the aortic pressure curve (the *incisura, or dicrotic notch*), as well as by the second heart sound.

ISOVOLUMETRIC RELAXATION (INLET VALVE CLOSED, OUTLET VALVE CLOSED)

Once more the ventricle is a closed chamber (as in the phase of isovolumetric contraction), in which the volume cannot change (the shape can, and does). The pressure falls very rapidly as the tension in the ventricular muscle decreases. The pressure eventually falls to below the atrial pressure, causing the opening of the atrioventricular valve and ending this phase in less than 0.1 sec. [►This remarkably rapid fall of ventricular pressure in isometric relaxation was for many years a physiological puzzle, for the relaxation of tension in strips of cardiac muscle after contraction did not appear to be nearly as fast as this. The idea of "active relaxation" began to be promulgated, although it was accepted with great reluctance because no one could see how a muscle "pushed itself out" to its relaxed length. Rushmer (1) supplied what is probably the explanation. The ventricular muscle was said to be in three layers. The outer layer of fibers (superficial bulbospiral muscle) swirls around the ventricle clockwise, as we look from base to apex. The middle layer (ventricular constrictor muscle) is circular; the inner (deep bulbospiral muscle) swirls counterclockwise. Actually this division into three distinct muscular layers is quite arbitrary. Streeter *et al.* (2) rapidly fixed the ventricular wall of the dog heart, either in systole or in diastole, and studied histologically the orientation of the muscle fibers throughout the thickness of the wall. The result (Fig. 15–2) shows that the angle changes smoothly from the outside to the inner surfaces, and we must think of a very large number of successive "layers" of fibers, which are linked by elastic fibers. Because the direction of the fibers changes, contraction must cause a sliding movement of each fiber over its neighbors, i.e., a *"shear strain,"* in which the elastic connective tissue is stretched. Elastic potential energy is stored during the isovolumetric contraction phase, and its release during the isovolumetric relaxation phase

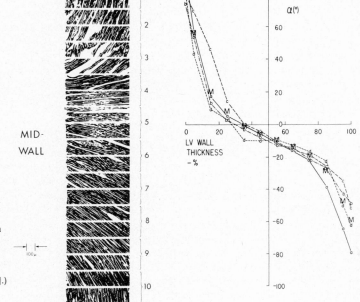

Fig. 15-2.—Left, sequence of photo-micrographs showing fiber angles in successive sections taken in systole of a dog's heart (sections are in planes parallel to the ventricular surface). **Right,** measured fiber angles at four sampling sites plotted vs per cent distance through the wall. (From Streeter *et al.*[2].)

supplies the force which increases the rate of relaxation.◄] Further consideration of the elastic component in the ventricular muscle is given in Chapter 19.

Valvular Incompetence; Regurgitation

It will be noted that at no time in the normal heart are both the inlet and the outlet valves open. If they were, great inefficiency of pumping would result. In disease, calcification of the valvular tissue or scarring due to bacterial lesions leads to *incompetence* of the valves, so that, although they have closed, blood can still pass through them. Aortic incompetence leads to *aortic regurgitation.* After the aortic valve has closed, because the aortic pressure exceeded the ventricular pressure, blood will flow back into the relaxing heart, as well as out through the peripheral resistance. As a consequence, much of the work of the heart is wasted, and the actual stroke output of the left ventricle must greatly exceed the stroke volume that effectively flows in the system. Similarly with incompetence of the pulmonary valve. Incompetence of either of the inlet valves leads to backflow into the atria, which may be greatly

distended under abnormally high pressures. The same acquired valvular lesions of disease often cause *valvular stenosis* as well as incompetence; that is, the opening is smaller than normal when the valves are open, offering a considerable resistance to the flow in or out of the ventricles. In *muscular subaortic stenosis,* narrowing in the outflow tract behind the valve is due to hypertrophy or malformation of the septum. The outflow tract may narrow greatly during systole when the hypertrophied septal muscle contracts and "bulges."

Recognition of incompetence and of stenosis of the cardiac valves is an important part of cardiac diagnosis. It is based on simple logic and knowledge of the mechanical events of the cardiac cycle.

Synchrony and Asynchrony of Events in the Two Sides of the Heart

While, as pointed out already, the exact synchrony of the two sides of the heart has little or no importance in the pumping, the timing of the events on the two sides can give valuable information in cases of cardiac dysfunction. The timing is measured against the waves of the

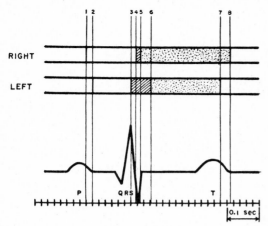

Fig. 15-3.—Diagrammatic representation of the average timing of electrical and mechanical events on both sides of the heart during atrial and ventricular systole in normal persons. *1,* onset of right atrial contraction. *2,* onset of left atrial contraction. *3,* onset of left ventricular contraction. *4,* onset of right ventricular contraction. *5,* onset of right ventricular ejection. *6,* onset of left ventricular ejection. *7,* end of left ventricular ejection. *8,* end of right ventricular ejection. The hatched areas represent ventricular isometric contraction. The stippled areas represent ventricular ejection. (From Braunwald *et al.* [3].)

electrocardiogram and the heart sounds. For such use in medical diagnosis, in man, all of the excellent work on the timing of events in the hearts of dogs and other animals is, of course, not conclusive. Fortunately, Braunwald, Fishman and Cour-

nand (3) were able to record (by catheters) pressures in the chambers of the heart and in the great vessels of 13 human beings during exposure of the heart in chest surgery. The patients had no evidence of cardiovascular disease. Figure 15–3 is a diagram reproduced from the work of these investigators.

Atrial contraction occurs earlier in the right atrium than in the left, presumably because the pacemaker is on the right side. In contrast, ventricular contraction starts earlier on the left side, even though the start of significant electrical activity occurs later. As one might expect from the lower pressure that must be reached before the outlet valve opens on the right side, ejection is considerably earlier on the right than on the left (even though contraction started later). The end of ejection is earlier on the left than on the right. This is signaled by the closure of the outlet valves and the second heart sound, which is consequently double (from aortic and pulmonary valves). If the difference in time of closure between the two ventricles is sufficient, the second heart sound is *split*, with the aortic valve closing first. During inspiration, the split becomes wider, as the pulmonary resistance decreases during inspiration and the ejection period is lengthened.

Table 15–1 shows how priority alternates in the electrical and mechanical events of the cardiac cycle.

TABLE 15–1.—TIME SEQUENCE OF EVENTS BETWEEN
LEFT AND RIGHT SIDES OF HEART

	LEFT SIDE	RIGHT SIDE	REMARKS
	ELECTRICAL		
Beginning of depolarization	1	2	
Full depolarization	2	1	Less tissue to depolarize
Full repolarization	1	2	
	MECHANICAL		
Beginning of atrial contraction	2	1	Right atrium contains pacemaker
Beginning of ventricular contraction	1	2	Almost coincidental
Closure of arterial valves	1	2	First heart sound. Mitral first
Opening of arterial valves	2	1	Ejection. Right heart less pressure required
Closure of arterial valves	1	2	Split second heart sound. Aortic valve first
Opening of atrio-ventricular valves	?	?	Third heart sound

Systole and Diastole

The many definitions to be found in different books as to *systole* and *diastole* are a source of confusion to students. The terms were originally descriptive of the period when the heart was pumping versus the period when it was filling, or periods of "activity" versus "rest." Obviously, the mechanical "ventricular systole" is different from the "aortic systole," and "electrical systole and diastole" are something else. The one fact without disagreement in the use of these terms is that "systolic pressure" means the maximal arterial pressure reached in the pulse, and "diastolic pressure," the lowest pressure reached, just before the next beat. [►It can readily be seen that completely unimportant hairs can be split as to whether ventricular systole includes only the ejection period or includes the isometric contraction period also. Why waste time over words as long as we understand the sequence of events in the cardiac cycle?◄]

Why Are There Sounds in the Circulation?

Without the use of the stethoscope to listen to the heart sounds, cardiovascular diagnosis would be very severely handicapped. *Auscultation* is an ancient art; yet knowledge of why there should be sounds at all, and of how they reach the bell of the physician's stethoscope on the chest from their point of origin, has only very recently been acquired (Faber and co-workers [4, 5, 13]).

In general, we should expect the circulation to be silent because the flow of blood through the blood vessels is, at most points and in most circumstances, *streamline* or *laminar flow*. Adjacent laminae (layers) of blood, which travel at different velocities down the vessels (a maximal rate on the axis, zero at the wall), slide silently over one another, interchanging energy from layer to layer (this is why there is viscous resistance) but doing so smoothly and continuously. In laminar flow there is nothing periodic that could cause vibration or sounds. Heart sounds and murmurs therefore must be due to disturbances of the normal pattern of flow, as by turbulence (see Chapter 11) or otherwise.

The two heart sounds which are always audible—the first and second sounds—do not necessarily involve turbulence of flowing blood, for they are due to the *closure* of the valves (mitral and tricuspid for the first, aortic and pulmonary

for the second), and it is to be expected that closure will cause vibrations in the valves themselves, in the wall of the arteries and in the blood. The sounds are analogous to the noise of a door shutting. The attempts in different languages to imitate the first and second heart sounds (onomatopoeia) are interesting. Students taught in English learn that they sound like *lub-dup* or *lub-tup*. In French, it is (translating into English) *frou-ti,* or *frou-ti-ti,* where the second *ti* is for an "opening snap" of mitral stenosis; in German, students are taught *doop-teup;* in Turkish, *r-rupp-ta*; and one colleague's Russian professor taught what might be written as *htah-ta.*

Heart Vibrations or Heart Sounds?

What follows was kindly written by J. J. Faber, whose research on the mode of transmission of heart sounds has greatly elucidated this problem. The "sounds" originate as vibrations, travel over the surfaces of the ventricles and of the great vessels, and over the surface of the chest, not as longitudinal vibrations, as would sound waves through tissues, but as transverse vibrational waves at much slower velocities. When these vibrations reach the diaphragm or bell of the stethoscope, they cause a true longitudinal vibration in the column of air in the stethoscope tubes and here are truly "sound." Up to that point, both as they originate and during their transmission through the body, it would be more suitable to speak of "heart vibrations" instead of "heart sounds."

Details of the Heart Sounds

The mechanical activity of the myocardium causes the heart to vibrate. These vibrations cover a wide range of frequencies, from about 1 to over 1,000 cycles per second (cps). The ear does not respond to frequencies under 30 cps. The apex beat of the heart and the slow movements of the body due to the recoil when the blood is ejected fall in this range. Frequencies over 30 cps are audible if loud enough; but the ear is not very sensitive to frequencies below 100 cps, and more than 95% of the energy of the audible vibrations (i.e., the heart sounds) is contained in frequencies below 100 cps.

In normal persons, at least two heart sounds can be heard when the ear is applied to the surface of the body or when the heart sounds are conducted to the ear via a stethoscope; in some

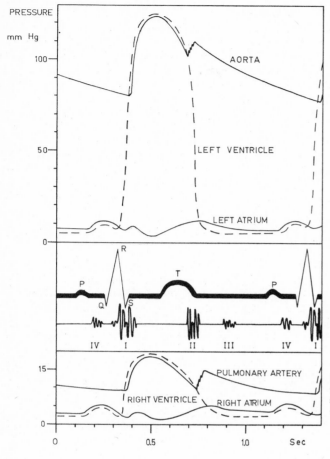

Fig. 15-4.—The timing of the heart sounds in the cardiac cycle with respect to the ventricular, atrial and arterial pressures, and the corresponding electrocardiogram.

persons, three or four heart sounds may be heard in each cardiac cycle. The numbering of the four heart sounds is conventional. The first and the second heart sounds are the loudest, and they occur at the moment of closure of the atrioventricular valves and arterial valves, respectively. The interval between the first and the second sound is shorter than the interval between the second and the next first sound (Fig. 15–4).

First Heart Sound

The first sound is caused by the closure of the atrioventricular valves, the inlet valves of the ventricle. This fact determines the place of the sound in the cardiac cycle. The ventricular contraction which begins during the QRS complex of the electrocardiogram causes the pressure in the ventricle to rise. As soon as the pressure in the ventricle exceeds the pressure in the atrium, the

blood begins to flow back into the atrium and forces the valve to close. The sudden deceleration of the blood sets the valve in vibration, and this vibration is transmitted along the wall of the ventricle with a velocity of a few meters per second. The mitral valve of the left ventricle and the tricuspid valve of the right ventricle close almost simultaneously and generally give rise to a single sound, which follows immediately after the QRS complex of the electrocardiogram.

The conclusive experimental evidence (7) that the first heart sound is caused by the closure of the atrioventricular valves is the temporal relation between the two events and the abolition of the first sound when the atrioventricular valves are excised in experimental animals. Further, the first sound has been shown to travel from the base of the ventricle to the apex. When the heart sounds are recorded with small microphones in the blood stream, the first heart sound is found to be louder in the ventricle than in the atrium or in the aorta (8).

A small contribution to the first heart sound is made by the *initial vibration*, a vibration of low amplitude and low frequency which precedes the valve-closure sound. The initial vibration is a movement in the ventricular wall when the ventricle starts to contract (9).

[►It is conceivable that the opening of the aortic valve, the increasing tension of the wall of the great vessels and the movement of the blood at the beginning of the ejection constitute the last part of the first heart sound, but the evidence for this view is far from conclusive. (10).◄]

SECOND HEART SOUND

The second sound is caused by the closure of the aortic and pulmonary valves, just after the T wave of the electrocardiogram. At the end of systole, when the pressure in the ventricle falls below the arterial pressure, the reversed pressure gradient closes the outlet valves of the ventricles. The aortic and the pulmonary valves do not close simultaneously; the degree of asynchronism depends on the respiratory cycle. In expiration the two sounds merge, whereas in inspiration the second sound is split into an aortic component and a later pulmonary component (11).

The arrest of further backflow into the ventricles by the closure of the valves causes a sudden change in arterial pressure, which can be seen in recordings of the arterial pressure, as the *dicrotic notch* (Fig. 15–4). The dicrotic notch consists of vibrations of various frequencies; the frequencies over 30 cps are audible and constitute the origin of the second heart sound. The second sound, being a part of the dicrotic notch, is conducted along the arteries with the velocity of the pulse wave and is audible over the carotid arteries. The second sound cannot be seen in the dicrotic notch of most recordings of arterial pressures because the amplitude of these higher frequencies is low and because the "frequency response" of most pressure recorders is limited. The second heart sound is conducted through the tissues and can be heard on the surface of the thorax.

When intravascular sound recordings are made, the second sound is found to be louder in the ascending aorta and in the pulmonary artery than it is in the left and the right ventricles, respectively (8).

THIRD HEART SOUND

A third heart sound can be heard in some normal persons. It occurs when the blood from the atrium suddenly rushes into the ventricle after the atrioventricular valves open at the beginning of the diastole. The third heart sound comes about 0.2 sec after the second sound.

[►Two mechanisms are considered to be responsible for the production of the third heart sound (10): (1) the vibration of the ventricular myocardium under the impact of the blood flowing into the ventricle and (2) the reclosure of the atrioventricular valve by the vortices that follow in the wake of the inflowing jet through the valve.◄]

FOURTH HEART SOUND

The fourth heart sound, not present except in states of elevated left ventricular end-diastolic pressure, has its place between the P wave and the QRS complex of the electrocardiogram. It precedes the first heart sound by about 0.1 sec. The fourth heart sound is caused by the contraction of the atrium. This is shown by the disappearance of the fourth sound from its normal place in the cardiac cycle when the normal sequence of cardiac activation is disrupted by a disease process of the conduction system.

MURMURS

The use of the term "heart sound" is often limited to those sounds which have an abrupt beginning and end and a short duration. Murmurs are sounds produced by turbulence. It is almost always easy to distinguish murmurs from heart sounds by their gradual beginning and end, their duration and their higher pitch. Since streamline flow is silent, a murmur always indicates turbulence in the blood stream. Common in normal persons is a systolic murmur produced by turbulence in the outflow tract of the ventricle. But often a murmur is evidence of a disease process, for instance, the diastolic murmur produced by the (turbulent) backflow through a leaking aortic valve.

THE AUSCULTATORY AREAS

Although the heart sounds can be heard over a large area of the thoracic surface, there are spe-

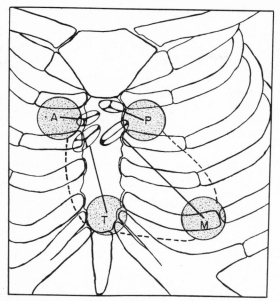

Fig. 15-5.—The auscultatory areas on the chest, showing that they are certainly not those closest to the heart valves from which they originated. A, aortic; P, pulmonary; T, tricuspid; M, mitral areas.

cific points on the precordium where the sound from a particular valve can be heard best. These "points of maximal intensity" are shown in Figure 15–5. The aortic and pulmonary areas lie quite close to the aortic and pulmonary valves because the sounds are transmitted to the surface from those parts of the arteries that are closest to the chest wall. The mitral and tricuspid sounds which arise in the atrioventricular valves are conducted along the ventricles to the points where the left and the right ventricles are in close contact with the thoracic wall; these are not the points on the surface closest to the valves. Note that the auscultatory areas of the arterial valves lie on the contralateral side of the chest.

The auscultatory areas can be established with the help of heart-sound recordings made on persons with clearly split heart sounds in whom the mitral and tricuspid sounds and the aortic and pulmonary sounds can be distinguished (3) in the first and second heart sound.

It has been shown experimentally (4) that these auscultatory areas are the areas where the heart sounds reach the surface first. The heart sounds then spread from these areas to other points on the chest wall with a low velocity. The velocity increases with the square root of the frequency;

the velocity of a vibration of 100 cps is about 15 meters per second.

The loudness of the heart sounds varies much from person to person, but in any one person the relative loudness with which the various heart sounds are heard is important. A heart sound is louder if the valve is wide open at the moment it is forced to close, and also when the force that closes the valve is greater than normal. The effect of a decrease of the filling of the right heart, and later the left heart, on the loudness of the heart sounds can readily be observed during a Valsalva maneuver (a forceful expiratory effort against a closed glottis) (12).

The Use of Phonocatheters*

In recent years, cardiac catheters that carry a microphone at their tip, as well as providing means of injection or withdrawal of blood samples, have been available. It has been hoped that these catheters would enable the point of origin of heart sounds and murmurs to be determined and would give better detail of these sounds than does auscultation on the surface of the body. These hopes have been only partly fulfilled. It is now known (work of Faber) that heart sounds and murmurs travel in the great vessels, not to any extent in the blood stream, but along the wall, like pulse waves. The *microphone at the tip of catheters is normally picking up vibrations that had traveled in the wall.* This explains some peculiar features already noted in phonocardiography; for example, murmurs due to a valvular stenosis are picked up only when the microphone is downstream from the valve, not to any extent when it is on the upstream side of the valve. The vibration travels on the wall in both directions from the area of turbulence downstream from the valve but is damped out almost completely by the weight of tissue at the valvular ring. In addition, there seems to be little advantage in using a microphone (necessarily very small and therefore relatively insensitive) at the catheter tip, rather than recording from a larger, more sensitive microphone at the other end of the catheter (as Luisada has shown). The time lag in conduction of the sound in the catheter is constant and can be made as a correction.

This knowledge of how heart sounds and murmurs are transmitted on the body should explain

*This section of this chapter has been added by A.C.B.

the otherwise inexplicable location of the best areas for hearing some abnormal circulatory sounds (e.g., the murmur of patent ductus arteriosus is often heard best just beneath the clavicle and to the left of the sternum).

REFERENCES

1. Rushmer, R. F.: Functional Anatomy of Cardiac Contraction, *Cardiovascular Dynamics* (2d ed.; Philadelphia: W. B. Saunders Company, 1961), chap. 2.

2. Streeter, D. D., Jr.; Spotnitz, H. M.; Patel, D. P.; Ross, J., Jr., and Sonnenblick, E. H.; Fiber orientation in the canine left ventricle during diastole and systole, Circulation Res. 24:339, 1969.

3. Braunwald, E.; Fishman, A. P., and Cournand, A.: The relationship of dynamic events in the cardiac chambers, pulmonary artery and aorta in man, Circulation Res. 4:100, 1956.

4. Faber, J. J., and Burton, A. C.: Spread of heart sounds over chest wall, Circulation Res. 11:96, 1962.

5. Faber, J. J., and Purvis, J. H.: Conduction of cardiovascular sound along arteries, Circulation Res. 12:308, 1963.

6. Roberts, L. N.; Smiley, I. R., and Manning, G. W.: A comparison of direct and indirect blood-pressure determinations, Circulation 8:232, 1953.

7. Orias, O.: The genesis of heart sounds, New England J. Med. 24:763, 1949.

8. Lewis, D. H.; Deitz, G. W.; Wallace, J. D., and Brown, J. R., Jr.: Present status of intracardiac phonography, Circulation 18:991, 1958.

9. Counihan, T.; Messe, A. L.; Rappaport, M. B., and Sprague, H. B.: The initial vibration of the first heart sound, Circulation 3:730, 1951.

10. McKusick, V. A.: *Cardiovascular Sound in Health and Disease* (Baltimore: Williams & Wilkins Company, 1958).

11. Boyer, S. H., and Chisholm, A. W.: Physiologic splitting of the second heart sound, Circulation 18:1010, 1958.

12. Leatham, A.: Auscultation of the heart, Lancet 2:703, 1958.

13. Faber, J. J., and Burton, A. C.: Biophysics of heart sounds and its application to clinical auscultation, Canad, M.A.J. 91:120, 1964.

16

The Law of the Heart

Starling's Law of the Heart

E. H. STARLING, in the Linacre Lecture of 1915 (published in 1918), enunciated a law which is of the greatest importance in cardiac physiology. It has been discussed critically by physiologists ever since. Some have set up a "house of cards," restating the law in a way that Starling never would have approved, and then have proceeded to knock down their own version. Others have, correctly, pointed out that the law, as it was experimentally demonstrated, applied only to the isolated heart (or heart-lung preparation) and that, in the intact animal, nervous and hormonal influences on cardiac output could greatly modify the law. Nevertheless, the law remains operative from beat to beat of the heart of the living animal, and functioning of the heart according to the operation of this law is probably essential to the maintenance of a steady state of the circulation.

Starling stated that "the energy of contraction (i.e., of the ventricular muscle) is a function of the length of the muscle fiber." Therefore, if the ventricles were filled to a greater extent (i.e., the end-diastolic ventricular volume were increased), the subsequent systolic contraction would be more vigorous and a greater stroke volume would be ejected. Starling felt that in this way the heart automatically controlled its output by the degree of filling of each ventricle.

Experimental Evidence of Starling's Law

Starling's law is based on evidence derived from a "heart-lung preparation," consisting of a heart, deprived of all nervous connections, pumping its blood through isolated lungs (or an artificial oxygenator) to be reoxygenated, and through some artificial peripheral resistance and the coro-nary circulation, to supply the energy to the heart muscle. A great number of different "preparations" have been devised by cardiac physiologists to satisfy these essentials by different means. The degree of filling and the stroke volume of the ventricles can be manipulated by changing the atrial or the arterial pressure levels, for example, by altering the level of a venous reservoir or the pulmonary and peripheral resistances. The stroke volume is measured by the use of flowmeters in the aorta or by the change in volume of the ventricles, and the pressures in the cardiac cycle in the various vessels are measured by manometers.

The results may be plotted in a variety of ways; for example, systolic pressure or mean arterial pressure might be plotted versus atrial pressure, which might be considered to be proportional to the degree of filling. However, the most direct and relevant plot is that of stroke volume versus the end-diastolic volume of the ventricles. Other more indirect tests of the law, as, for instance, using the atrial pressure instead of ventricular volume, have the disadvantage that the latter is not necessarily proportional to the "filling pressure," for the distensibility of the ventricle may alter—and, in any case, it would be the atrioventricular pressure *gradient* (or better, the total energy gradient) that mattered. [►Thus, to show, as many physiologists have done, that, even in a heart-lung preparation, the stroke volume may not always increase with an increase in atrial pressure really has no bearing on the validity of Starling's law.◄]

The results of experiments which have been reported many times for the different ways of doing the experiments are illustrated diagrammatically in Figure 16–1. As the diastolic volume increases, so does the stroke volume—up to a point. If the heart is filled beyond a critical point, the curve ceases to rise and further increase in volume leads to a decrease, rather than an increase, of stroke volume (the stage of *decompensation* is reached).

Explanation of the Law

Undoubtedly, the curve of Figure 16-1 depends on a fundamental property of cardiac ventricular muscle, in that the strength of its contraction increases, up to a point, with the initial length or the initial tension of the fibers. [►Which of these is the real determinant of the force of contraction has not been settled.◄]

[►Direct experimental evidence of this property, on isolated ventricular muscle, has been very scanty. Since the fibers in the ventricle are arranged with different orientation, cutting a strip of ventricle inevitably cuts across many fibers. It is much more convenient to use the papillary muscles of the chordae tendineae in the experiments. It is an assumption, of course, that their behavior would be identical. Lundin (1) found with the fibers of the frog ventricle that the contractile force increased to a maximum of six to eight times the initial unstretched value at about twice the unstretched length. However, further increase of stretch did not produce a decrease in tension; that is, the curve was flat, rather than falling, beyond this maximum. In contrast, the corresponding graph for skeletal muscle shows an abrupt decline (Fig. 16-1) after the maximum.

Fig. 16-1.—Schematic diagram illustrating Starling's law of the heart. The inset shows how the tension of skeletal muscle is related to its initial stretch. Cardiac muscle *(broken line)* does not follow the same law but reaches a relatively constant force at high degrees of stretch. The decline of the stroke volume can be attributed to the increased size of the heart and its mechanical disadvantage (law of Laplace).

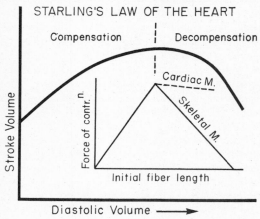

STARLING'S LAW OF THE HEART

We no longer have to rely (insecurely) on data from isolated papillary muscles, or on the analogy to striated muscles, for the relation between initial stretch of ventricular muscle and the tension developed in contraction. Sonnenblick and his colleagues (2), by rapid injection of gluteraldehyde into the coronary arteries of a beating heart, were able to fix the ventricular muscle at any stage of systole or diastole and then measure the sarcomere (contractile unit) length microscopically for different regions of the ventricular wall in dogs. The increase in active tension developed with increasing sarcomere length (the rising phase of the Starling's law curve) is well shown, the decline after a critical degree of stretching is present but not so well demonstrated. The method has also been used to study passive changes in length of the sarcomere with stretch and in permanently dilated ventricles, as in "heart failure." Active tension is zero at sarcomere length of about 1.5 μ, rises to a maximum at initial sarcomere length of about 2.2 μ and declines for further initial stretch.

It must not be forgotten that the production of pressure in the ventricle to expel the stroke volume depends not only on the tension developed in the muscle but on the "mechanical advantage," by the law of Laplace (Chapter 12, Fig. 12-4). As the ventricular volume increases, the pressure developed by a given tension decreases (the radii of curvature increase). Adding this factor to the curve of tension vs. volume will explain the *phase of decompensation* found in the intact ventricle.

Starling's Law in the Intact Animal

If experiments relating cardiac output or stroke volume to the degree of ventricular filling had been made on the intact animal only, it would be most unlikely that Starling's law of the heart would have been discovered. For example, in comparing rest and exercise, the cardiac output is found to be greatly increased during exercise, and the stroke volume may be increased (although the increased heart rate in exercise is more important), yet the heart in diastole may actually be smaller.

Sarnoff (3), in a series of studies using a modified heart-lung preparation, has greatly elucidated the difference in "ventricular performance curves," as those similar to Figure 16-2 are called, in different physiological conditions. Stimulation of the vagus (parasympathetic) or sympathetic nerves to the heart greatly alters the performance

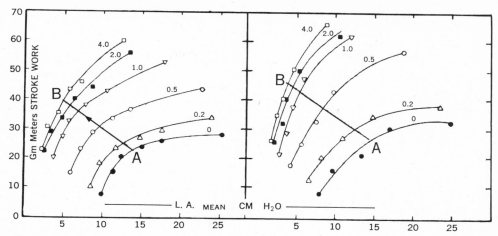

Fig. 16-2.—A family of ventricular performance curves produced by stimulation of cardiac sympathetic nerves at the frequencies indicated (0–4.0 cps). In the intact animal, the operating point may move from *A*, at rest, to *B*, in heavy exercise, and so provide an apparent contradiction to Starling's law. (Slightly modified from Sarnoff and Mitchell [3].)

of the ventricular muscle (vagus decreases the force, sympathetic increases), so that the curve of tension versus initial stretch is completely shifted to a new level. There has been a change in "ventricular contractility." *We should think, then, not of one curve of Starling's law, but of a whole family of curves, according to the contractility of the heart muscle under the influence of nervous impulses (via noradrenaline) and of circulating hormones like adrenaline (Fig. 16–2).*

The decrease in the force of contraction, at the same diastolic ventricular volume, under vagal stimulation (the so-called *inotropic vagal effect*) is a matter of controversy. In contrast to the marked effect of sympathetic stimulation, Sarnoff found no vagal effect when stroke work was plotted against left ventricular end-diastolic pressure, although, if plotted against atrial (filling) pressure, vagal effect was apparent. This may be a vagal effect on the relation between atrial pressure and the filling of the heart rather than a true change in contractility of the heart, that is, a true shift of the Starling's curve. Thus, when we pass from one physiological state of the heart to another physiological state, as from rest to exercise, we may pass from one point on a particular Starling curve to another point, not on this curve, but on another curve (*A* to *B*, Fig. 16–2). The over-all picture would apparently be an exception to Starling's law.

In view of this, it might be thought that Starling's law did not have importance in the intact animal. On the contrary, it remains all important. Its importance in health does not lie in the adjustment of the cardiac output to the varying needs of the body (as Starling thought), for this is accomplished very adequately by the control of the contractility of the heart by nervous and hormonal influences. In disease, Starling's law may operate as Starling suggested (Hamilton [4]). *As Hamilton (5) has pointed out, the function of Starling's law is to ensure that in any period the output of the left and that of the right ventricle are approximately equal, and that the total blood volume remains distributed in the proper way between the systemic and pulmonary circulations.* This function is independent of the shift of performance curve under nervous and hormonal influences, because both ventricles are under the same influences and shift from curve to curve together.

The Trouble with Two Pumps in Series

Consider two pumps whose stroke volumes (or output) can be adjusted to some chosen value but are not automatically varied by some such device as Starling's law (Fig. 16–3). The pumps are arranged in series with two "vascular beds," corresponding to the pulmonary and systemic circuits, between the pumps. In spite of every effort that might be made to have the two outputs exactly equal, this would be impossible. One pump might have an output, say, of 5.00 L per min; the other, 5.01 L per min, or, if the adjustment possible was less exact, of 5.1 L per min. In the latter case, 0.1 L of the fluid in the system would be transferred every minute from one circuit (say the systemic) to the other (the pulmo-

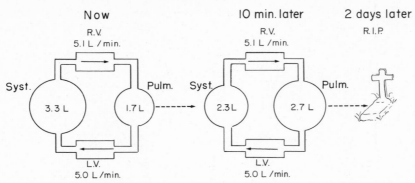

Fig. 16-3.—Illustrating what would happen to the systemic blood volume *(syst.)* and the pulmonary blood volume *(pulm.)* if Starling's law, or some other mechanism, did not keep the mean outputs of the left ventricle *(LV)* and right ventricle *(RV)* the same, but instead, the mean output of the right was only 2% greater than the left. The 2 days is an allowance for the undertaker and the parson; death would ensue in less than 10 min.

nary). In 10 min, the shift would amount to 1 L. In the circulation, the blood volume is normally divided with two thirds in the systemic circuit (about 3.3 L) and one third in the pulmonary circuit (about 1.7 L). If the output of the left heart exceeded that of the right heart (say 5.1 L per min versus 5.0 L per min), in 10 min 1 L of blood would be transferred to the pulmonary circuit, with now 2.7 L in the pulmonary and 2.3 L in the systemic circuit. This would amount to an impossible degree of *pulmonary congestion,* with rise in pressure of the pulmonary vessels and consequent pulmonary edema.

It is absolutely essential, then, that there should be some automatic feature of cardiac action to keep the partition of blood volume between the two circuits. This is what Starling's law accomplishes. The outputs of the two hearts are seldom identical in any one beat. In fact, during inspiration, owing mainly to a decrease in pulmonary vascular resistance when the lungs are expanded, the output of the right heart is considerably greater than that in expiration and exceeds the output of the left heart. However, this increased output of the right heart soon (a few beats later) increases the filling of the left heart, and by Starling's law its output increases correspondingly, preventing any piling-up of blood volume in the pulmonary circuit.

An engineer faced with this problem of maintaining volume distribution when two stroke pumps are in series might use a simple device to maintain the steady state. He would provide a "bleeder" circuit (or shunt) across one of the pumps. If a progressive shift of volume into one circuit occurred, the mean pressure there would rise and the flow through the shunt would alter in such a way as to compensate. This device would

prevent gross, progressive shifts of fluid but would not, of course, maintain the partition or the pressures in the circuits within very narrow limits. [►It is interesting that in the circulation this safeguard, additional to Starling's law, is provided by the bronchial circulation (Chapter 6, Fig. 6–1). This is a route from the aorta to the pulmonary veins and left atrium, and so constitutes a shunt of the kind described, across the left heart. How important the bronchial circulation may be in stabilizing the partition of blood volume has not been determined. In cases where the automatic control by Starling's law ceases to operate (see discussion on heart failure below), the consequences may possibly be of vital importance.◄]

Limitations of Starling's Law: Cardiac Decompensation and Heart Failure

In the condition known as *heart failure,* the output of one heart (either left in *left heart failure* or right in *right heart failure*) tends to be reduced, usually because of damage to the ventricular muscle. As a consequence, that ventricle will fill more completely (ventricular dilatation, visible often on x-radiographs of the heart). By Starling's law, this increases the output of the failing ventricle, so that there is *compensation.* However, if the dilatation exceeds the critical value corresponding to the maximum in Starling's curve, the situation becomes desperate. On the descending limb of the curve, further filling (dilatation) of the ventricle will result not in an increased but in a decreased stroke volume. The automatic adjustment of blood-volume partition now works in reverse, and in failure of the left heart, pulmonary congestion is rapidly produced. [►In addition, the regulation of the total blood volume, which in health is very accurate, seems to be impaired in heart failure, and patients in chronic left heart failure tend to retain fluid excessively. The reason for this may be that this control depends on some receptor (where, is not yet known) the stimulation of which is governed by the blood flow of that region. An increase of blood flow might produce a reflex release of hormones, which have a tendency to reduce the blood volume. As long as, in general, increased blood volume is associated with increased cardiac output, the control of blood volume would function. In decompensation, however, an increase of blood volume may, on the contrary, cause a decreased cardiac output, and so cause retention of blood volume and further increase the congestion. Whatever the reason, patients in heart failure show a loss of regulation of blood volume, and treatment to reduce it (e.g., by diuretics) is called for.◄]

Right heart failure is characterized by a piling-up of blood in the systemic venous vessels and a rise in venous pressure, easily seen in the neck veins (Chapter 10, Fig. 10–3). The accompanying rise of capillary pressure upsets the fluid balance in these vessels and leads to peripheral edema, particularly in the dependent vessels.

The treatment of decompensation and heart failure is to strengthen the failing heart muscle (digitalis helps greatly—we still do not know just how) and to reduce the blood volume (diuretics) so that the ventricular function curve may be on the "compensation," rather than on the "decompensation," portion of the curve.

In view of the disastrous consequences of decompensation, *giving transfusions, which will increase the blood volume, in cases of cardiac shock or failure can be very dangerous unless it is certain that cardiac dilatation will not result.*

LOW-OUTPUT AND HIGH-OUTPUT FAILURE. —The term "cardiac failure" must not be taken as indicating, necessarily, a reduced cardiac output, although this is often so. A weakened ventricle, by dilatation in the compensation phase, may have a normal, or even a higher than normal, output. Thus, "heart failure" should be defined, not in terms of whether cardiac output is low, but in terms of *the cardiac output considered in relation to the size of the heart.* This was illustrated by the work of Starr many years ago. He measured the cardiac output of a number of normal persons and of patients in heart failure and plotted the output versus the size of the heart, as estimated from the x-ray shadow. The points for those in failure all lay below the line on the graph denoting normal cardiac function.

Attempts to study cardiac failure in experimental animals have not been very successful in imitating the condition of patients. [►One conclusion has been that a complete clinical picture can be produced experimentally only if the ventricular muscle is damaged. Some physiologists have confused everyone by defining "forward" and "backward" failure. Apparently the protagonists in the arguments about this understood what they meant by the terms, but not what their opponents meant, and no one else understood any of them.◄]

Poetical Summary

So subtle and important a law as Starling's law of the heart deserves a summary in verse, for it is far from being prosaic.

WHAT GOES IN, MUST COME OUT

The great Dr. Starling, in his Law of the Heart
Said the output was greater, if, right at the start,
The cardiac fibers were stretched a bit more,
So their force of contraction would be more than before.
Thus the larger the volume in diastole
The greater the output was likely to be.
But when the heart reaches a much larger size,
This leads to Heart Failure, and often, Demise.
The relevant law is not Starling's, alas,
But the classical law of Lecompte de Laplace.
Your patient is dying in Decompensation,
So reduce his Blood Volume, or call his Relation.
If the right heart keeps pumping more blood than the left,
The lung circuit's congested; the systemic—bereft.
Since no one is healthy with pulmo-congestion,
The law of Doc. Starling's a splendid suggestion.
The balance of outputs is made automatic
And blood-volume partition becomes steady-static.

REFERENCES

1. Lundin, G.: Mechanical properties of cardiac muscle, Acta physiol. scandinav. (supp. 20) 7:7, 1944.
2. Spotnitz, H. M.; Sonnenblick, E. H., and Spiro, D.: Relation of ultrastructure to function in the intact heart, Circulation Res. 18:49, 1966. This is followed by a series of papers on this topic by these authors, (e.g., Circulation Res. 28:49, 1971).
3. Sarnoff, S. J., and Mitchell, J. H.: The Control of the Function of the Heart, in Dow, P. (ed.): *Handbook of Physiology*, Sec. 2, Vol. I: *Circulation* (American Physiological Society) (Baltimore: Williams & Wilkins Company, 1962), pp. 489–532.
4. Hamilton, W. F.: The Lewis A. Connor Memorial Lecture: The physiology of the cardiac output, Circulation 8:527, 1953.
5. Hamilton, W. F.: Role of Starling concept in regulation of the normal circulation, Physiol. Rev. 35:160, 1955.

17

Coronary Circulation and Metabolism of Cardiac Muscle

Coronary Arterial Supply

TWO MAIN CORONARY ARTERIES, the left and the right, arise from the sinus of Valsalva, near the aortic valvular ring. The left coronary artery supplies the left ventricle plus the anterior half of the septum; the right coronary artery supplies the right ventricle and the posterior half of the septum. There are many *anastomoses* of the two systems at the apex, so that the circumflex branching of the left coronary artery can supply the apex of the right ventricle also (Fig. 17–1). The anastomoses provide a safety factor, reducing the area of ischemia when a branch artery is occluded *(myocardial infarction)*. The left coronary artery also supplies the vasa vasorum of the root of the pulmonary artery. The volume of blood flow in the two arteries is comparable, about 80 ml per 100 Gm of left ventricle per minute. The total flow may amount to 5% of the resting cardiac output.

In passing through the coronary circuit, the blood gives up an unusually large part of its content of oxygen. The arterial content of 20 vol% is reduced to about 5 vol%; that is, the "extraction" of oxygen is high. This extraction remains remarkably constant in the face of large changes in rate of cardiac oxygen consumption, indicating that the coronary blood flow is accurately regulated to the oxygen needs of the heart.

The capillary network which the arteries supply is unusually rich, so that each muscle cell is very close to a capillary. Venous drainage follows the usual pattern of venules, collecting veins and, finally, the single coronary veins reaching the right atrium at the coronary sinus, where more than 80 or 90% of the coronary flow empties.

Fig. **17-1.**—Casts of the coronary arterial system of the dog heart, made by injecting vinyl acetate and then dissolving the tissue away. In the cast at the right, the left coronary artery was ligated at its origin (point *X*), yet its branches were filled by a retrograde flow *(arrow)* from other coronary arteries. (Photographs of casts supplied by D. Busby, Department of Surgery, University of Western Ontario.)

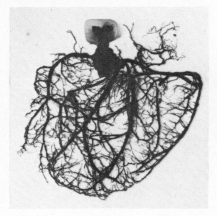 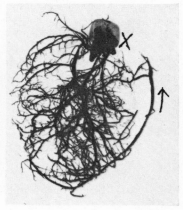

Other veins empty separately into the atrium. There is no doubt of the existence of the *thebesian veins*, connecting the coronary vascular bed directly with the ventricular chambers, but these are considered to play an insignificant part in venous drainage. [►It is much more likely that they play an arterial role, supplying, in the left ventricle, oxygenated blood to the inner layers of muscle, at a time in the cardiac cycle when the coronary arterial supply is occluded by the muscular contraction. In the ventricle of lower forms (fish), the inner layers of the ventricular wall are spongelike, with ventricular blood freely passing through small channels between the muscle fibers. The thebesian veins may be, to a small degree, analogous. Certainly the pressure gradient is positive from ventricular pressure to coronary artery pressure through all of the ventricular systole and the ejection period, so that in this period any flow in the thebesian veins would have to be retrograde.◄]

Changes in Coronary Arterial Flow in the Cardiac Cycle

The investigation of coronary flow and hemodynamics has proved to be one of the most difficult studies undertaken by physiologists (1), although it is of the greatest importance to medicine. The obstacle has been the very marked mechanical effect of ventricular contraction on the caliber of the small coronary vessels that run within the contracting muscles. Contraction must be accompanied by a rise of tissue pressure to some fraction of the ventricular pressure, depending on how deep within the wall the vessels lie (2). This increase in tissue pressure surrounding the small vessels reduces their transmural pressure, even to below zero for the left coronary vessels, and they are temporarily occluded. The resistance to flow of the coronary vascular bed therefore changes greatly throughout the cardiac cycle.

This complication makes the interpretation of the direct effects of hormones, drugs, etc., on the coronary vessels very difficult. Most of the agents of interest alter the heart rate and blood pressure. Both of these factors greatly affect the mechanical effects on the vessels. Changes in coronary flow must, therefore, be interpreted as primary effects on the vessels only after the secondary effect of changes in cardiac dynamics has been assessed, or in cases where heart rate and blood pressure have not been significantly altered.

The availability, in recent years, of small elec-

Fig. 17-2.—Series of curves relating variations in left coronary inflow, coronary sinus and anterior cardiac vein flow to aortic pressure, ventricular pressure and peripheral coronary pressure. The numbers on the curves indicate pressures in mm Hg. (In error, the aortic pressure during the ejection phase is shown as slightly above, instead of slightly below, the ventricular pressure.) (From Gregg [1].)

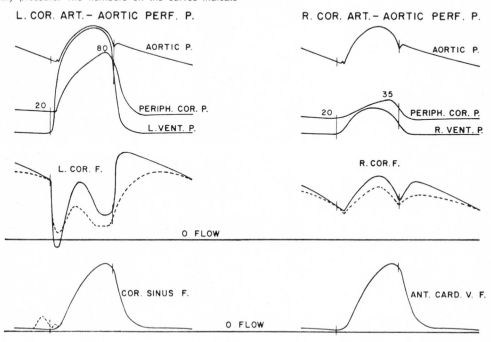

L. COR. ART. – AORTIC PERF. P.

R. COR. ART. – AORTIC PERF. P.

tromagnetic flowmeters that can be implanted in the course of coronary arteries has, in the hands of such devoted research workers as Gregg, begun to give reliable information as to the profile of coronary flow during the cardiac cycle (Fig. 17–2). Flow in the left coronary artery falls precipitously as soon as the ventricular muscle begins to contract (at the start of the isometric contraction period) and even is retrograde for a short time, indicating that the closure of the capillary bed can force blood back up the arteries. During the ejection period, the flow rises to a subsidiary maximum, only to fall in a period when the perfusion pressure (coronary artery pressure) may still be rising. Probably this fall occurs because the ventricular pressure, and therefore the tissue pressure, is also still rising at that time and producing more "squeezing" of the minute vessels. Only after the ventricular pressure has fallen in the isometric relaxation period is the flow curve at all parallel to the curve of perfusion pressure, indicating that in diastole the coronary resistance to flow is relatively constant. As would be expected from the lower right ventricular pressure, these mechanical effects are less marked on the flow in the right coronary artery.

As a consequence, most, although by no means all, of the coronary flow occurs in diastole (estimated as 70–90%). *The level of diastolic pressure may therefore be more important than that of systolic pressure in governing coronary flow.* Slowing of the heart (without changes in cardiac ventricular dynamics) would be expected to increase coronary flow because of the increased duration of diastole; and speeding of the heart, to reduce coronary flow. In the intact heart, these expected changes are complicated by chemical factors altering coronary resistance in accordance with the changes in cardiac dynamics that usually accompany any changes in heart rate.

Chemical Factors; Autoregulation of Coronary Flow

As already mentioned, in spite of large changes in the oxygen consumption of the heart (as between rest and exercise, decrease or increase of heart rate, etc.), the oxygen content of the coronary venous outflow remains remarkably constant, indicating that the coronary blood flow is automatically adjusted to the needs for oxygen. Explanation for this has been sought in terms of the dilator effects of metabolites that accumulated in states of anoxia, as of metabolic carbon diox-

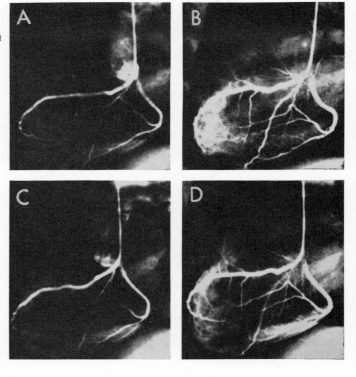

Fig. 17-3.—Effects of oxygen lack and carbon dioxide excess on coronary vessels. Catheter in the left descending branch. **A,** control: blood pressure 175/120; heart rate 80. **B,** within 30 sec after inhalation of low oxygen (5%): BP 187/125; HR 75. **C,** control: BP 172/120; HR 80. **D,** within 30 sec of inhaling 15% carbon dioxide in 21% oxygen: BP 175/122; HR 80. In each case, 5 ml of contrast material was injected. (From West and Guzman [3].)

ide. A decrease in coronary resistance can be demonstrated if the blood perfusing the coronaries is increased in carbon dioxide pressure (P_{CO_2}) (to a very high P_{CO_2}) or if the pH is decreased (3) (Fig. 17–3), but this effect is not sufficient to explain the automatic increase in flow when the energy consumption of the heart increases. Short periods of ischemia, or perfusion with blood low in oxygen pressure (P_{O_2}), do, however, produce marked increases in coronary flow, even if the oxygen consumption remains constant (1). It is therefore postulated that the coronary vessels respond, by vasodilation, to very small degrees of local hypoxia and that this is the mechanism of autoregulation of coronary flow. [▶In *chronic anemia*, if not too severe, there is a sustained increase in coronary flow, partly, of course, because of the decreased viscosity of the blood. If the anemia is severe (less than 8 Gm of hemoglobin per 100 ml of blood), cardiac oxygen consumption increases and a further, maximum, coronary dilatation results. Although the P_{O_2} of the arterial blood is normal in anemia, the oxygen-carrying capacity is reduced, and the venous coronary outflow may have a saturation as low as 2 vol% (normal about 5 vol%); so anoxia of the cardiac tissues may be responsible for the vasodilation even though arterial P_{O_2} is normal.◀]

Nervous Influences

Both parasympathetic (vagal) and sympathetic innervation of the heart is rich, but this does not necessarily mean that these nerves control the caliber of the coronary vessels in addition to their well-known function of controlling heart rate (via the pacemaker) and the strength of heartbeat (by effects on ventricular muscle).

[▶*Vagal stimulation* results in an increase in coronary flow, but probably indirectly by the slowing of heart rate; there is no conclusive evidence of a direct vagal vasodilation of coronary vessels. However, adding acetylcholine, the neurohumor released by stimulation of the vagus (it was originally called *Vagus-Stoff*), produces an increased coronary flow, even in cases where changes in heart rate and blood pressure are minimum (3).◀]

Stimulation of the cardiac sympathetic nerves (stellate ganglion) produces much more marked effects, with direct dilatation of the coronary vessels (their resistance to flow decreases even though the heart rate increases). Oxygen consumption of the cardiac muscle also increases,

and this could also contribute to the vasodilator effect. [▶There is little or no direct evidence of sympathetic constrictor activity in coronary vessels (1). On the other hand, there is abundant evidence of reflex spasm of coronary vessels, experimentally and clinically (e.g., *angina pectoris*).◀]

Coronary Spasm and "Intercoronary Reflexes"

Many patients die suddenly of coronary infarction, yet the infarcted area, at postmortem, seems less important than that in other patients who survive. This has led to the theory that occlusion of a single coronary arterial branch by a thrombus or an embolus might lead to widespread spasm of other coronary arteries. [▶Leroy and Snider (4) put the concept very positively: "The sudden death of a patient with infarction of the myocardium is due to reflex coronary vasoconstriction whose stimulus is the infarct, whose afferent pathway is the cardio-sensory innervation and whose efferent pathway is the vagus. The result of this reflex vasoconstriction in a susceptible person is fatal ventricular fibrillation."◀]

Agress and his colleagues (8) produced emboli in the coronary vessels by injection of glass spheres of different sizes, which resulted, in many cases, in profound cardiac shock and death. Spheres of intermediate size (325 μ) were fatal more often than were smaller (190 μ) or larger (450 μ) spheres, as if there were specific areas in the arterial system which could "trigger" reflex spasm in other vessels. Spasm in coronary arteries, not embolized, have been demonstrated by angiography when another branch was blocked. [▶On the other hand, the existence of these "intercoronary reflexes" has been challenged (6). The work of Manning and his co-workers (5) certainly favors the theory of reflex vasoconstriction, for when a coronary artery or branch was suddenly ligated in dogs, ventricular fibrillation and death often followed; but the incidence of this was significantly lowered by prior sensory denervation of the heart, by deep anesthesia and by blocking agents, particularly by atropine (which blocks cholinergic effects). The evidence is strong that the cardiosensory fibers can make the effects of coronary infarction more drastic by eliciting reflex spasm. Yet infusion of both adrenaline and acetylcholine, the neurohumors one would associate with efferent nervous activity to the heart, results in coronary vasodilation. The matter requires further elucidation.◄] Meanwhile, giving atropine or other blocking agents to patients as soon as possible after an acute coronary attack has some physiological justification.

Effect of Hormones

The circulating hormone *adrenaline*, present in the blood in excitement and in heavy exercise, produces a coronary vasodilation directly. With higher concentrations, the dilation is further increased because of the added effects of increased aortic pressure (the perfusion pressure) and myocardial oxygen consumption. *Thyroxin*, as in hyperthyroidism, produces an increase in coronary flow consistent with the increased metabolic rate of the cardiac muscle, comparable to the increased rate in other tissues. *Pitressin* decreases coronary flow, probably by a direct vasoconstrictor effect. Among the drugs, *nitroglycerin* and *nitrites* (e.g., amyl nitrite) are most useful coronary dilators.

Metabolism of Cardiac Muscle

Mommaerts (7) points out that the biochemical and biophysical organization by which cardiac muscle transforms chemical to mechanical energy must be such that it proceeds at a high rate without interruption. In contrast, skeletal muscle functions in short bursts of intense activity, beyond the capacity of the oxidative enzymes present, but utilizing anaerobic metabolism (glycolysis) and accumulating an "oxygen debt," which is repaid in subsequent periods of relative inactivity. In cardiac muscle, and in striated muscles that have to maintain sustained activity (e.g., the pectoral muscles of long-flying birds), there is a much more developed oxidative phosphorelative system, characterized by the presence of more *mitochondria*, known to carry the relevant enzymes.

Cardiac muscle has some oxidative reserve, in that it is provided with *myoglobin*. The affinity of myoglobin for oxygen is such that it remains undissociated at normal values of oxygen tension, but can release O_2 in conditions of anoxia. In spite of this, the heart tissues cannot survive periods of complete ischemia for more than a few minutes. Bing (6) calculates that the maximal oxygen debt that a ventricle can tolerate is equivalent to the supply of oxygen in only 65 ml of arterial blood. Again, since the extraction of oxygen from the blood by the heart is so nearly complete (about

75%), the supply cannot be greatly increased by further reducing the venous content.

Qualitative Aspects of Cardiac Metabolism

Only about one third of the oxygen consumption of the heart is derived normally from the oxidation of carbohydrate (cf. 0–15% for skeletal muscle in physiological conditions and close to 100% for the brain). The carbohydrate metabolism is unusual in that *lactate* and *glucose* are utilized about equally, even though the concentration of lactate in the blood is usually lower than that of glucose. This ability of the heart muscle to utilize lactate is obviously most advantageous, for in conditions of heavy exercise, where cardiac activity must be greatly increased, an increased supply of lactate in the blood results from its diffusion from the working skeletal muscles, where lactic acid is an end-product of anaerobic metabolism.

Table 17–1, from the work of Bing, using arterial-venous differences in the blood, indicates the preferential use of fatty acids by the human heart. There is also older evidence that, in isolated mammalian hearts deprived of all nutritive supply and allowed to beat until they stop, the content of carbohydrate (glycogen) is not significantly reduced, compared with the store of lipids. The utilization of glucose depends on the blood concentration and reaches a maximum of about 100 mg%. When the blood glucose is low, the heart utilizes lipid metabolism almost exclusively. [►This is one more reason why the current deprecation, by some experts on atherosclerosis, of lipid in the diet seems rather illogical and uninformed.◄]

TABLE 17–1.—RELATIVE CONTRIBUTION OF CARBO-
HYDRATES AND NONCARBOHYDRATES TO TOTAL
MYOCARDIAL OXYGEN USAGE*

CARBOHYDRATE		NONCARBOHYDRATE	
Glucose	17.90%	Fatty acids	67.0%
Pyruvate	0.54%	Amino acids	5.6%
Lactate	16.46%	Ketones	4.3%
Total	34.90%†	Total	76.9%†

*From Bing (6).

†The total is more than 100% because some of the substrates removed from the blood, in amount measured by the arterial-venous differences, were stored by the heart or not completely metabolized.

Disturbances of Cardiac Metabolism

Very little research has been done on myocardial metabolism in heart disease. Whether cardiac dysfunction is due to a depletion of the enzymes, like cocarboxylase, which is concerned with the supply of energy-rich compounds (e.g., adenosine triphosphate [ATP]), or to disturbances in the utilization of these compounds in producing mechanical energy in the last step of muscular contraction (e.g., with actomyosin) is not known, although the latter is the prevailing view.

Attempts to Improve Coronary Circulation

Many attempts, in animal research and in a few patients, have been made to increase the coronary circulation, in the case of myocardial insufficiency, by surgical intervention. One method is to stimulate the heart to develop new collateral vessels by pericardial irritation (e.g., by talcum powder). Another is to graft arteries from some other system (e.g., the mammary) on to the surface of the heart; still another is the removal of the epicardium. These measures have had varying success.

It is important to realize that the total coronary blood flow might be increased by such methods without a significant increase in the "nutritive flow" carrying oxygen to the cardiac muscle fibers. This would be so if the collateral circulation lacked the capillaries intimately associated with the muscle fibers which characterize the normal coronary system, that is, if the new vessels acted as *nonnutritive shunts*. For this reason, the result should be assessed by *clearance* rather than on the basis of total blood flow. A radioactive tracer such as I^{131} is injected into the heart muscle. The rate at which the local concentration falls, as it is washed away by the blood stream, is a measure of true nutritive flow.

Meanwhile, the techniques of microsurgery are advancing so rapidly that surgical repair of coronary arterial occlusion (e.g., by end-to-end anastomosis of small arteries) may soon be considered as an emergency measure in acute coronary crisis.

REFERENCES

1. Gregg, D. E.: Coronary Circulation, in Luisada, A. A. (ed.): *Cardiovascular Functions* (New York: McGraw-Hill Book Company, Inc., 1962), Chap. 23, pp. 198–212.

2. Burton, A. C.: Appendix to Physical Principles of Circulatory Phenomena: The Physical Equilibrium of the Heart and Blood Vessels, in *Handbook of Physiology*, Vol. I, *Circulation* (1962), Chap. 6, pp. 85–105.

3. West, J. W., and Guzman, S. V.: Coronary dilation and constriction visualized by selective arteriography, Circulation Res. 7:527, 1959.

4. Leroy, C. V., and Snider, S. S.: The sudden death of patients with few symptoms of heart disease, J.A.M.A. 117:2019, 1941.

5. Skelton, R. B.; Gergely, N.; Manning, G. W., and Coles, J. C.: Mortality studies in experimental coronary occlusion, J. Thoracic & Cardiovas. Surg. 44:90, 1962.
   This is the most recent of a series of papers citing earlier references.

6. Bing, R. J.: Myocardial metabolism, Circulation 12:635, 1955.

7. Mommaerts, F. H. M.: Metabolism of the Heart, in Luisada, A. A. (ed.): *Cardiovascular Functions* (New York: McGraw-Hill Book Company, Inc., 1962), p. 2.

8. Agress, C. M.; Rosenberg, J.; Jacobs, H. I.; Bonder, M. J.; Schneiderman, A., and Clark, W. G.: Protracted shock in the closed-chest dog following coronary embolization with graded microspheres, Am. J. Physiol. 170:536, 1952.

18

The Pulse and Its Interpretation

Introduction

FROM THE BIRTH OF MEDICINE, there has been great interest in the pulse and its "shape," or "contour," as well as in its rate. It is said that a Chinese treatise on the pulse was written more than 4,000 years ago. The pulse remains, particularly in Eastern medicine, a valuable aid to cardiovascular diagnosis. The first application that Galileo made of his discovery of the isochronism of the pendulum (from watching the great braziers swing in the cathedral instead of listening to the sermon) was to make a device for counting the pulse rate (called the *pulsilogium*). A pendulum was shortened by winding the string on a reel until it was approximately synchronous with the pulse felt at the wrist. A dial on the winding apparatus then indicated the average pulse rate.

The Aortic and Central Arterial Pulse

If the events of the cardiac cycle are understood, the shape of the aortic pulse contour can be interpreted (Fig. 18–1). At the moment when the aortic valve opens and cardiac ejection begins, the aortic pressure rises rapidly. The steeply rising part of the pulse curve is called the *anacrotic limb* (Greek, "upbeat"). Until the maximal pressure is reached, there has been very little outflow of the stroke volume through the peripheral resistance, and most of this volume (some 80 ml in resting conditions) is "stored" by an increase in capacity of the whole distensible central arterial system (not just of the root of the aorta). The descending limb of the curve is called the *dicrotic limb* (Greek, "double beat"). The pressure decreases mainly because the cardiac muscle is relaxing rapidly but also, of course, because the blood is running out of the arterial system through the

peripheral resistance. The decrease of pressure is interrupted by the *dicrotic notch* (or *incisura* [Latin, "cutting into"]) and an upswing called the *dicrotic wave*. This interruption is the result of the abrupt closure of the aortic valve, when the ventricular pressure falls below that in the aorta. The elastic recoil of the aorta and of the valve itself creates the rise of pressure. Beyond the dicrotic wave, the pressure descends at a decreasing rate, as the runoff into the peripheral circulation continues under the pressure created by the

Fig. 18-1.—**Top,** the normal profile of the pulse at the root of the aorta and at the femoral artery, which is usually spikier, with both systolic and diastolic pressures higher, although the mean pressure is the same or lower. **Bottom,** the corresponding flow pulses.

Symbols on the curves are: *a,* Anacrotic limb; *b,* dicrotic limb; *c,* dicrotic notch, or incisura; *d,* dicrotic wave with vibrations that correspond to the second heart sound; *e,* reflected waves; *f,* reverse, or regurgitant, flow in the aorta, which is not seen in the femoral flow because of the *Windkessel* effect; *M,* true mean pressures.

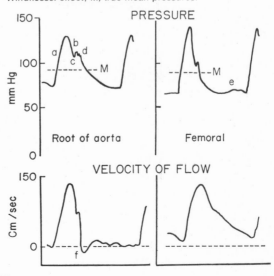

stored elastic energy of the central arteries. If there was no subsequent heartbeat, the pressure would continue to fall to very low values, until

closure of arterioles under vasomotor tone might stop the further outflow or a uniform pressure throughout the system had been reached. (If the heartbeat is arrested, this final pressure, in animals, seems to be about 25 mm Hg. It is obviously dependent on the vasomotor tone, on the total blood volume and on the elasticity of the whole vascular system.) The diastolic level of pressure reached is dependent on (a) the rate of outflow from the arteries (i.e., on the mean pressure divided by the total peripheral resistance) and (b) the time before the next heartbeat (i.e., the cardiac period).

This temporary storage of much of the stroke volume during the ejection period (called the *Windkessel* effect by the German hemodynamicists, such as O. Frank) serves to smooth out the flow of blood in the circulation, so that flow

continues during diastole. Without it, the blood would reach the tissues in spurts with each heartbeat. The pulsatile character is present down to the very small vessels, but capillary and venous flow are almost continuous. Modern measurements of the velocity of flow in the root of the aorta indeed show that flow here occurs only during systole and that the velocity falls to zero, or may even be backward, briefly during diastole (Fig. 18–1). Farther downstream, the flow persists later into diastole, since more "storage" by arterial elasticity has occurred before the point of measurement. The *Windkessel* role is not to be thought of, then, as played by the root of the aorta alone; rather, it is a function of distensibility of the whole of the arterial tree.

What Determines the Pulse Pressure?

If we ignore (or make some correction for) the escape of blood from the arterial tree during the period in which the aortic pressure is rising (i.e., the anacrotic limb), we can see that the amount of rise of pressure in the arterial system that will occur depends on (a) the *stroke volume* which the

arteries have to "store" by increasing the arterial volume and (b) the arterial *distensibility*. Absolute *volume distensibility* is defined as:

$$\text{Absolute volume distensibility } (D) = \frac{\text{Increase in volume } (\Delta V)}{\text{Increase in pressure } (\Delta P)}$$

Some investigators prefer to work with the *per cent volume distensibility,* defined by:

$$D\% = \frac{100 \, \Delta V/V}{\Delta P}$$

For the argument that follows, let us use the absolute distensibility defined. Then,

$$\Delta P = \frac{\Delta V}{D}$$

Now ΔP is the difference between systolic and diastolic pressures, that is, the *pulse pressure*. (If the blood pressure is 120/80, the pulse pressure is $120 - 80 = 40$ mm Hg.) And ΔV (if we ignore "runoff" in this period) is the stroke volume. We then arrive at the simple approximate relation:

$$\text{Pulse pressure} = \frac{\text{Stroke volume}}{\text{Arterial distensibility}}$$

or

$$\text{Stroke volume} = (\text{Pulse pressure} \times \text{Arterial distensibility})$$

Long before other, more modern, methods of measuring cardiac output were easily available, Erlanger and Hooker [1] suggested that this relation provided an estimate of stroke volume in man. Bazett and his colleagues [2] and Hamilton and Remington [3] developed this into a method for cardiac output called the "pulse contour method." They made a correction for the runoff during systole and used standard values for the arterial distensibility, based on some measurements of this in different parts of the arterial tree of dogs and on measurement of pulse-wave velocity in man (see later, p. 163). In man, he assumed value for arterial distensibility could be corrected for age. The method gives results that, at least in dogs, agree with results of other methods for cardiac output much better than would be expected. However, the method is of little use clinically, for the arterial distensibility of the patient in question may be very different from the standard value for his age.

As long as we deal with one individual man or dog, the relation between pulse pressure and stroke volume gives a most useful index of changes in cardiac output. For:

Cardiac output = (Stroke volume × Heart rate) = D (Pulse pressure × Heart rate)

where D can be regarded as approximately constant for the given individual. Thus, at rest, with a blood pressure of 120/80 and a heart rate of 70 beats per min, the product

(Pulse pressure × Heart rate) = 40 × 70 = *2,800*

In heavy exercise, say, the blood pressure is 180/90 and the heart rate is 100 beats per min, then,

(Pulse pressure × Heart rate) = 90 × 100 = *9,000*

The product has increased threefold, which would be about the increase of cardiac output. The rule would be very useful, for example, in following the recovery of a patient with chronic anemia (where the cardiac output is increased) from day to day under therapy. Hamilton gives the rule that *each millimeter of mercury of the pulse pressure corresponds to about 1 ml of stroke index* (i.e., stroke volume divided by body surface area).

The simple relation between pulse pressure and distensibility, for the same stroke volume, would predict that in *arteriosclerosis,* where the distensibility is reduced, the pulse pressure would be correspondingly increased. This is so, and a high, but short-lived, spike of systolic pressure with a normal diastolic pressure is the sign of arteriosclerosis.

Abnormal Pulse Contours in Disease

Figure 18–2 shows several characteristic abnormalities in disease. The rate of rise of pressure of

Fig. 18-2.—Some abnormal shapes of central arterial pulse in disease. **A**, normal. **B**, aortic stenosis. **C**, arteriosclerosis. The shape is much the same in essential hypertension, but there the systolic pressure is higher and the diastolic pressure much higher **D**, aortic insufficiency.

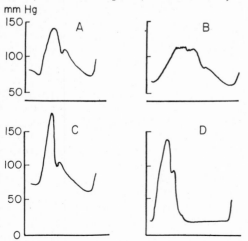

the anacrotic limb is an indication of how freely the blood is ejected into the root of the aorta. In *aortic stenosis* (Fig. 18–2, *B*), the high resistance at the aortic valve slows the rate of rise of pressure in the arteries beyond.

The steepness of fall of the pressure from the peak to the dicrotic notch is, on the other hand, an index of arterial distensibility, for example, in the contour of *arteriosclerosis* (Fig. 18–2, *C*). This contour of the pulse, felt at the wrist, is usually described in books on medicine as the *water-hammer pulse* or *Corrigan's pulse.* The former term is no longer helpful because students have never heard of water hammers, which evidently occurred in early British or Irish plumbing (and probably still do). The *collapsing pulse* of *aortic insufficiency* is also sometimes described as a water-hammer pulse.

The decline of pressure in diastole is, of course, an index of total peripheral resistance in the normal condition and of the amount of *aortic regurgitation* where the aortic valve is incompetent (insufficiency). With aortic regurgitation, the diastolic pressure is greatly reduced, approaching zero in some cases (Fig. 18–2, *D*).

In *essential hypertension* (blood pressure may be as high as 240/160), the pulse contour looks like that of the arteriosclerotic patient. Because the arteries are distended by a higher pressure, their distensibility is reduced, for it is a characteristic of arteries that they become less distensible the more they are stretched (Chapter 7).

Changes in the Pulse as It Travels

The distention of the root of the aorta stretches the wall there, and this pulls on the adjacent arterial wall, so that a *pulse wave* travels down the arteries, much as the wave of a plucked violin string travels down the string. The velocity with which the wave travels must not be confused with the velocity of the blood flow in the artery, with which it has nothing to do (the pulse-wave velocity is many times faster than the maximal blood velocity).

PULSE-WAVE VELOCITY

As the arterial pulsation is recorded from different points down the length of the arterial system (e.g., from the carotid, subclavian, brachial and radial arteries), there is an increasing lag before the beginning of the upstroke (the electro-

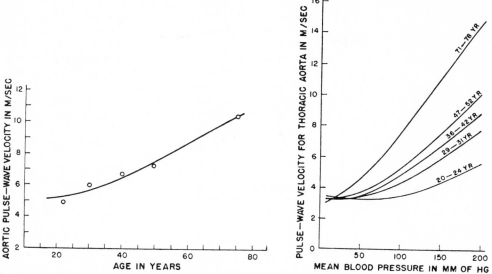

Fig. 18-3.—**Left,** pulse-wave velocity versus age. **Right,** pulse-wave velocity versus blood pressure. (From King [5].)

cardiogram is used to give a reference time). Dividing this time interval by an estimated length of artery between the two points of recording gives the pulse-wave velocity.

physics for the velocity of propagation of transverse elastic waves. It was applied first by Moens (1878) and was modified by Bramwell and his associates (6, 7). In practical units it is:

$$\text{Pulse-wave velocity } (V \text{ in m/sec}) = \frac{3.57}{[\text{Distensibility } (D)]^{1/2}} \text{ or Distensibility} = \frac{12.7}{V^2}$$

Measurements of pulse-wave velocity in man, starting with the classic work of Hallock (4) (on 500 persons, aged 5–85), have shown that the velocity increases with age, from an average of 4 meters (m) per sec in the young person to 10 m per sec in the old person. (The values are for the aorta from heart to subclavian artery.) The velocity in the smaller distributing arteries is considerably faster (King [5]), so that, when the pulse at a distant artery is compared with the central pulse, the velocity calculated is really a mixture of a number of very different velocities of many different segments. There are probably large changes in velocity at every branching of the aorta. The level of blood pressure—that is, the degree of distention for the arteries—also affects the velocity (Fig. 18–3).

The determination of pulse-wave velocity would remain rather academic except that it is one of the few ways that the arterial distensibility, as an index of the aging of arteries, can be measured conveniently in man. The connection between the pulse-wave velocity and the volume distensibility of the arteries is based on a classic calculation in

where "distensibility" is defined as the percentage of change in volume per 1 mm Hg rise of pressure. A pulse wave velocity of 5 m per sec, by the formula, gives a distensibility of about 0.5% per 1 mm Hg rise of pressure, while a pulse-wave velocity of 10 m per sec (old age) corresponds to a distensibility of 0.13% per 1 mm Hg rise.

CHANGES IN CONTOUR OF PULSE AS IT TRAVELS

In addition to the increased lag in arrival, there is a change in the pulse as it travels.

1. In the large and long arteries, surprisingly enough, the pulse pressure tends to increase and the systolic wave to become more "spiky." Indeed, the femoral pulse pressure is usually considerably greater than the aortic 18–1. One would think that "damping" would produce the opposite effect. [►The explanation lies in the dependence of the pulse-wave velocity on the distensibility, and the distensibility on both the "frequency" (i.e., the rate of rise of distending pressure) and on the degree of distention (i.e., on the level of blood

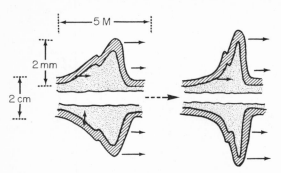

Fig. 18-4.—Illustrating how the "dispersion" of pulse-wave velocity (i.e., the peak of the pulse wave traveling faster than the lower parts of the wave) leads to an increased pulse pressure. The displacement of the arterial wall is not nearly so great as it appears in this diagram, unless one were to use a very distorting lens (note the great disparity between the vertical and horizontal scales) and the arterial system were to be extended for several meters.

pressure). The distensibility decreases, and therefore the pulse wave increases, with rate of rise of pressure (dynamic elasticity versus static elasticity) and with increased pressure. The latter is due to the fact that the more an artery wall is stretched, the stiffer it becomes. As a result of these two factors, the peak of the pulse wave travels faster than the lower parts of the wave (Fig. 18–4).◄] (The pulse-wave disturbance that is traveling appears "backward" from the way we usually draw it [i.e., the pressure versus the time at a given point].) If the top of the wave travels faster, the wave front becomes steeper and the maximum reached is higher. A similar explanation is given for the "breaking" of a wave on the sea as it approaches the shore. The low-amplitude parts of the wave are slowed down more by the shallow

water than by the high-amplitude crest of the wave. [►Former explanations were based on reflected waves, or *"standing waves" in the arteries,* but it is now realized that true standing waves cannot exist in the system, for two reasons. First, the wavelength of the pulse wave is very much greater than the length of the arterial system; that is, in the 1 sec between heartbeats the wave would have traveled more than 5 m. Second, to maintain a system of standing waves requires a periodic generation of waves with a very regular rhythm, whereas the cardiac period fluctuates from moment to moment. Reflections of the pulse wave, when the resistance to flow and total cross-sectional area of the bed change abruptly at the termination of the arterial tree, can, however, produce additional variable waves in the pulse curve near the end of diastole.◄]

2. The expected damping of the pulse wave as it travels does occur in the smaller arteries, and it is seen best by comparing the pulse recorded from arteries down to very small size. This now has been done in vessels of only 200 μ (8). The damping is due to the distributed distensibility of the tree plus the viscous resistance to flow, particularly of the arterioles beyond the arterial tree. In hypotensive shock, the damping is very markedly increased, presumably because the arterial walls are less distended (Fig. 18–5).

Capillary Pulsation

In spite of the great damping of the pulse wave in the arterioles, pulsation in the capillary bed can be observed normally (as in the capillaries), although it is usually slight. It is seen in aortic

Fig. 18-5.—**A,** records of the pulse from arteries of diminishing size in the dog, showing the damping of the pulse pressure and smoothing of the contours. **B,** the very greatly increased damping when the blood pressure is lowered. (From Saigiura and Fries [8].)

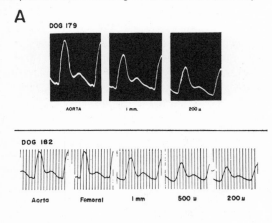

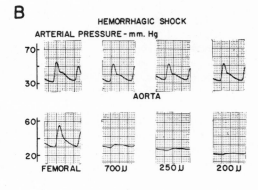

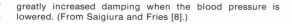

insufficiency by the rhythmic reddening of the nail bed. It increases greatly in conditions where there is maximal arteriolar dilatation, as produced by heating the body or the tissue concerned. The pulsation of the volume of a finger, easily recorded by a plethysmograph (Chapter 24), is also evidence that some pulsation of pressure survives to the capillaries and venules, for the contributions of arterial pulsation to this *finger-volume pulse* would be much too small to explain its magnitude, and, also, the size of the finger-volume pulse is greatly affected by level of venous pressure (i.e., by the degree of filling of the venous vessels).

The Venous Pulse

The pressure in the great veins (e.g., vena cava, jugular vein) is markedly pulsatile (Fig. 18–6). The fluctuation in pressure reflects the events in the right atrium and right ventricle, plus some artifactual waves transmitted to veins by the systolic pulsation of adjacent arteries. The waves from different veins are not very similar. Three main waves (*A, C* and *V;* see Fig. 18–6) are distinguished, with additional small waves such as the *A-V* wave. The *A* wave is indisputably associated with atrial contraction, and this is consistent with its occurrence a little later than the *P* wave of the electrocardiogram. The *C* wave, prominent in the jugular venous pressure, is probably almost entirely transmitted to the vein from proximity to the carotid artery, and partly from aorta to vena cava at the level of the heart. The *V* wave occurs in early diastole and reflects the opening of the tricuspid valve and the rise of pressure at the beginning of right ventricular filling. It is exaggerated in cases of right heart congestion. The *A-V* wave, which can often be distinguished between the *A* and *C* waves, is due

to the closure of the atrioventricular valve and the beginning of isometric ventricular contraction. It therefore could be regarded as being the first part of the first heart sound, transmitted along the walls of the atrium and veins (the same vibration travels also over the ventricle to emerge on the chest at the mitral auscultatory area). A similar notch between the *C* and *V* wave represents the closure of the aortic valve (i.e., as the component of the second sound). The inconstancy of the form and of the exact timing of the waves in the venous pulse, when recorded from the neck veins, is to be expected in view of the fact that the pulse-wave velocity in veins depends so much on their degree of distention (venous distensibility decreases abruptly as the veins are filled), and this is changed with posture and in the respiratory cycle.

Measurement of Pulse Rate

It is a fact that a very high percentage of all physicians measure the pulse rate of their patients incorrectly. The author discovered this in a research project where he measured heart rate from records of the blood pressure for the same times at which a clinical colleague measured it by palpation at the wrist. The clinician's values were consistently 4 beats per min higher than those from the records.

When asked to explain exactly how he counted the pulse, the clinician explained that he placed his fingers over the radial artery, looked at his watch and counted "one, two, three, etc.," until 15 seconds had elapsed, and then multiplied by 4. This explained the discrepancy. How? (Make every effort to think out the answer for yourself before consulting the inverted footnote immediately below.*)

REFERENCES

1. Erlanger, J., and Hooker, D. R.: An experimental study of blood-pressure and of pulse-pressure in man, Johns Hopkins Hosp. Reports 12:145, 1904.
2. Bazett, H. C.; Cotton, F. C.; Laplace, L. B., and Scott, J. C.: The calculation of cardiac output and effective peripheral resistance from blood-pressure measurements, with an appendix on the size of the aorta in man, Am. J. Physiol. 113:312, 1935.

Fig. 18-6.—**Top,** the venous pulse as recorded from the jugular vein. See text for explanation. **Middle,** the heart sounds. **Bottom,** the electrocardiogram.

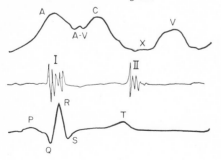

*When timing any periodic event (e.g., the swing of a pendulum or the pulse), one should count "zero." For the first occurrence, "one," for the next, not "one," "two," etc., for the first "cycle" has not occurred until the second "signal" is noted. The point may be academic; but if we measure something in physiology or medicine, why not do so correctly?

3. Hamilton W. F., and Remington, J. W.: The measurement of the stroke volume from the pulse-pressure, Am. J. Physiol. 148:14, 1947.

4. Hallock, P.: Arterial elasticity in man in relation to age as evaluated by pulse-wave velocity method, Arch. Int. Med. 54:770, 1934.

5. King, A. L.: Circulatory System: Arterial Pulse; Wave Velocity, in Glasser, O. (ed.): *Medical Physics,* Vol. II (Chicago: The Year Book Publishers, Inc., 1950), pp. 188–191.

6. Bramwell, J. C.; Hill, A. V., and McSwiney, B. A.: The velocity of the pulse wave in man in relation to age as measured by the hot-wire sphygmograph, Heart 10:233, 1923.

7. Bramwell, J. C., and Hill, A. V.: The velocity of the pulse-wave in man, Proc. Roy. Soc., London, Ser. B, 93:298, 1922.

8. Saigiura, T., and Fries, E. D.: Pulse pressure in small arteries, Circulation Res. 11:838, 1962.

19

The Measurement of Cardiac Output and of Cardiac Mechanics

The Fick Principle: A Fable

IN A TELEVISION BROADCAST of one of the 1963 World Series games, there was an embarrassing moment for the producer. For reasons not explained, it is considered of the greatest importance that the exact paid attendance should be announced before the game is over. To the consternation of the officials, it was found that the counting mechanism at one of the turnstiles at one of the entrance gates had failed to function. What was to be done? In desperation, a call was made over the public address system: "Is there a circulation physiologist in the house?" There was.

The physiologist explained that it was very simple, by the Fick principle. He had noticed that, as he left the gate, he had $5.00 less in his pockets than when he entered, and he assumed that this was true for everyone passing through that gate.

representative sample of the blood flowing into, and of the blood flowing out of, the system. (Or to measure the concentration of an indicator, such as oxygen, without obtaining the sample, as by the ear oximeter.)

2. The blood must carry an *indicator*, or "marker," X, the *concentration* of which in these samples can be measured. The indicator may be something normally carried by the blood (e.g., oxygen, carbon dioxide) or something not normally present but added to the blood (e.g., foreign gases such as carbon monoxide, acetylene, indicator dyes, radioactive serum albumin, or altered temperature).

3. The *total exchange of the indicator,* either added to the blood or removed from the blood in its passage through the system, must be measurable (e.g., the total oxygen consumption, carbon dioxide evolved, etc.).

The Fick principle (1870) is, then:

$$\text{Blood flow (in L/min)} = \frac{\text{Total exchange (in units of indicator } X\text{/min)}}{\text{Conc. of } X \text{ entering (in units of } X\text{/L)} \sim \text{Conc. of } X \text{ leaving}}$$

Why not count the money collected at that gate, divide by $5.00 (the arterial-venous difference), and get the number of persons entering?*

The principle is identical with what the physiologist uses to measure the blood flow through any region of the body (e.g., a limb, or an organ such as the heart or lungs). The requirements for applying the Fick principle are:

1. The investigator must be able to obtain a

---

*It is possible that the choice of this particular analogy had something to do with the fact that I decided to stay at home to write this chapter on the day the first World Series game of 1963 was played.

The symbol $\sim$ means "the difference between" and is used because, in different cases, the denominator, which is the arterial-venous difference, may be positive or negative.

Errors of Sampling

The major difficulty, through the years, in attempts to apply the Fick principle to the measurement of cardiac output has been with requirement 1, above, regarding the *representative venous sample.* While samples of blood from any artery are closely the same, samples from different veins may differ in concentration of indicator (e.g., of oxygen) very greatly indeed. For instance, the flow, which is equal to the cardiac output. The equation becomes:

$$\text{Cardiac output (ml/min)} = \frac{\text{O}_2 \text{ consumption (ml/O}_2 \text{ min)}}{\text{Syst. art. O}_2 \text{ conc. (ml/O}_2 \text{ ml blood)} - \text{Pulm. art. O}_2 \text{ conc. (ml/O}_2 \text{ ml blood)}}$$

oxygen concentration in a peripheral vein will depend on the metabolism of the tissue which it serves and will be far from that of the *mixed venous sample* required. Before the availability of cardiac catheterization, there were many ingenious attempts to obtain the value for the mixed venous sample indirectly. For example, in the "acetylene method," the subject rapidly inhaled (and mixed in his lungs) a mixture of gas containing acetylene, then held his breath and finally exhaled the gas in his lungs for analysis. The concentration of the blood leaving the lungs at the end of the period of breath holding was assumed to be in equilibrium with the measured concentration in the gas. Since there was none of the gas in the blood entering, before there had been a *recirculation*, this gave the arterial-venous difference, and the gas analysis gave the total gas absorbed. There were many variations of this sort of method. All of them were limited by the fact that recirculation, by the short routes in the peripheral circulation, can begin as early as 10 sec after the absorption of the indicator. This short time of recirculation still is a limitation in many indicator-dilution methods (see below).

It is now easy to introduce a catheter into a peripheral vein and to advance its tip into the heart. It is not sufficient to take a sample from the vena cava, atrium or even the right ventricle to obtain a truly mixed venous sample, for, until the pulmonary artery is reached, there are still separate streams (laminae) of blood with concentration of indicator different from that of adjacent laminae. To withdraw a sample of blood from the pulmonary artery, the curved tip of the catheter is therefore manipulated until it has passed through the pulmonary valve. For the systemic arterial sample, the femoral or brachial artery is used. Where the indicator is oxygen, consumption is measured by the many methods available (e.g., a "metabolism machine").

As a particular example, in the *direct-oxygen-Fick method*, the organ, or system, is the lungs, and we are measuring the pulmonary blood

In this application, there is no difficulty about the recirculation of the indicator, for in the *steady state* it is removed in the systemic circuit by the metabolism of the tissues. *In the nonsteady state, as in a transition between rest and exercise, the calculation is not really valid.*

There are numerous possibilities of varying the application of the Fick principle, and new methods will undoubtedly be published before this book is in print. Radioactive indicators (like radioactive krypton dissolved in saline solution) make the measurement of concentrations easy even for very small concentrations of indicator. The many methods have been reviewed by Hamilton (1), and description or enumeration is not appropriate here. If the medical student thoroughly understands the application of the Fick principle in the example given here of the direct-oxygen-Fick method, he is in a position to evaluate these newer methods as they appear.

The Slow- or Continuous-Injection Indicator-Dilution Method

The so-called indicator-dilution methods are usually discussed as being different from those based on the Fick principle, but in reality the steady-injection method uses the same principle, whereas the rapid-injection indicator-dilution method (see p. 169) differs. The indicator-dilution methods were first used by G. N. Stewart in 1896.

An indicator (e.g., a dye in solution) is injected (or infused) at a steady rate into a vein, or from a catheter tip in the desired *site of injection*, and simultaneously the concentration of samples withdrawn from an artery or from another *sampling site* is measured from serial samples or recorded continuously. The mean concentration of indicator at the sampling site is calculated. This is a Fick method, with the constant infusion of indicator substituted for the constant uptake of oxygen by the lungs in the oxygen-Fick method, and the vascular bed between the point of injection and the point of sampling taking the place of the lungs. Then, obviously:

$$\text{Blood flow (ml/min)} = \frac{\text{Units of indicator injected per min}}{\text{Conc. of indicator in sample (in units/ml)}}$$

If the indicator is not removed in the peripheral circuit, recirculation will again be a complication. The sites of injection and sampling can be chosen to give the flow in a limb, through the heart and so on. The same precautions as to adequate mixing and representative samples must be taken as in the other Fick methods. When applied to measurements of limb circulation, the difficulty is to obtain a mixed venous sample, for Zierler has shown that the concentration of indicator may be very different in different veins draining the limb unless "jet injection," creating turbulence, is used (and this can cause hemolysis). If mixing is adequate at the arterial injection site, the concentration in all the veins is the same.

Basic Errors in Applying the Fick Method to Pulsatile Flow

The logic of the Fick principle seems so simple and direct that there has been a tendency to think that the resulting values for flow must be correct as long as the sampling errors are not important. *This is true only for steady flow*, and there can be a very serious error when the flow is pulsatile, as it is in the arterial circulation. This has been pointed out by Visscher and Johnson (2). The concentration at the sampling site fluctuates with the fluctuation of flow. It is still true that the concentration (C_t) in any period of time is related to the rate of flow (F_t) at that time by the equation:

$$F_t = \frac{\text{Rate of injection of indicator}}{C_t}$$

The total volume that has flowed over a longer time, say a cardiac cycle, is given by:

$$V = \int_0^T F_t \cdot dt = (\text{Rate of injection of indicator}) \times \int_0^T \frac{1}{C_t} \cdot dt$$

The mistake is that, instead of averaging the reciprocal of the concentration in the sample, the average of the concentration C_t itself has been used, and then the reciprocal of this average used in the equation. With a large degree of pulsation of flow, the error could easily be 40 or 50%, although Wood and his associates (3) consider that it is much less than this. Once the source of error has been recognized, it should be easy to eliminate it (especially with modern methods of computing) by using the proper kind of mean (the harmonic mean) of the concentrations (4).

The Rapid-Injection Indicator-Dilution Method

Instead of continuous injection, rapid injection of a known quantity of indicator may be used.

Here the principle is more difficult to understand. The idealized curve of concentration at the sampling site is shown in Figure. 19–1. After a delay, representing the time taken from the point of injection by the shortest route, the concentration rises abruptly to a maximum, then falls in an exponential-like curve, which is interrupted by the arrival of recirculated blood containing indicator.

If it were not for the complication of recirculation, the total volume of blood that has flowed between the point of injection and the point of sampling, up to the time the concentration approaches zero, could easily be calculated, accurately in the case of steady flow. The concentration arriving at any time (t to $t + dt$) multiplied by the constant flow (F) would give the total indicator emerging in that interval of time. The area under the curve, $\int C_t \, dt$, multiplied by F, must be the grand total of indicator emerging, which must equal the known total amount of indicator (I) that was injected. That is,

$$F = \frac{I}{\int C_t \, dt} = \frac{I}{\text{Area under concentration curve}}$$

The difficulty due to the recirculation obscuring the last part of the curve, so that the total area cannot be accurately measured, is removed by the fact that the fall of the concentration before recirculation (and it would be all the way if there was no recirculation) is exponential (contains e_{-kt}). (The reason for this is given below.) By plotting the "logarithm of the concentration versus time" instead of "concentration versus time" a straight line is obtained in that part of the curve

(Fig. 19–1) from which the bottom part of the curve that would be recorded, if there had been no recirculation, can be deduced, and the area correctly estimated.

Unfortunately, the curve of decay of concentration often is so distorted in patients with cardiac abnormalities, in whom the measurement of cardiac output is most desired, that there is too short a portion of the curve that is a straight line on the semilogarithmic plot for any accuracy in making this correction for recirculation. The newer method, called *thermal dilution*, where heat (or negative heat) is the indicator, has the advantage of removing the effects of recirculation. Instead of dye, cold saline solution or cold blood is injected, and the curve of blood temperature at the sampling site versus time takes the place of

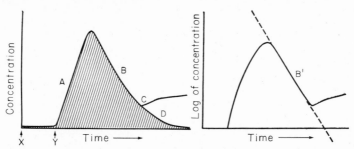

Fig. 19-1.—The concentration curve at the sampling site in the rapid-injection indicator-dilution technique. *X,* time of injection at the injection site. *Y,* time of first arrival at sampling site. *A,* rising part of concentration curve as more indicator arrives. *B,* exponential decay part of curve. *C,* beginning of recirculation. *D,* continuation of curve if there had been no recirculation. The shaded area gives the con-centration, from which the flow rate can be calculated. At the right, the semilogarithmic plot gives a straight line *(B')* for the exponential part of the curve, *B.* Extrapolation of this line allows the part *D* of the curve to be calculated, and thus the total area, free from the recirculation error. The calculation is strictly valid only for steady flow.

concentration of dye versus time. By the time the blood has recirculated, it has regained the body temperature. However, thermal-dilution methods have the disadvantage that heat (or cold) may leak from the blood vessels between the point of injection and the point of sampling (especially if this included the lungs). Dow (5) has thoroughly reviewed the various applications of the method of indicator dilution.

As in the Fick and continuous-injection methods, there is a basic error if the flow is pulsatile, representing each systolic ejection. To understand this, think of the ventricle into which the dye is injected, and in which it is very rapidly and uniformly mixed, as a bucket of water containing mixed dye. The water in the bucket is to be cleared by the process of dipping into it a cup, throwing the cupful out and replacing the volume removed by a cupful of clear water. After the first "cycle" of these two operations, the concentration of dye in the bucket will be reduced by the ratio:

$$\text{New concentration} = \text{Old concentration} \times \frac{\text{Volume of bucket} - \text{Volume of cup}}{\text{Volume of bucket}}$$

and this has not been adequately recognized. Unfortunately, this cannot be corrected, as it can be easily for continuous-injection methods. The method also yields the *volume of the vascular bed between the point of injection and the point of sampling,* from the mean time taken for dye to arrive at the sampling site, multiplied by the calculated flow rate. This is how the end-systolic volume of the ventricle has been measured, as compared with the stroke volume. This is explained below, and the explanation also serves to show why the decline of concentration, in the rapid-injection method, should be exponential.

Ratio of Stroke Volume to End-Diastolic Volume

Take the case where the site of injection is the ventricle itself and the sampling site is in the artery, as in the work of Rapaport and his associates (6, 7) and as illustrated in Figure 19–2. Here the dye curve declines in a series of steps

For example, if the cup volume was $^1/_4$th that of the bucket, after one pair of operations (removing a cupful and replacing with clear water) the concentration will be reduced to $^3/_4$ths of what it was. The next cycle of operations reduces it to $^3/_4$ths of this, and so on. Thus the concentration of indicator on the blood sampled in the artery (aorta or pulmonary artery) will fall in the steps of a geometrical series, each step representing a reduction in the ratio:

$$1 - \frac{\text{Stroke volume}}{\text{End-diastolic ventricular volume}} : 1$$

Such a geometrical series, when the steps become very small (in the limit, with steady outflow), passes into a curve of exponential decay (the characteristic of experimental decay is that the rate of fall is proportional to the amount that remains). This is the reason why the ratio of stroke volume to end-diastolic ventricular volume can be determined from Figure 19–2, and why the decay curve in the rapid-injection indicator-

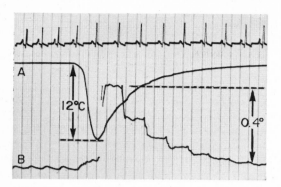

Fig. 19-2.—Records of a thermal-dilution experiment where cooled blood was injected into the right ventricle of a dog and a thermistor recorded the change of temperature in the pulmonary artery. *Top line,* the electrocardiogram. *A,* temperature at the injection site. *B,* temperature in the artery. From the series of "steps" in *B,* the ratio of stroke volume to end-diastolic ventricular volume may be calculated. Note the almost complete absence of a recirculation artifact with the thermal-dilution method. (Courtesy of Elliott Rapaport. References 6,7).

dilution method can be assumed to be an exponential decay curve. If the injection site to the sampling site includes a much bigger volume, including much more than the single ventricle in the example above, the constant of the exponential decay curve gives the ratio of the rate of flow to the total volume between injection and sampling. The method illustrated has shown that the stroke volume remains close to 40–50% of the end-diastolic ventricular volume in a variety of physiological circumstances, that is, *a normal ventricle ejects about half of its contents with each beat.* The dilated heart of heart failure of course ejects a much lower proportion, although the absolute stroke volume may be no less.

Different Methods for Measuring Cardiac Output: Accuracy and Correlation

Unfortunately, as new methods for measuring cardiac output are devised, too few "calibrations" are made versus the known output in models where this could be measured unequivocally. Instead, reliance has been placed on comparing the results of one method with another. When each may contain serious errors, it is not surprising that very serious discrepancies between them have been found.* Indeed, physiologists have come to regard agreement to within ±25% as "satisfac-

---

*If the blind lead the blind, both shall fall into the ditch.

tory," *faute de mieux.* Certainly, no one of the methods in living animals should be regarded as so free from major errors that it deserves to be used as a check on any other method.

Other (Non-Fick) Methods for Measuring Stroke Volume or Cardiac Output

X-ray cinematography of the cardiac shadow can give an estimate of the stroke volume (or twice this, on the average, when the shadow of both ventricles is used) as the difference between maximal and minimal volumes. The difficulty is that, even when both of two shadows, taken at right angles, are used, the estimate of volume is still uncertain, for the heart changes shape so greatly in the cardiac cycle. The use of a radioactive tracer in the blood and of scanning of the whole heart (or the concentration included in the beam) by a collimated counter is a modern variation. The difficulty, again, is the changing thickness of the heart in the "beam" as the heart beats.

There are other methods of measuring "something" relating to the cardiac pump for which claims of correlation with cardiac output have been made. Of these, the *ballistocardiograph* (8) deserves mention, for, *although it cannot measure cardiac output, it may well measure something else (the cardiac "impulse" or "impact") that is of diagnostic value on its own merits.* In the earlier apparatus, a bed platform on which the subject lay was suspended so that the bed's movements on a horizontal plane could be sensitively recorded almost isometrically; that is, the record of the force exerted on the bed was recorded. With the ejection of blood from the heart, there is, by Newton's third law, an equal and opposite reaction—a force on the body acting toward the feet (giving the I wave) (Fig. 19–3). When the blood rushes around the arch of the aorta, a high proportion of it has its momentum reversed (some continues toward the head). This gives a headward force on the body greater than the initial downward force (the J wave). Later waves in the record are hard to interpret, for by that time the momentum of the blood in different parts of the body is in a variety of directions and of many different magnitudes. The amplitude of the initial I and J waves has been used as an index of cardiac output. A more convenient type of ballistocardiographic machine was developed by Dock; this consisted of an apparatus strapped to the body (e.g., the thigh). The inertia of a weight in the

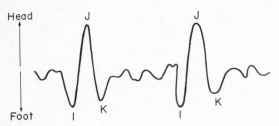

Fig. 19-3.—The waves of a ballistocardiogram. For explanation see text.

apparatus itself allowed it to record the acceleration of the body (such as the accelerometers used in aviation medical research). A quite similar record can be recorded simply by pressing a physiologist's pressure tambour, recording on a smoke drum, to the cranium of a subject lying on a bed.

Now, by Newton's second law, force is equal to *rate of change of momentum*, that is, to the rate of change of (mass of blood ejected times its velocity). The cardiac output is directly related to the momentum, not to its rate of change. Obviously, if the heart pumped blood continuously, the ballistocardiogram would record no deflections at all. The method cannot, therefore, measure cardiac output reliably. A patient who ejects the same stroke volume more forcefully and rapidly will have ballistocardiographic waves of much greater amplitude. [▶Integration of the ballistocardiogram might yield something correlated with the cardiac output (the integration constant would still be unknown), but the difficulty would remain that, even during ejection, the blood would be changing its momentum in other parts of the body.◀] The movement of the cardiac walls makes a considerable contribution of momentum. The proper view would seem to be that the ballistocardiogram measures, not the cardiac output, but the cardiac "force" or "impulse," which

may well be of considerable intrinsic diagnostic value.

Measurements of "Myocardial Mechanics"

Just as the ballistocardiogram may measure not the cardiac output but something about cardiac function that is valuable, so the newer concepts of studying how the ventricular muscle functions, *as a muscle rather than as a pump,* may provide new aids to diagnosis. The model worked out by A. V. Hill, in 1938, for striated muscle is taken as the analogy. On the basis of experiments on isolated skeletal muscle in which the muscle, when stimulated to contraction, was held at a fixed length until the tension rose to a given value (preloading) and then was able to shorten against a second load (afterloading), Hill interpreted the data in terms of a contractile element (the sarcomeres) which had an elastic element in series, and a parallel elastic element (Fig. 19–4). Thus, even though the total length of the muscle might be constant during an apparently "isometric" contraction, the contractile element might shorten, while the series elastic element lengthened.

Hill's work revealed two outstanding features of muscle behavior. First, the maximal isometric force developed by the stimulated muscle increased with the initial length (this is the basis of Starling's law for heart muscle). Second, for a given length, the force developed depends on the velocity of shortening, when this is allowed in the isotonic contraction under constant "afterload." The force diminishes as the velocity increases, in a "force-velocity curve" that is characteristic of the muscle. (Although the first thought is that this curve is due to an "internal viscosity" of muscle, the true explanation is in terms of the thermodynamics of muscle contraction and the existence of a "shortening heat.")

Fig. 19-4.—Schematic diagram of the contractile and elastic elements in the ventricular wall. (After Fry [9].) The conventional "elastic model" is shown at the right.

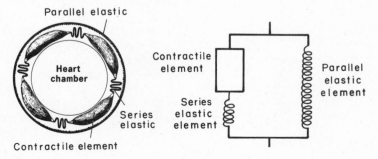

How can the analogous properties of cardiac ventricular muscle be studied in the intact, beating heart of animals? The matter has been clearly explained by Fry *et al.* (9), and the method has been developed in a series of researches by Sonnenblick and his colleagues (10). In the isovolumetric contraction phase of the cardiac cycle, we have something analogous to the isometric contraction of striated muscle, under different "preloading," i.e., with different degrees of initial stretch, measured by the end-diastolic volume of the ventricle. In the "ejection phase," the ventricular muscle is shortening with varying velocity, under an "afterload" corresponding to the aortic pressure (which, however, is not constant during the ejection phase). At all times, the force excited by the muscle can theoretically be deduced from the pressure developed in the ventricle, with the curvatures of the wall, by the law of Laplace. Unfortunately, the shape of the ventricle changes during the isovolumetric phase, becoming more spherical as the pressure rises, but ellipsoidal or spherical "models" allow approximate estimates of muscle force to be made.

The analysis is complicated, and approximate only, but the data have established the same two features: an increase in force with initial stretch, and a decrease of maximal force as the velocity of shortening increases. It is hoped that the study of force-velocity relations in the failing heart, or one affected by various drugs, will give us more precisely defined measures of what has been often called "*ventricular contractility*." The term has been used without any real definition, meaning different things to the different individuals who have used it.

Although the analysis is difficult, it emerges that measurement of the maximal rate of rise of ventricular pressure, dP/dt, or perhaps this divided by P (a consequence of considering the role of the law of Laplace), i.e., $d(\log P)/dt$, might be a useful measure of the contractile status of the ventricular muscle. This can be relatively easily computed from pressure recordings from a small catheter thrust through the aortic valve into the left ventricle of the patient. As with the electrocardiogram, the usefulness of the results will depend on ultimate clinical correlation, rather than the basic analysis. At any rate, we might have, in the rate of rise of ventricular pressure, an index of ventricular performance alone, whereas the measurement of cardiac output tells us the result of two combined factors, action of the heart muscle plus the resistance to flow in the peripheral vascular bed. Attempts to apply similar analyses to the ejection period have not been successful because the complicating factors are many.

Results of Cardiac Output Measurements; the Cardiac Index

The cardiac output at rest naturally depends on the size of the individual. As with metabolic rate, this is taken into consideration by expressing it as liters per minute divided by the surface area of the body in square meters (the average man has about 1.7 m² of body surface). This is called the *cardiac index*, and its normal value at rest is about 3. Heavy protein meals will increase cardiac output by up to 30%.

CARDIAC OUTPUT IN EXERCISE

It used to be taught that in normal physiology the cardiac output was increased in exercise, excitement, etc., by two cardiac adjustments: (1) an increase in *stroke volume* and (2) an increase in *heart rate;* the earlier measurements of stroke volume seemed to indicate that this was so. Recent investigations seem to show clearly that in most normal subjects there is no consistent change in stroke volume and that the burden of increase in output is on the increase of heart rate. Rushmer has reviewed the subject (11) and put together the results of many others with his own (Fig. 19–5). The exception may be well-trained athletes, in whom the stroke volume may increase. In cardiovascular disease (e.g., valvular insufficiency), an increase in stroke volume does occur in exercise. The apparent discrepancies in earlier work may possibly be explained on the basis of the effect of posture on the stroke volume. In the lying position, stroke volume is greater than when sitting or standing (cardiac output is also greater). If the lying posture is maintained in performing the exercise, there is no consistent change in the stroke volume. However, in the sitting and standing position, the lower stroke volume at rest rises, at the start of exercise, to the greater stroke volume characteristic of lying. *There is, therefore, in this case an increase in stroke volume at the start of exercise, but no consistent increase with the severity of exercise.*

Patients with complete heart block (e.g., Adams-Stokes syndrome) can now be kept alive by providing an artificial pacemaker, an electrical device delivering periodic electrical stimulation to the ventricle. Study of their cardiac output with

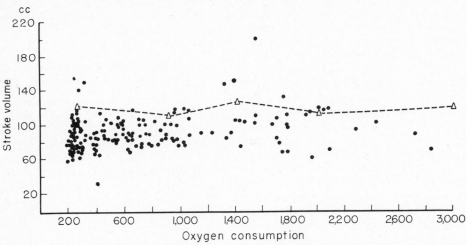

Fig. 19-5.—Showing how the stroke volume does not consistently increase with the severity of exercise. The data, collected by Rushmer, are from six different groups of research workers, using two different methods of measurement of cardiac output. The broken line joins points for an individual subject. (Adapted from Rushmer and Smith, Jr. [11].)

increasing rates of artificial stimuli has given new insight into the normal increase with exercise (12). If the patient is at rest, increasing the rate increases the cardiac output to a maximum of only about 30%, reached at a rate of about 80 beats per min, because the stroke volume decreases correspondingly. When the patient is exercising, stroke volume is higher than at rest for each value of the ventricular rate.

Thus the statement that increases in cardiac output in exercise normally depend almost entirely on the increased heart rate must not be misunderstood. Without the reflex effects in exercise, such as the inhibition of the negative inotropic effect of the vagal tone, and possibly positive inotropic effects of the conduction system and of the humoral agents in exercise, the stroke volume would decrease with increased heart rate instead of remaining constant, and cardiac output would not be increased markedly. *The maintenance of the constant stroke volume in exercise, in reality, is evidence of the important reflex and humoral regulations in exercise.*

Provision of an artificial pacemaker at a fixed rate of 70–80 beats per min probably provides as adequate a substitute for the normal conduction system as one whose rate could be voluntarily increased by the patient in exercise. There is some evidence that the location of the stimulus in the ventricle affects the output achieved.

The almost total reliance on increases in heart rate imposes a severe limitation on the maximal increase in cardiac output that is possible, for, when the heart rate reaches 160–170 beats per min, diastole is so shortened that adequate filling of the ventricles and adequate coronary flow are seriously impaired. If the resting rate is 70 beats per min, this would suggest that an increase of cardiac output of $2^{1}/_{2}$–3 times the resting level would be the maximum.

Yet, in trained athletes, increases up to 5 times the resting value have been measured. This is explained, to a large degree, by the fact that their stroke volume in the resting state is increased (ventricular hypertrophy) and the resting heart rate is abnormally low (as low as 40 beats per min) in some cases (13). (It is said that an intercollegiate champion miler was twice rejected by medical boards of the United States Navy because his heart rate at rest was less than 40 beats per min) Increasing the heart rate alone to 160 beats per min would, in these athletes, give a fourfold increase in cardiac output.

EFFECTS OF POSTURE ON CARDIAC OUTPUT

There is, perhaps surprisingly, a *decrease* in cardiac output (up to 20%) from lying to sitting or standing, explained mostly by a decrease in stroke volume. The ventricular volume correspondingly decreases. The redistribution of blood volume under the effect of gravity and the change in blood pressure at the site of the baroreceptors that control important cardiovascular reflexes must be responsible, although the explanation is difficult. Indeed, after acclimatization to heat, the output when standing may be greater than when lying.

This fact is largely ignored by clinicians in charge of the management of cardiac patients, in that many insist that the patient remain absolutely flat on his back, when sitting up would actually reduce the work of his heart, as well as reduce the psychological stress on the patient and his visitors. Again, the effort of trying to defecate in the supine position can put a very serious strain on the heart, compared with allowing the patient to move slowly to a more physiological posture for this function. Even in the normal posture in the bathroom, the act of defecation, accompanied by the Valsalva maneuver (raised abdominal pressure with a closed glottis) can impose a severe load on the heart. Cardiac patients often die at stool. *Ban the bedpan!*

Possible Differences in Cardiac Output Measured at Different Sites

It is a good exercise in physiological thinking to consider how the results of measuring output at different places may differ. Some of the methods really measure the blood flow in the pulmonary artery (i.e., of the lungs); others measure the aortic blood flow. The aortic flow measured directly, as by a flowmeter in the aorta, will be less (even averaged over a long period) than the pulmonary flow, by the amount of coronary blood flow. The indicator-dilution method using samples from the aorta or central arteries will, however, include the coronary flow. On the other hand, the blood flowing in the aorta must include that which will flow through the bronchial circulation, while the pulmonary flow will not include this item (since bronchial drainage is in part into the pulmonary veins). Bronchial flow is probably normally only from 1 to 3% of the cardiac output (14).

While the accuracy of present methods is not sufficient to allow the use of such differences for estimating, for example, coronary or bronchial flow in normal persons, comparisons becomes significant in cases of congenital or acquired circulatory shunts, as in the case of patent ductus arteriosus. The differences in concentration of indicator, such as oxygen content, in different sites (e.g., right ventricle versus pulmonary artery and aorta) are the basis of estimating the amount of flow through such shunts, which may be left to

right or right to left, in the various conditions. Full discussion of the methods and results in the case of shunts is inappropriate in this book. The medical student and the intern are referred to the classic monograph by Cournand and his co-workers (15) (Cournand received the Nobel Prize for work in this field) and to the very complete discussion by Wood and associates (16).

REFERENCES

1. Hamilton, W. F.: Measurement of the Cardiac Output, in *Handbook of Physiology*, Sec. 2, Vol. I: *Circulation* (1962), Chap. 17, pp. 533–584.
2. Visscher, M. B., and Johnson, J. A.: The Fick principle: Analysis of potential errors in its conventional application, J. Appl. Physiol. 5:635, 1952.
3. Wood, E. H.; Bowers, D.; Shepherd, J. T., and Fox, I. J.: Oxygen content of mixed venous blood in man during various phases of the respiratory and cardiac cycles in relation to possible errors in measurement of cardiac output by conventional application of the Fick method, J. Appl. Physiol. 7:621, 1954.
4. Cropp, G. J. A., and Burton, A. C.: Theoretical considerations and model experiments on the validity of indicator dilution methods for measurement of variable flow, Circulation Res. 18:26, 1966.
5. Dow, P.: Estimates of cardiac output and central blood volume by dye dilution, Physiol. Rev. 36 (supp. 2): 77, 1956.
6. Bristow, J. D.; Ferguson, R. E.; Montz, F., and Rapaport, E.: Thermodilution studies of ventricular volume changes due to isoproterenol and bleeding, J. Appl. Physiol. 18:129, 1963.
7. Rapaport, E.; Weigand, B. D., and Bristow, J. D.: Estimation of left ventricular end-diastolic volume in the dog by a thermodilution method, Circulation Res. 11:803, 1962.
8. Starr, I.; Rawson, A. J.; Schroeder, H. A., and Joseph, N. R.: Studies on the estimation of cardiac output in man, and of abnormalities in cardiac function, from the heart's recoil and the blood's impacts: The ballistocardiogram, Am. J. Physiol. 227:1, 1939.
9. Fry, D. L.; Griggs, D. M., and Greenfield, J. C., Jr.: Myocardial mechanics: Tension-velocity-length relationships of heart muscle, Circulation Res. 14:73, 1963.
10. Sonnenblick, E. H.; Parmley, W. W.; Unshel, C. W., and Brutsaert, D. L.: Ventricular function: Evaluation of myocardial contractility in health and disease. Prog. Cardiovas. Dis., 12:449, 1970.
11. Rushmer, R. F., and Smith, O. A., Jr.: Cardiac control, Physiol. Rev. 39:41, 1959.
12. Beregard, S.: Observations on the effect of varying ventricular rate on the circulation at rest and during exercise in two patients with an artificial pacemaker, Acta med. scandinav. 172:615, 1962.
13. Hall, V. E.: The relation of heart rate to exercise fitness: An attempt at physiological interpretation of the bradycardia of training, in Symposium on ex-

ercise fitness tests, Pediatrics 32 (no. 4, part 2, supp.):723, 1963.

This is an excellent collection of papers on the adjustment of the heart and peripheral circulation to exercise.

14. Aviado, D. M.; de Burgh Daly, M.: Lee, C. Y., and Schmidt, C. F.: The contribution of the bronchial circulation to the venous admixture in pulmonary venous blood, J. Physiol. 155:602, 1961.

15. Cournand, A.; Baldwin, J. S., and Himmelstine, A.: *Cardiac Catheterization in Congenital Heart Disease* (New York: Oxford University Press, 1949).

16. Marshall, H. W.; Helmholtz, H. F., Jr., and Wood, E. H.: Physiologic Consequences of Congenital Heart Disease, in *Handbook of Physiology*, Sec. 2, *Circulation* (Washington, D. C.: American Physiological Society, 1962), pp. 417–487.

The Regulation of the Circulation

20

General View of Homeostatic Control Mechanisms and of Overriding Controls

"The brain may devise laws for the blood, but a
hot temper leaps over a cold decree." *The Merchant of Venice,*
Act. I, Scene 2.

Cybernetics

THE SECRET of operation of fantastically complicated machines, such as the modern airliner, is that a maximal number of the separate functions are provided with automatic controls which keep some chosen variable constant. For example, the posture of the aircraft is automatically stabilized. Any tilt of the wings results in a signal (the "error signal") to a computer, which responds by sending out a signal to an "effector system" that immediately corrects the "error" and brings the posture back to normal. Dozens of different variables, such as altitude, engine temperature, air speed, etc., are simultaneous but separately kept at chosen constant levels by such feedback mechanisms in the automatic pilot.

Of course, this set of homeostatic mechanisms must also be "overridden," when necessary, by the pilot, who may "command" the computer to suppress one homeostasis in favor of another or to reset the level of the variable concerned to a new control point (e.g., to keep the nose down to a glide angle instead of level).

Actually, the human organism is vastly more complicated in function than an airliner; but its control mechanisms are organized on the same pattern with a set of homeostatic mechanisms, which tend to keep a variety of physiological variables at a constant level, and an overriding control over these feedback controls by the brain.

Some of the concepts and some of the terms used in cybernetics (the science of control mechanisms) are useful in studying physiological regulations, such as circulatory control. Excellent books on the subject of control systems in biology are available. The chapter in the book by Randall (1) is highly recommended to the readers of this book, and for those wishing to go more deeply into the analysis, the book by Bayliss (2).

Essential Components of a Homeostatic Control System

The essential components of a homeostatic control system are illustrated in Figure 20–1. They are as follows:

The *controlled variable*—the variable which is automatically kept to some standard level. One of the dominant regulations in the circulation is that of the central arterial blood pressure. In this control system, then, this blood pressure is the controlled variable.

A *specialized sensor*, which responds specifically to changes in the controlled variable and can report to the system the degree of deviations from the standard level (this deviation is called an *error*). In the control of the blood pressure, the sensors are the *baroreceptors*, strategically placed in the walls of central arteries and elsewhere.

An *input loop*, or, in physiology, an *afferent reflex arc*. The sensor sends an error signal by this arc to the computer, or coordinating center. The baroreceptors signal the error by the number of

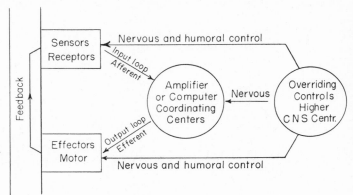

Fig. 20-1.—Basic components of a feedback homeostatic mechanism, such as that of the carotid sinus reflux. See text for discussion.

nervous impulses traveling by afferent nerves to the vasomotor and cardiac centers in the brain.

The *coordinating center,* or *computer.* On receiving the error signal, this center responds by sending out a correcting signal, via—

The *output,* or *feedback, loop* (or efferent reflex arc), to—

The *effector mechanism* (or "autonomic motor system"), which then produces a change in the controlled variable in a direction such as to reduce the error which started the whole process. In our physiological example of homeostasis of blood pressure, the effector system achieves a change in cardiac activity and in the caliber of the peripheral blood vessels. The effector action may be relatively direct on the controlled variable, or indirect, so long as it results in a restoration to the standard level. In the physiological case, the connection between the effector mechanism (e.g., the transmission of pressure from the ventricle in systole to the site of the receptors for pressure in the carotid artery) may also be said to be part of the feedback loop.

This is *negative feedback,* in which a change in the controlled variable (error) results in an effect on it in the opposite direction. *Positive feedback* would increase any deviation (error) of the controlled variable and therefore lead to instability rather than stability. Physiological systems that show positive feedback must be extremely rare, although they do exist. One such system is the generation of the action potential in nerve tissue, for if the normal "resting potential" is reduced beyond a certain critical level, depolarization proceeds all the way, even to reversal of the potential. [▶We may encounter positive feedback when great sensitivity of response and explosive reactions (all or nothing) are desirable. In the circula-

tion, reflex control is probably almost exclusively of the negative feedback kind, producing automatic stability. Only in disease is there instability.◀]

The *gain* of the control system is measured by the magnitude of the corrective effector action in response to a unit change (error) in the controlled variable. The greater the gain, the more closely the controlled variable is held to the standard level. It must not be thought, however, that any control system can hold the controlled variable exactly at the constant level in the face of great demands on the system. What is called the *load error* must exist, although it is small if the over-all gain is high. For example, a feedback control system operates to hold the arterial blood pressure constant. If the tendency for blood pressure to rise is very great, the effector system will have to work harder continuously to maintain the control level. This requires that the stimulus to the system, the error signal, which is a rise of blood pressure above the standard level, must remain correspondingly greater. Thus, we could not expect the blood pressure to remain exactly at the same level in exercise as at rest. Many of the control systems of the body, however, possess so great a gain that this load error is hard to detect. For example, the respiratory center is so exquisitely sensitive to the carbon dioxide level in the blood, responding by increased respiration to any rise in Pco_2, that large sustained increases of respiration may give evidence of strong action of the effector mechanism, yet with hardly detectable increases in the controlled level of carbon dioxide. The gain of the blood pressure control system is much less, and the load error greater.

For this reason, the mechanism of physiological feedback systems often remains obscure until some part of the system is interrupted by the cutting of afferent or efferent arcs or by the effector system being rendered inoperative. The resultant large fluctuation of the controlled variable then reveals the homeostatic mechanism that had operated. A good example of this is provided by the way in which the chief homeostatic mechanisms of the circulation were discovered—by isolation of the receptors from the effector mechanism.

The Controlled Variables of the Circulatory Regulation

If the definition of the function of the circulation given in Chapter 1 is accepted, one might expect to find circulatory control systems that maintained constant the amount of oxygen carried to the tissues, or perhaps the Po_2 at the tissues (or the Pco_2). Such systems are found, but they appear to be those regulations which are local and autonomous controls, rather than the general controls of the whole circulation. In the central control, the variable that is controlled directly is usually more indirectly concerned with the oxygen supply of the tissues. In the later chapters of this section, many reflex circulatory regulations are described. Some of these, classified according to the particular variable which they serve to keep constant, are listed below:

Homeostasis of Po_2.—Autoregulation of the kidney blood flow: Autoregulation of coronary blood flow. Reactive hyperemia in muscle (to some extent). Autoregulation of blood flow to specific lobes of the lungs.

Homeostasis of Pco_2.—Reactive hyperemia in muscle: Regulation of brain blood flow.

Homeostasis of arterial blood pressure.—This is the dominant circulatory reflex, mediated by the carotid sinus and aortic reflexes. [▶The postulated *myogenic reflex of Bayliss* would also depend on fluctuations in arterial blood pressure, but it is hard to believe in because it would represent positive feedback instead of negative feedback, tending toward instability in the circulation rather than homeostasis (this was recognized by Bayliss). The myogenic reflex is a constriction of arteries in response to a stretching of their wall, as by a rise of the arterial pressure.◀]

Homeostasis of heart rate.—This regulation (also called the *Bainbridge reflex*), whose existence and function has so long been a matter of debate, probably represents a mechanism keeping the heart rate within normal limits.

Homeostasis of rate of blood flow.—The reflexes that have been described from receptors in the veins, affecting arteriolar tone (the venous-arteriolar reflexes) tend to keep the rate of flow constant. They may also represent a *direct homeostasis of venous pressure.* Autoregulation in the kidney circulation, in the range of high blood pressures, might also be placed in this category.

Homeostasis of cardiac output.—Starling's law of the heart might be said to achieve this, as far as keeping the equality of output of the two ventricles, but its mechanism is more direct than the reflex feedback system here described. There seems to be no homeostasis of cardiac output itself, which is rather the instrument of other homeostatic mechanisms, as of blood pressure.

[▶A number of other cardiovascular reflexes have been described, such as the *Bezold and Jarisch reflexes* elicited by certain drugs on receptors in the ventricular walls. Evidence for receptor areas in the atria and pulmonary artery has also been advanced. As yet, the function of these reflexes in keeping constant any particular physiological variable has not been suggested, and definite evidence that they are elicited by physiological stimuli, rather than "exotic" drugs, is often lacking.◀]

The Nature of Overriding Controls

In engineering control systems, overriding control is often applied to the sensor, as when we turn "up" or "down" the thermostat in the living room. It may be applied equally well to the coordinating center or to the effector system (we may turn off the hot water entering the radiator). In circulatory control, we usually think of overriding control through the influence of higher brain centers on the vasomotor centers in the medulla, but already we know of mechanisms of overriding that work on the receptors or on the effector systems. The humoral agent adrenaline is an example. This is liberated from the adrenal medulla in excitement and in heavy exercise and circulates in the blood. There is good evidence that it produces an effect on the *sensitivity* of the baroreceptors in the carotid sinus and aorta, thus changing the level of the controlled variable (i.e., the central blood pressure). Its abundant effects on the effector system are well known, in that it increases the tone of the peripheral resistance vessels and the strength of the heartbeat. [▶Neurophysiologists are discovering that overriding control, by the brain, of other functions occurs by modification of peripheral receptors (e.g., the reticular formation may modify the sensitivity of auditory receptors in the ear itself), not merely by facilitation and inhibition in the coordinating brain centers. More of this type of overriding control in the circulatory system may be waiting for discovery. For example, the hormones of the adrenal cortex may play their role by changing the "reactivity" of blood vessels, which would be an action on part of the effector system.◄]

Details of the homeostatic mechanisms of the circulation are given in the chapters that follow.

An excellent research article on the carotid sinus reflex from the cybernetic point of view has been published by Scher and Young (3).

REFERENCES

1. Randall, J. E.: *Elements of Biophysics* (2d ed.; Chicago: Year Book Medical Publishers, Inc., 1962), Chap. 4, p. 91.
2. Bayliss, L. E.: *Living Control System* (London: The English University Press, Ltd., 1966).
3. Scher, A. M., and Young, A. C.: Servoanalysis of carotid sinus reflex effects on peripheral resistance, Circulation Res. 12:152–162, 1953.

21

Homeostasis of Arterial Blood Pressure; The Carotid Sinus and Aortic Reflexes

Historical

THERE IS NO DOUBT that the most important and notable automatic control of the circulation is the carotid sinus, aortic arch reflex. Claim for participation in the discovery may be made for a large number of physiologists, going back to the turn of the century and even earlier; but the full elucidation of the mechanism of the reflex was due to the work of Hering and of Heymans and his collaborators between 1925 and 1930. A history of the matter, and very exhaustive review of all the subsequent research, is to be found in the monograph by Heymans and Neil (1).

A classic law taught to students of physiology was *Marey's law*, which stated that blood pressure and heart rate bear a reciprocal relation; that is, a rise of blood pressure was usually associated with a slowing of the heart, and vice versa. There are so many obvious exceptions to this rule in normal physiology (e.g., in exercise both heart rate and blood pressure rise) that one wonders how the generalization could have been made. As early as 1806, Cyon and Ludwig discovered the *depressor nerve* in the neck, an afferent nerve running with the vagus (separate from it in the rabbit), and noted that stimulation of the cut (peripheral) end produced bradycardia and hypotension. Others confirmed this and also found that section of the depressor nerves produced an increase in heart rate and blood pressure, that is, that there were "tonic" discharges in these afferent nerves that were depressing cardiac activity.

The effects of carotid arterial occlusion in ac-

celerating the heart were also well known, but this was earlier attributed to an effect of ischemia on brain centers. We now know that the nerve endings of the depressor nerve are receptors, specifically sensitive to rise of arterial blood pressure, which are located in a special region at the bifurcation of the carotid arteries and also (for the aortic nerve) in the arch of the aorta.

The clear localization of the receptor areas, and the nerves involved, depended on the famous cross-circulation technique used by Heymans (Fig. 21–1). Modifications of this technique have been used ever since to discover the location of sensory areas of cardiovascular reflexes. The head and neck of a recipient dog were completely isolated from its body, except for the vagus nerves, and were supplied with blood from a donor animal by connecting the two carotid arteries and the two jugular veins. The head of the donor animal survived, supplied by the collateral circulation through the vertebral arteries. Injection of a pressor agent (adrenaline) into the body of the donor dog produced, as expected, a rise in pressure in that body, but it also produced a bradycardia and hypotension in the body of the recipient dog. Since the only way the injection could have affected the heart of the recipient dog was via the still intact vagus nerves, the rise of pressure in the region of the perfused neck or head must have elicited a reflex from that region. Section of the remaining nerve connections to the recipient dog's body abolished the reflex bradycardia.

Later it was shown that there must be barore-

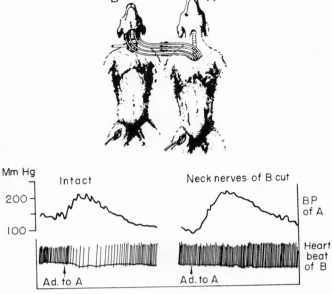

Fig. 21-1.—Illustrating the famous cross-circulation technique of Heymans and his associates, by which the carotid sinus reflex was elucidated. The records at the bottom show the arterial blood pressure of the donor *(dog A)* with the heartbeat of the recipient *(dog B)* below. At the left, intravenous injection of adrenaline into *dog A* was followed, not only by a rise in blood pressure (to be expected), but also by a slowing of the heart of *dog B*. At the right, after section of the nervous connections in the neck of *dog B*, the bradycardia was no longer seen. (From Heymans and De Vleeschhouwer: Arch. internat. pharmacodyn. 84:401, 1950.)

ceptors in the aortic arch as well as in the carotid sinus region, because injection of pressor agent into the body of the recipient produced, not only the expected rise of pressure in the body, but bradycardia of its heart; this bradycardia was abolished by cutting the vagi, which were the only connection of the body to the brain of the recipient dog.

Later experiments used perfusion, from a donor dog, of the carotid sinus or aortic arch regions alone, with these regions hemodynamically isolated from the rest of the circulation of the recipient dog. Inflatable balloons in the great vessels also were used to stimulate the receptors.

The Baroreceptors

Baroreceptors had long been noticed by histologists, and the action potentials in their afferent nerves had been recorded before their function was fully known. The region in the bifurcation of the common carotid artery into the external and internal carotids is a richly innervated "bulb," full of nerve endings in boutons, coils and latticework (Fig. 21–2). There is no doubt that these receptors, although we call them "baroreceptors," are really stretch receptors similar to those of the muscle spindle and tendon receptors. They do not respond directly to pressure (like piezoelectric crystals) but to the deformation and stretch that occurs because of their attachment to

the wall, which is distended by a rise of blood pressure (2). Langren (3), by detailed study of the action potentials in single fibers of the carotid sinus nerves, has shown that some receptors may be strung in parallel, some in series with the elastic elements of the wall, and that their response to rise of pressure is correlated with the distensibility of the arteries of this region. If the distensibility is reduced, there is less stretch of the wall for a given rise of pressure and less discharge from the receptors.

Heymans emphasizes that the sinoaortic receptors are by no means the only sensory area involved in the reflex. There is probably a host of "outposts," notably in the *Pacinian corpuscles* distributed through the visceral circulation, as in the mesentery. These, however, may control local circulation, or local blood volume, rather than the central blood pressure. Pressor or baroreceptors participating in the reflex have been reported even in such unlikely places as the pancreas. As Heymans puts it, the carotid sinus and aortic areas represent the "headquarters" of the homeostatic control, which has widespread minor "stations."

[►Similar receptor areas have been found at the junction of the thyroid arteries and the common carotids, but it has been suggested that these have a special role in controlling, not the central blood pressure, but the release of the hormone aldosterone by the adrenal cortex, through centers in the cerebral cortex. The homeostasis here would be more directly concerned with blood volume than with blood pressure.◀]

The action potentials in the carotid sinus nerve and in the aortic nerve, when the pressure is raised, have been beautifully recorded by Bronk and his co-workers and also by Neil. Details are given in the monograph by Heymans and Neil (1). Figure 21–3 shows the discharges in a single nerve fiber of the aortic nerve that occur in the systolic peak of pressure in each cardiac cycle. The threshold appears to be a pressure of about 40 mm Hg, so that, with normal blood pressures, the receptors fire throughout all of the cardiac cycle. Like most receptors, the baroreceptors "adapt" and respond to rate of change of pressure as well as to the level of pressure. For example, Figure 21–3 shows that the rate of firing, at a given level of pressure, is greater when the pressure is rising than when it is falling. Therefore, the response to a pulsatile pressure is greater than to a static pressure of the same mean value (4). When the carotid sinus is perfused with a steady pressure, close to the threshold level, the total discharge of these receptors is very slight compared with that

Fig. 21-2.—A baroreceptor from the wall of the carotid sinus of an adult man. *A*, large myelinated nerve fibers; *g* and *f*, terminal nerve endings. (From De Castro, F.: Tr. Lab. Invest. biol. Univ. Madrid 25:331, 1928.)

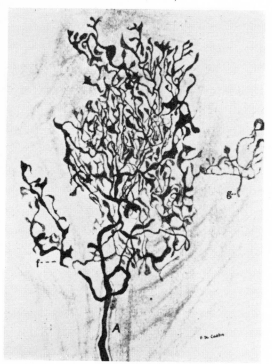

when the pressure is pulsatile with the same mean value. The true picture of the role of the reflex cannot, therefore, be obtained in experiments with steady perfusion. At high pressures (about 200 mm Hg), the discharge of the receptors reaches a maximal value, and it is not increased by further elevation of pressure.

These receptors are, then, continuously directing messages to the brain regarding the level of arterial pressure at these locations in all normal circumstances. Only when—for instance, in hemorrhagic shock—the arterial pressure is far below physiological levels is the precise "information" lacking.

The threshold pressure, below which these baroreceptors do not respond, can be affected by a change in the distensibility of the arterial wall where they reside. For example, it has been shown that wrapping the carotid sinus and aortic arch areas with an external cuff of cellophane or other plastic will produce a systemic hypertension in the animal. A rise of pressure no longer produces the same stretch of the wall or the same deformation of the receptors; so they do not send as many impulses in the reflex control. One of the few certain features of *essential hypertension* in humans has been rather neglected. In patients with this disease, the blood pressure is maintained at levels much higher than normal (say, 240/160 instead of 120/80). Yet, if the posture is changed in such patients, there is evidence that the carotid sinus reflex is still just as active as ever in homeostasis of arterial blood pressure; that is, standing after lying horizontally does not reduce the blood pressure, and a compensatory increase in heart rate is seen in hypertensives as in normotensives. The homeostatic, buffer reflex is still operating but at a very different level of the controlled variable. [►There must have been a change in the threshold and in the operating range of the baroreceptors. A thickening or increased stiffness of the wall in the receptor regions may be responsible. This is not suggested as primary in the etiology of essential hypertension, but as a necessary accompaniment to explain why the buffer reflexes are not keeping the blood pressure normal.◀]

Another example of the change in the responsiveness of the baroreceptors is the effect of topical application of pressor and depressor drugs to the carotid sinus region. Topical application of adrenaline or other drugs causes local vasoconstriction (i.e., contraction of vascular smooth muscle) and increases the discharge for a given

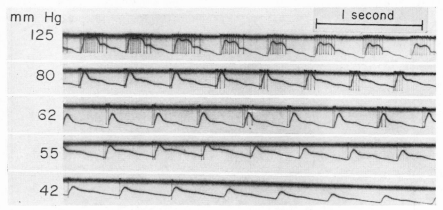

Fig. 21-3.—Impulse activity in a single fiber of the left aortic nerve, with the blood pressure recorded from the left common carotid artery. The figures at the left give the mean level of pressure; vasodilators such as sodium blood pressure. (From Neil, E.: Arch. Middlesex Hosp. 4:16, 1954.)

level of pressure; vasodilators such as sodium nitrite decrease the discharge. These effects are probably due to changing the mechanical stretch of the receptors, that is, the distensibility of the wall. [►Acetylcholine, in very small amounts, increases the sensitivity of the receptors to pressure, probably directly rather than through a change in distensibility (5). Such effects may (or may not) occur from the use of physiological concentrations of systemic drugs or vascular hormones. If they do, this would be one form of overriding control, by the brain, of the reflex through the release of circulating hormones.◄]

The baroreceptor area of the carotid sinus must not be confused with the *chemoreceptors of the carotid body,* which lie very close by (on the other side of the carotid artery). Similarly, the aortic baroreceptors must not be confused with the *aortic body,* in which there are chemoreceptors. The innervation of the chemoreceptor areas is equally rich, but they are more richly vascularized. The chemoreceptors are concerned with the homeostasis of blood gases, by control of the respiration. It is true that strong stimulation of the chemoreceptors has an effect on the circulation, but this is a secondary effect, mediated probably through connections between the respiratory centers and the vasomotor center.

The carotid baroreceptors may be stimulated directly by pressing on the tissue in the angle of the neck, causing a discharge similar to that of an increased blood pressure. (Carotid occlusion lower in the neck, on the contrary, lowers the pressure in the sinus and decreases the discharge.) The heart is dramatically slowed by this manipu-

lation, and fainting results if the pressure is continued. In the days of our grandfathers (or great-grandfathers), when high, starched collars were worn by all "gentlemen," there were cases of syncope (fainting) from this cause.

The Afferent Areas and the Vasomotor Center

Figure 21–4 shows the different pathways of the discharges from the baroreceptors in the aortic arch and those in the carotid sinus, as well as the pathway for the chemoreceptor impulses from aortic and carotid bodies. Both baroreceptors and chemoreceptors of the carotid region send impulses up the carotid sinus nerves to join the glossopharyngeal nerve, whereas the aortic receptors fire up the depressor branch of the vagus in the same sheath as the rest of the vagus (separate in the case of some animals [e.g., rabbits]). The pathway of baroreceptor impulses from Pacinian corpuscles in the viscera is not established but is probably also up the vagus. The *vasomotor center,* or, better, the "medullary vasomotor centers," on which the baroreceptor impulses impinge, is a functional rather than a strictly anatomical term, although sectioning the midbrain at different levels shows the limited area concerned. Section at the level of the first cervical segment destroys the reflex control of blood pressure, but section at the upper border of the pons leaves the control intact. Within this broad area of the medulla, studies with the Horsley-Clarke stereotactic apparatus, allowing electrical stimulation or punctate destruction of specific areas, have shown that there is ge-

BARORECEPTOR SYSTEM

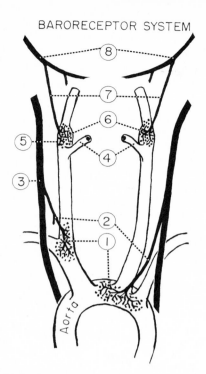

CHEMORECEPTOR SYSTEM

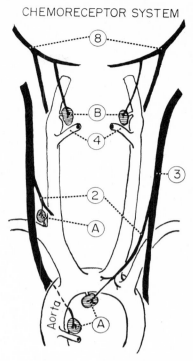

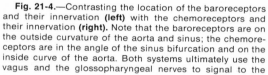

Fig. 21-4.—Contrasting the location of the baroreceptors and their innervation **(left)** with the chemoreceptors and their innervation **(right)**. Note that the baroreceptors are on the outside curvature of the aorta and sinus; the chemoreceptors are in the angle of the sinus bifurcation and on the inside curve of the aorta. Both systems ultimately use the vagus and the glossopharyngeal nerves to signal to the respective brain centers (i.e., to the vasomotor centers for the baroreceptors and to the respiratory centers for the chemoreceptors). *1*, Aortic baroreceptors; *2*, aortic nerves (depressor branches of vagi); *3*, vagus nerve; *4*, external carotid artery; *5*, carotid sinus; *6*, carotid baroreceptors; *7*, carotid sinus nerves; *8*, glossopharyngeal nerves. *A*, aortic bodies; *B*, carotid bodies. (Kindly drawn by R. H. Phibbs.)

ographical separation of a pressor area (rostral two thirds of the medulla) and a depressor area (caudal one third of the medulla). Destruction of the pressor centers abolishes vasoconstrictor effects of the carotid sinus reflex but leaves intact the depressor effects on the heart, while destruction of the depressor centers leaves the pressor reflex mechanism intact. However, although there may be an anatomical separation of those pressor and depressor areas, there is no doubt that the two centers are reciprocally innervated and that, physiologically, excitation of the pressor area is accompanied by inhibition of the reciprocal center.

[▶It must not be thought that the vasomotor center is active only in response to the afferent impulses of the buffer reflexes or to impulses from higher centers. It is believed that the cells of the center are in continuous rhythmic activity, which is merely modified by the arrival of afferent impulses concerned with vasomotor reflexes. This is a very usual concept about brain centers, although it becomes very difficult to prove that any center or centers would be in spontaneous activity if all impulses from outside of them were cut off. The volume on neurophysiology* in this series deals more adequately with this matter. Certainly, with regard to the buffer reflexes of blood pressure, it is clear that there is continuous depressor efferent activity in the vagus which is increased if the baroreceptors fire more often in response to a rise of blood pressure. Would there be any cardiac vagal tone if there were no firing at all from the baroreceptors, when the arterial pressure was below the threshold level? The answer is not really known or, if it were known, interpretable, for reflex activity of the chemoreceptors and a host of other contributory reflexes would have to be considered.◀]

_____
*Eyzaguirre, C.: *Physiology of the Nervous System* (Chicago: Year Book Medical Publishers, Inc., 1969).

The Efferent Areas and Effector Mechanism of the Reflex

The efferent response of the vasomotor center to the baroreceptor sensory input is multiple but can conveniently be divided into two categories: the cardiac and the peripheral vasomotor effects (Fig. 21–5).

CARDIAC EFFECTOR MECHANISM

The cardiac effector mechanism is mainly depressor, through the vagal fibers to the heart; but it is also depressor through reciprocal activity of the cardiac sympathetic accelerator nerves, for the *cardioinhibitory center* and the nearby *cardioaccelerator center* (parts of the general medullary vasomotor area) are reciprocally connected, increased activity of one being accompanied usually by decreased activity of the other. While in the normal physiology of an animal at rest there is always cardioinhibitory activity in the vagus (cutting the vagi produces an increased heart rate), there appears to be little tonic activity in the cardiac accelerator fibers (cutting them does not usually slow the heart). The efferent impulses from the buffer reflex travel down the vagi, through the cardiac branches of the nerve, to the heart itself. Their relay station is in minute parasympathetic ganglia in the walls of the two atria. The relatively short postganglionic fibers end in the heart tissue of the atria, sinoatrial node and ventricles. Their action on the heart is by slowing the intrinsic rhythm of the cardiac pacemaker. As one might expect, from the position of the pacemaker in the right atrium, stimulation of the right vagus is more effective in slowing the heart than stimulation of the left vagus.

The mechanism by which impulses in the cardiac vagus nerves decrease the heart rate is of great historical importance in physiology, for here is where Otto Loewi (in 1921) discovered the first neurohumoral transmitter, in *acetylcholine*, which he noncommittally called *Vagus-Stoffe*. Later research by Sir Henry Dale and his many coworkers has given us a great deal of information on this and on other chemical substances liberated at nerve endings.

Loewi worked with isolated beating hearts of frog and of toad, perfused with Ringer's solution. Electrical stimulation of the attached vagus nerve produced a slowing, and a decrease in amplitude, of the heartbeat. He collected the perfusing solution that had been in contact with the heart during a period of vagal stimulation and found that when substituted later for new Ringer's solution it produced a slowing of the heartbeat (without any more vagal stimulation). Obviously, some substance had diffused out into the fluid (presumably from the parasympathetic nerve endings) which later could produce a depression of heart rate and force, and Loewi postulated that it was through

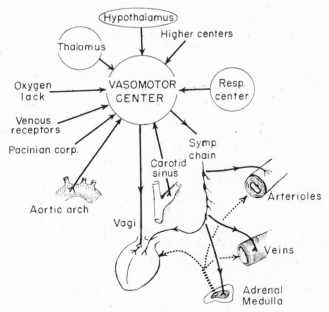

Fig. 21-5.—Schematic diagram of the pathways of the carotid sinus-aortic reflex. Only the pathways are shown, not the details of the neuronal connections.

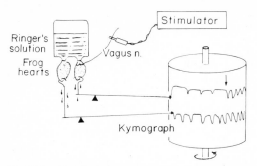

Fig. 21-6.—Sketch of the method used by Loewi to demonstrate the chemical transmission of vagal effects. On stimulation of the vagus of one heart, the other also shows a slowing.

this chemical mediator that the normal activity of the nerves produced their effect. A later, dramatic demonstration of this is illustrated in Figure 21–6, where two frog hearts are connected to outlets of the same reservoir of Ringer's solution. Stimulation of the vagus nerve to one heart slows not only that heart but also the second heart. It is only by diffusion of a humoral substance from the stimulated heart into the reservoir that this could have occurred.

We can today identify the *Vagus-Stoffe* of Loewi as acetylcholine, and we know that this is the mediator of parasympathetic nervous action. It is present in the nerve endings, probably in submicroscopic vesicles (seen in electron micrographs) whose contents, when the nerve impulse arrives, are liberated from the nerve endings to act on the tissue (e.g., the pacemaker cells) in the area. Acetylcholine is liberated at the endings of the parasympathetic postganglionic nerves (such as the vagus) and at the motor endplates of skeletal muscle, and it also is the transmitter in sympathetic ganglia (i.e., liberated from the preganglionic sympathetic endings). It may play the role of transmitter in many other places not yet demonstrated.

It is interesting that physiologists have found it very difficult to demonstrate to students the simple, dramatic experiments of Loewi exactly as he performed them. Acetylcholine, when liberated, is rapidly destroyed by a specific enzyme *(cholinesterase)*, which is always found in the tissues at the parasympathetic endings. In fact, the presence of cholinesterase, demonstrated by histological staining, is taken to indicate that nerve endings are *cholinergic*. The physiological role of cholinesterase is to terminate the action of the released acetylcholine so that it is not unduly prolonged

and moment-to-moment effector control is possible. The presence of cholinesterase makes the liberation of acetylcholine into the perfusate difficult to detect, unless there is either a very short time for the destructive enzyme to work or the enzyme is inhibited by adding the drug *neostigmine* or *eserine*. Later workers always used such cholinesterase inhibitors, so that quantitative assays of the amounts of acetylcholine released by known amounts of stimulation, or in reflex activity, could be made. *Atropine* blocks the action of the liberated acetylcholine and therefore produces an increase in heart rate of a resting human subject, another proof that there is normally vagal depressor tone.

The cardiac effector mechanism of the carotid sinus reflex, by vagal control, is both *chronotropic* (altering the heart rate) and *inotropic* (altering the strength of the heartbeat). The latter is obvious when the effects of vagal stimulation on isolated frog hearts are observed; but in the intact mammalian heart it is more difficult to prove, since the effects of change of heart rate on the filling of the heart, by Starling's law, will themselves alter the strength of the heartbeat. However, when these factors are separated, as in the work of Sarnoff on the ventricular performance curves, the negative inotropic effect (weakening) of vagal impulses is proved (Chapter 16, Fig. 16–2). The weakening of the ventricular contraction on vagal stimulation is due to the release of acetylcholine at the parasympathetic endings in the ventricular walls.

The efferent pathway of the cardiac reflex via the sympathetic system is from the medullary cardiac accelerator center via the spinal cord, emerging at different levels to synapses in the sympathetic chain. Thence the postganglionic fibers proceed by the cardiac accelerator nerves to end in the heart tissue. Their action there is mediated by the release of *noradrenaline*, which is the neurohumor of sympathetic nerve endings *(adrenergic)*, just as acetylcholine is the neurohumor of parasympathetic endings. Again there is a double effect—chronotropic in an acceleration of the pacemaker and positively inotropic in an increased force of ventricular contraction (by action on ventricular muscle).

The sympathetic outflow also is to the adrenal medulla, and if the blood pressure falls markedly there is, by the carotid sinus reflex, a discharge of *adrenaline* (with some noradrenaline) from the gland into the venous circulation, which carries it to the heart and there produces cardiac acceleration and increased strength of heartbeat. Probably the direct action on the heart of cardiac accelerator nerves is the important effector mechanism (with the vagal tone) in homeostasis of blood pressure in the normal range of physiological regulation, but it is reinforced by circulating adrenaline in severe hypotensive crisis. [▶No controlling destructive enzyme for the noradrenaline released by the cardiac sympathetics (analogous to cholinesterase for acetylcholine) has been completely identified, although the enzymes *monoamino oxidase* and *O-methyl transferase* have often been suggested. The matter is still controversial.◀]

NONCARDIAC EFFECTOR MECHANISM

The noncardiac effector mechanism affects the activity of the sympathetic outflow on the blood vessels (vasoconstriction), increasing the peripheral vascular resistance in response to a threatened fall of arterial blood pressure. A strong vasoconstriction in the arterioles of the digits is seen when a subject is tilted from the horizontal toward the vertical; this vasoconstriction, with the increase of heart rate and force, may actually overcompensate, so that the blood pressure rises instead of falling. The administration of a chemical vasodilator drug, such as sodium nitrite under the tongue or sniffing amyl nitrite, produces a complete temporary cessation of blood flow in the fingers. These are evidences of the peripheral effector mechanisms of the carotid sinus reflex. Details of the control of peripheral blood vessels are given in Chapter 23.

In discussing the carotid sinus and aortic reflexes, it is a mistake to think of only the sympathetic vasoconstriction of the arterioles as increasing the peripheral resistance. Heymans and Neil (1) emphasize that the increase in tone of the walls of the venous system (venimotor tone), preventing shifts of blood volume rather than changing peripheral resistance, is just as important in the carotid sinus reflex, particularly in compensating for postural changes in blood pressure. Most of the blood volume is in the veins, and a very slight change in their tone will be as effective in preventing pooling of blood in the dependent limbs as a large change in the caliber of the arteries and arterioles. The venous vessels are richly innervated by the sympathetic system, although detailed study of their activity is still lacking. (The venimotor system is still the neglected field of research on the circulation.)

Relative Importance of Cardiac and Peripheral Effector Systems

There is no doubt that, in the homeostasis of blood pressure, the relative importance of the effector mechanisms on the heart and on the peripheral blood vessels is very different in different species. In animals that do not assume the upright posture, the cardiac effects are probably the more important; in man, the peripheral effects are probably just as important. It is easy to misinterpret the result of research on this point in man unless the whole homeostatic, cybernetic mechanism is kept in mind. [▶For example, Shepherd and Roddie (6) ingeniously investigated the effect of stimulation of the carotid sinus reflex in man by blowing up a pneumatic cuff round the neck of their subjects and by manual compression of the carotid arteries, so lowering the pressure in the carotid sinus. There were marked increases in heart rate but insignificant changes in forearm blood flow, which they were measuring plethysmographically. It must not be concluded from this that, in the normal buffer reflex, an increase in peripheral resistance and of tone of the veins is not important. The information to the brain as to the level of blood pressure comes from two main sources—the carotid sinus baroreceptors and the aortic baroreceptors—as well as from many widely scattered "outposts" of the reflex. What is the homeostatic mechanism to do when contradictory information arrives at the center (e.g., that the blood pressure has fallen [from the signals of the carotid sinus], yet that it has risen [from the aortic arch receptors])? We never get a true picture of the operation of a complicated homeostatic mechanism by dissecting it into isolated parts. Also, muscular blood flow is not a good index of vasoconstrictor activity, which is much greater in the skin vessels.◀]

Influence of Higher Centers: Temperature Regulation, Emotions, Response to Startle

The vasomotor center is influenced continuously by impulses from the *temperature-regulating center* in the *hypothalamus,* for a large part of the mechanism of regulation of deep-body temperature to a remarkably constant level is the adjustment of the peripheral circulation by vasomotor control. The skin temperature is thus altered, rising with an increase in blood flow to the skin, falling with a vasoconstriction of skin vessels; the *heat loss of the body* correspondingly increases or decreases. It is remarkable that these two homeostases, of arterial blood pressure and of deep-body temperature, which make use of a common effector mechanism of vasomotor control of peripheral vessels, are yet able to achieve independently the constancy of their particular controlled variable. The mean resting arterial blood pressure is very little altered in hot environments versus cold environments, in spite of a great difference in vasomotor tone of the skin, which are fully dilated in the hot environment and greatly constricted in the cold. A difference in the arterial pressure is seen in the pulse pressure, which tends to increase, mainly by a decrease in the diastolic level in thermally induced dilatation (e.g., 120/80 to 120/70). This reflects the decrease in peripheral resistance offered by the dilated vessels. A limitation in the capacity of the carotid sinus reflex to compensate for changes of posture is, however, seen, for in extreme heat, fainting from immobile standing, where the muscle pump is not operating, occurs much more often.

There is a close interaction between the vasomotor center in the medulla and the *respiratory centers.* Acute anoxia, which acts primarily through the chemoreceptors of the carotid and aortic bodies upon the respiratory centers, increasing greatly the respiratory rate and depth, also produces a marked pressor effect. [►This occurs probably via the interaction of respiratory and vasomotor centers.◄]

Emotion obviously affects the vasomotor center, although we do not know the details of the neurophysiology of emotion. [►Probably the *hypothalamus*, which is the center concerned with the manifestations of emotion (e.g., anger, anxiety), sends impulses to the vasomotor center.◄] The influence on the buffer reflex is so strong that it may be overridden to a considerable extent, and the rise of arterial blood pressure in anger, in excitement and in anxiety states is considerable. (See quotation from *The Merchant of Venice* at the beginning of Chapter 20). Indeed, *the overriding, by emotion, of the protection afforded by buffer reflexes of the blood pressure is a much greater hazard to cardiac and hypertensive patients than indulging in normal physiological activity, such as mild exercise.*

The operation of the carotid sinus reflex is beautifully illustrated by the changes in heart rate that accompany *startle*, as in the case of a subject lying quietly and suddenly hearing a loud noise (Fig. 21–7). The response in heart rate, although very different in different subjects, always shows three phases. There is (*A*) an immediate speeding of the heart, undoubtedly due to a direct influence of the accelerator nerves to the heart, accompanied by inhibition of vagal cardiac impulses by reciprocal innervation of the centers; and (*B*) a modification or reversal of this acceleration of the heart rate by a slowing, probably due to the carotid sinus reflex in response to the rise of blood pressure following (*A*). If the startle is great

Fig. 21-7.—Records **(bottom)** of the changes of heart rate (a fall on the record indicates cardiac acceleration) on startling three normal subjects (at the moment marked by the arrow). A triple response (*A* and *C*, accelerations; *B*, a slowing) is always seen. **Top,** record of voltage between palm and upper arm, the psychogalvanic reflex *(PGR)*, recording discharge of the nerves to the sweat glands. **Center,** respiration. (From unpublished work of G. E. Hobbs and K. Ingram of the University of Western Ontario.)

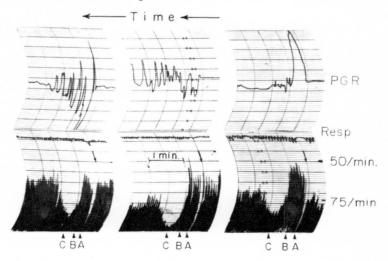

← T i m e ←

PGR

Resp

50/min.

75/min

C BA   C BA   C BA

enough, there is finally a long-lasting accelerator influence (*C*), strongly suggesting the effect of adrenaline released by the adrenal medulla from the sympathetic discharge in the splanchnic nerves.

The three phases can be of very different dominance, so that subjects can be found where cardiac slowing is actually the main response to startle. Presumably, these subjects have an extremely active carotid sinus buffer reflex. In others, the cardiac acceleration is so marked that the slowing phase (*B*) can hardly be detected.

Importance of the Buffering Action of the Reflex

Just how important the carotid sinus reflex is in reducing the large changes in arterial blood pressure that would otherwise occur is not appreciated until a patient who lacks the reflex is studied. Patients with the rather rare condition of classic orthostatic hypotension (7) show very little

change in vasomotor and cardiac activity upon change of posture, or the administration of peripheral dilator drugs (Figs. 21–8 and 21–9). In contrast, those with postural hypotension of other types, due to excessive vascular pooling of blood, show an exaggerated reflex response that still fails to maintain the level of the blood pressure (Fig. 21–9). A patient with the classic type (lacking the buffer reflex), if given a very minimal injection of adrenaline, will have a severe tachycardia and hypertension lasting many minutes, and, conversely, a profound hypotension when a dilator drug is given. Similarly, deeply anesthetized patients lack the buffering effect of the reflex, and changes in posture will produce very marked changes in arterial blood pressure. This is why operations under anesthesia (of the usual kind) are always done with the patient in the horizontal, or nearly horizontal, position, unless measures such as submitting the dependent legs to positive pressure, to prevent pooling of blood there, are used. Drugs having pressor or depressor effects

Fig. 21-8.—The response to change of posture from lying *(L)* to standing *(S)* in six normal subjects. The blood pressure changes very little, owing to the increase in heart rate and the increase in peripheral resistance, indicated by the de-

crease in finger blood flow (records of this by venous-occlusion plethysmograph are shown at top) and the narrowing of pulse pressure. (From Jeffers *et al.* [7].)

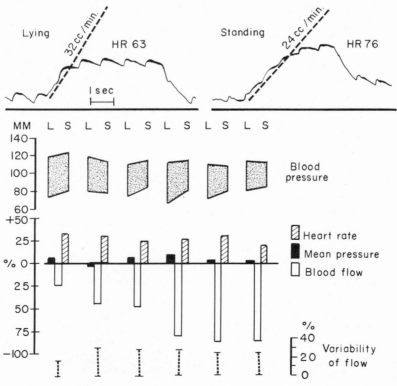

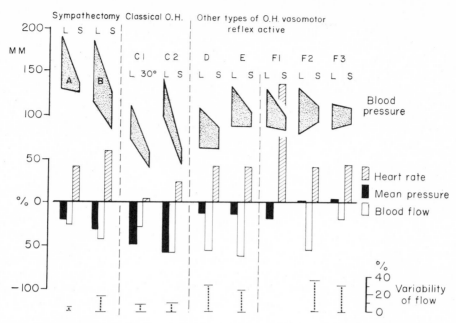

Fig. 21-9.—Similar to **Figure 21-8** but for different types of orthostatic hypotension. In sympathectomized patients *(A and B)* and in those with mechanical pooling of blood in the legs *(D, E* and *F)*, the cardiac reflex effects are exaggerated, yet the blood pressure falls. In the classic type *(C)*, the reflex is practically absent and the blood flow falls only in propor-tion to the fall of the blood pressure. **Bottom,** the per cent variability of flow (as the standard deviation of determina-tions made every 6 sec) also indicates the degree of activity of the sympathetic vasoconstrictor system. (From Jeffers *et al.* [7].)

should be given with great caution when the buffer reflexes are impaired. There is no adequate substitute for the reflex homeostasis of the circulation.

REFERENCES

1. Heymans, C., and Neil, E.: *Reflexogenic Areas of the Cardiovascular System* (London: J. & A. Churchill, Ltd., 1958).
2. Langren, S.: On the excitation mechanism of the carotid baroreceptors, Acta physiol. scandinav. 26:1, 1952.
3. Langren, S.: The baroreceptor activity in the carotid sinus nerve and the distensibility of the sinus wall, Acta physiol. scandinav. 26:35, 1952.
4. James, J. E. A.: The effects of altering mean pressure, pulse pressure and pulse frequency on the impulse activity in baroreceptor fibers from the aortic arch and right subclavian artery in the rabbit, J. Physiol. 214:65, 1971.
5. Langren, S.; Spoiekt, A. P., and Zotterman, Y.: Sensitization of baroreceptors of the carotid sinus by acetyl choline, Acta physiol. scandinav. 29:381, 1953.
6. Shepherd, J. T., and Roddie, I. C.: The effects of carotid artery compression in man with special reference to changes in vascular resistance in the limbs, J. Physiol. 139:377, 1957.
7. Jeffers, W.; Montgomery H., and Burton, A. C.: Types of orthostatic hypotension and their treatment, Am. J. M. Sc. 202:1, 1936.

22

Some Other Cardiovascular Reflexes

The Bainbridge Reflex

SOME GENERATIONS of medical students have been taught that of the cardiovascular reflexes the first to remember, if they wished to pass the course, was the carotid sinus reflex, and the second, the *Bainbridge reflex,* discovered in 1915. However, through the years since, repeated attempts to confirm the existence of the latter reflex—at least as its function was formerly interpreted—have failed, and only recently was the matter clarified.

Bainbridge showed that intravenous injection of blood or saline solution produced a tachycardia in dogs which was abolished by bilateral section of the vagi. This result was interpreted as evidence of a reflex, arising from stretch receptors on the venous side of the heart (probably in the atrium), which accelerated the heart and so relieved the venous congestion. As such, it seems an attractive "negative feedback" control mechanism. However, repeated studies on different species of animal failed to show the expected tachycardia consistently, while some studies even showed a bradycardia on distention of the vena cava and atria.

An article by Jones (1) finally elucidated the matter. It appears that venous distention from intravenous infusion may either increase or decrease the heart rate, depending on the existing level of that rate. Table 22–1 is taken from this article. If the heart rate of the dogs was below about 130 per min, which is said to be the optimal rate for maximal cardiac output in the dog, venous infusion caused acceleration of heart rate; if it were originally above 130 per min, then there was

TABLE 22–1.—CHANGE OF HEART RATE PRODUCED BY INTRAVENOUS INFUSIONS IN 47 DOGS WITH DIFFERENT INITIAL HEART RATES*

INITIAL HEART RATE (Beats/Min.)	NO. OF EXPERIMENTS SHOWING Tachy-cardia	No Change	Brady-cardia	% OF EXPERIMENTS SHOWING TACHYCARDIA	RATIO OF MEAN CHANGE OF HEART RATE TO RIGHT ATRIAL PRESSURE (Beats/Min. Cm H_2O)
<70	15	0	0	100	+5
70–90	24	4	0	86	+4
90–110	20	3	3	77	+3
110–130	18	10	3	58	+2
130–150	6	2	9	35	−1
150–170	6	10	9	24	−1
170–190	4	9	12	16	−2
>190	2	13	5	10	−2

The coefficient of correlation (r) of the initial heart rate with the percentage of experiments in which tachycardia occurred equals − 0.985.

---

*From Jones (1).

194

slowing. Thus, all the experimenters who found conflicting results can be satisfied that their experiments may have been valid.

The reflex, which must be very complicated, cannot be regarded as providing homeostasis of the venous pressure. Rather, it could represent a homeostasis of the heart rate, keeping it within the range where the heart is most efficient. Indirectly, if the cardiac output falls off at higher heart rates, there is a sense in which a homeostasis of venous pressure would result, for at high heart rates, venous distention slows the heart and would allow the more efficient pump to accept more blood from the veins and thus reduce the venous pressure. Students must still be taught about the Bainbridge reflex, but not in so unsophisticated a way.

Reflexes from Receptors in the Atria and Ventricles

The existence of receptors in the left atrium, pulmonary artery, pulmonary vein and both ventricles, which can, when stimulated by pressure (stretch) or by certain drugs, produce changes in heart rate and in peripheral resistance, cannot be doubted; but so far it has been impossible to suggest how these receptors function in physiological control of the circulation.

Aviado and his co-workers (2) (seven of them!) used cross-circulation techniques that isolated the right heart and the lungs, and they studied the effects on heart rate and cardiac output on changing the pressures. Increasing the perfusion pressure in the right heart caused bradycardia and systemic hypotension. The bradycardia was mediated by the vagus (inhibited by atropine), but the peripheral dilatation contributing to the hypotension was not inhibited. Vagotomy also abolished the reflex.

Increasing the pressure in the pulmonary artery also reflexly produced bradycardia, but not hypotension. However, other studies gave contradictory results. The evidence for pressoreceptors from the pulmonary veins and left atrium is more consistent and convincing (3). Rises of pressure produce bradycardia; that is, the reflexes are depressor.

Receptors also exist in the walls of the left ventricle, and increase in left ventricular pressure causes reflex slowing of heart rate and peripheral vasodilation. [►However, most of the work on these receptors, as of Dawes and Comroe (4), and of Paintal and his co-workers (if they are the same

reflexes), has been done using stimulation, not by pressure, but by alkaloid drugs (e.g., *veratrine*), and it is hard to see the physiological significance.◄]

Aviado has written a useful discussion (5) of these "controversial cardiovascular reflexes," pointing out that they share some common features: (*a*) that the organ containing the sensory receptors is also the responding organ (e.g., the names given to the reflexes could be "cardiocardiac," "intercoronary," "venoarteriolar," "interpulmonary" and "bronchobronchomotor") and (*b*) that there is a common pathway for the efferent and afferent arcs of the reflex. These features make the investigation of these reflexes difficult and the results hard to interpret.

[►It seems premature to discuss further the research being vigorously pursued, by many different workers, on receptors in the heart and lungs which can elicit reflexes changing cardiac activity and peripheral resistance (called *Bezold and Jarisch reflexes*). In many cases, these reflexes represent, apparently, cases of positive feedback. In our limited knowledge of the whole complicated system, it seems that they would tend toward instability, rather than stability, of the circulation. Again, some of the receptors found undoubtedly are concerned with regulation of blood volume rather than with regulation of the flow of blood and are dealt with in textbooks on kidney and body fluids. Local vascular reflexes from receptors in the lungs are important in the sequelae of embolism in small pulmonary blood vessels, where spasm of other pulmonary vessels and cardiac depression cause collapse of the systemic circulation and sudden death.◄] However, some cardiovascular reflexes from both deflation and inflation of the lungs have gained a new interest and importance because of modern work on diving and on high atmospheric pressures.

Reflexes from Inflation of the Lungs ("Selective Ischemia")

Studies of diving mammals by Irving and Scholander, and recently of diving man, have revealed cardiovascular reflexes that may be an important line of defense against death from asphyxia.

Irving (6) verified that seals can remain under water continuously for over 12 min, even with the vigorous muscular activity of swimming and the extra oxygen supply that this would demand. He measured the blood volume of the seal and its

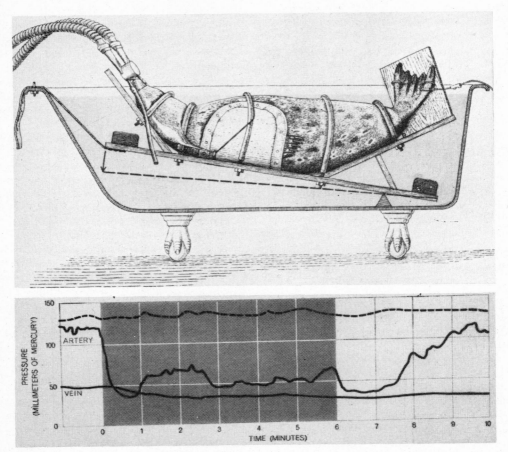

Fig. 22-1.—Top, apparatus for demonstrating the preferential ischemia reflex in a seal. **Bottom,** record showing that, when the board is lowered so that the head is under water, the pressure in a peripheral artery falls to a low level, while in a central artery it remains normal *(broken line)*. There is also a marked bradycardia. (From Scholander, P. F.: The master switch of life, Scient. Am., December, 1963, p. 92.) (Reprinted with permission. Copyright © 1963, by Scientific American, Inc. All rights reserved.)

oxygen-carrying capacity and was confronted with a mystery. The store of oxygen in the blood would suffice only for a few minutes at the normal metabolic rate of the animal; yet seals could easily remain, without any income of oxygen, for much longer periods than this.

The answer to the puzzle is that there is a drastic redistribution of cardiac output in diving mammals that takes place the moment the animal's head is under water (Fig. 22–1). Scholander (7) has written a popular account of this and suggests that, from modern work on divers, there is a similar set of reflexes in man. In the seal, the blood flow to the limbs and internal organs, such as the kidney and mesentery, is completely shut off, thus conserving the reserve of oxygen in the blood exclusively for the vital organs, the brain and heart. The heart simultaneously slows. The large oxygen debt incurred in the muscles by the underwater swimming is quickly made up when the animal comes to the surface. Curiously, a similar bradycardia develops in a flying fish when it is taken out of the water (diving in reverse).

In man, it has long been known that, when a deep breath is taken or the *Valsalva maneuver* is performed (expiratory effort against a closed glottis), the blood flow of the fingers and toes suffers an abrupt reduction, usually to zero, indicating a mass discharge of the vasoconstrictor system. Studies of pearl divers of northern Australia (8) have shown that they develop bradycardia in 20–30 sec after the dive. While the systolic pressure remains constant or rises, the absolute rate of fall of pressure in diastole greatly diminishes, indicating an increase in peripheral resistance (i.e., vasoconstriction). The lactic acid in the blood, an index of anaerobic metabolism of the muscles, does not rise during the dive (up to 2 min duration), but there is an acute rise during the recovery period. The blood flow in the calf of normal subjects abruptly decreases when the subject holds his breath—and more drastically if he puts his face in water. These facts strongly suggest that, in man, reflexes similar to those of diving mammals, elicited either by anoxia or by stretch receptors in the lungs, can shut off the circulation to the limbs. Scholander has given this the very descriptive name of *selective ischemia*. There is evidence that such shifts of circulation occur in asphyxia of the newborn, for, when breathing begins, lactic acid from the muscles suddenly floods the circulation.

It is to be noted that this pattern of reflex

circulatory adjustment, elicited by inflation of the lungs, immersion of the face in water and perhaps by anoxia, is very different from that of the buffer reflexes of the carotid sinus and aortic arch. In the former, peripheral vasoconstriction is accompanied by bradycardia, while in the buffer reflexes, peripheral constriction is accompanied by cardiac acceleration.

Local Reflexes from the Peripheral Venous System

Vascular surgeons dealing with arterial insufficiency in the limbs have long suspected that there must be some sort of reflex influence from the limb veins altering the vasomotor tone of the local arterial systems, because they encounter cases of pure spasm (e.g., of the femoral artery) where the only disease would appear to be in the

Fig. 22-2.—Mean blood flow in the toes of three supine subjects with change of posture of one leg *(solid line)* compared with other leg *(broken line)*, which was horizontal. Both raising above and lowering below the horizontal pro-

duce a decrease in flow. The decrease on lowering is interpreted as a reflex effect from distention of the veins. It was present after sympathectomy. From Gaskell and Burton [9].)

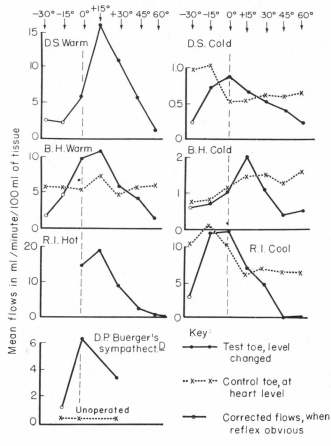

leg veins (phlebitis). There is a teleological argument for the existence of local control in the limbs, for, while the carotid sinus buffer reflex is well adapted to deal with changes of posture of the whole body (i.e., from lying to standing), it would not be suited to the situation where one leg was up, the other down (the *Folies Bèrgère syndrome*), which might result in inappropriate shifts of blood volume and of blood flow into individual limbs.

Evidence for these reflexes is supplied by study of the changes of flow in the toes when one leg only of a supine subject is elevated or lowered (9). Elevation of the limb results in a local decrease of flow (Fig. 22–2), which was expected because the transmural pressures of the resistance vessels (arterioles) are reduced by the hydrostatic factor (Chapters 9 and 10), and eventually *critical closure* occurs. However, one would expect that lowering the limb below the level of the heart might show either an increase in flow or no change—certainly not a reduction in flow. Yet there was consistent evidence of a decrease in flow on lowering the limb. Convincing evidence that the stimulus came from the distention of the leg veins was provided when it was noted that, in some subjects, returning the leg to the horizontal

did not restore the flow to normal until the leg was lifted momentarily and the veins were drained. Verification of the *venivasomotor effect* was provided in a study of the blood flow of the fingers, using negative tissue pressure (10) (negative pressure in the plethysmograph) as well as positive pressures (11) (Figs. 22–3 and 22–4). However the increase in transmural pressure and distention of the veins is accomplished, it elicits a vasoconstriction.

Such a *venous-arteriolar "reflex"* (or, better, "reaction") has been shown in dogs by Haddy and Gilbert. Again, in the kidney, any increase in venous pressure results in a marked decrease in blood flow, far greater than can be explained on the basis of the slightly reduced pressure gradient. [▶Although there can be no doubt as to the existence of these effects from veins to arterioles, their mechanism is not clear. In particular, the role of connections to the central nervous system is controversial; severing the central connections certainly modifies the effects, but they exist even when the tissues are isolated. A kind of *axon reflex* (i.e., transmission of an impulse from a sympathetic nerve ending up its parent nerve and retrogradely down another branch of this nerve to an ending elsewhere) is a possibility; but the axon

Fig. 22-3.—Change in blood flow of the fingers of four subjects when the tissue pressure is made negative (i.e., the transmural pressure is increased). The paradoxical decrease is attributed to a venivasomotor reflex. (From Yamada and Burton [11].)

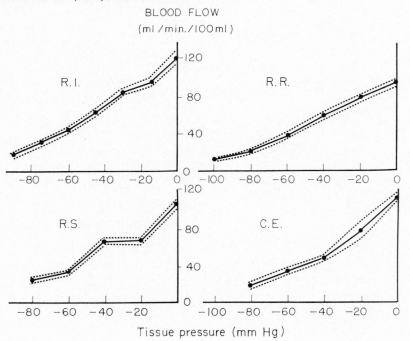

BLOOD FLOW
(ml /min./100ml)

Tissue pressure (mm Hg)

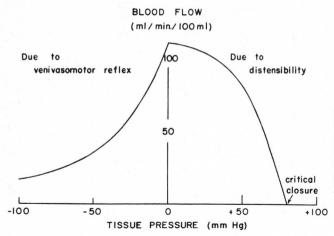

BLOOD FLOW
(ml / min./ 100 ml)

Due to
venivasomotor reflex

Due to
distensibility

100

50

critical
closure

-100   -50   0   +50   +100

TISSUE PRESSURE (mm Hg)

Fig. 22-4.—Schematic diagram showing the result of studies on effect of positive and negative tissue pressures on finger blood flow. Positive pressures lower transmural pressure and produce critical closure if the pressure is great enough. Negative pressures, by filling the veins, produce a reflex vasoconstriction, but never to the point of closure. (From Yamada and Burton [11].)

reflexes known to exist in the skin are dilator, not constrictor. One possibility is that the effects are mechanical rather than truly reflex. Any rise of venous pressure is accompanied by a very rapid increase in the formation of lymph from capillaries. If the microlymphatic channels around a tuft of capillaries come together in a lymphatic "cuff" around the metarteriole supplying that tuft, the rise of pressure here could reduce the size of that arteriole and be responsible for some of the effects seen. Probably this is the mechanism in the kidney, for, in such a rigidly encapsulated organ, any increase in edema fluid must "choke off" the arterial supply.◄]

Whatever the mechanism, venous-arteriolar local reflexes are well established. They are cybernetically most acceptable, as representing negative feedback, for if congestion of the veins increases the vasomotor tone of the arterioles, or mechanically reduces their radius, the congestion would be relieved as the outflow from the veins would exceed their inflow. A steady state would be quickly established. Moreover, it is the nature of such negative feedback that it can never lead to instability. For example, congestion of the veins could never, by this mechanism, close the arterioles completely. This feature was seen in the results cited. In contrast, complete critical closure of arterioles upon reduced transmural pressure does occur. Some investigators would interpret the results in terms of the *myogenic reflex of Bayliss*, but this reflex would show the characteristics of positive feedback rather than negative feedback.

[►Evidence is also being advanced of *veni-venomotor reflexes* (12). A segment of vein in the arms of human subjects was occluded by external clamping. Pressures in the occluded veins and in other, unoccluded veins were measured by using catheters connected to electromanometers. Venous congestion, produced by blowing up a cuff in the arm, evoked vasoconstriction (rise of pressure) in the hemodynamically isolated venous segment. Local anesthesia abolished the response. It is impossible that the results could depend on a myogenic reflex, for the isolated segment was not directly affected by the congestion of the remainder of the venous vessels.◄]

Local Reflexes from Sensory Endings (Axon or Lovén Reflexes)

Electrical stimulation of the cut central end of a sensory nerve from the skin often produces a local dilatation in the area which the nerve supplies, and it has been shown that impulses travel *antidromically* down other sensory nerves (emerging from the dorsal roots) to the specific area, producing the cutaneous vasodilation. A dilator substance—neither histamine nor acetylcholine, but possibly adenosine triphosphate (ATP)—is liberated at the sensory endings. This substance is a very powerful vasodilator of peripheral vessels. [►However, it is debatable that there is a physiological counterpart of this wrongway conduction in sensory nerves, produced by strong electrical stimulation.◄]

Antidromic conduction that is more local is indicated, however, in the famous *triple response of skin* to local injury, described by Sir Thomas Lewis. Local injury, such as is caused by stroking the skin, is followed by:

1. A line of pallor along the path of the instrument *(the white line)*. This is still said to be due to capillary constriction (although now no one believes that capillaries are capable of active vasoconstriction). The white line fades in about a minute.

2. Stronger pressure in the stroking produces a red line, followed by spread to neighboring areas of skin *(the red flare)*. [►This is due to arteriolar dilatation. It still occurs if the nerves to the skin have been cut, but not if there has been time for these to degenerate. It is therefore thought to be due to an axon reflex.◄]

3. If the stimulus is strong enough, a *wheal* due to local edema is later raised, and it persists for half an hour or more. [►This is thought to be due to the release of histamine or something similar (Lewis' H substance) by the injured tissue, which increases the permeability of the skin vessels to blood proteins.◄]

The triple response (line, flare, wheal) probably has little significance in normal physiology, but related phenomena are probably responsible for the increased local circulation in *inflammation*. Axon reflexes are probably involved, as well as Lovén-type reflexes elicited by sensory impulses (e.g., pain). [►While the classic interpretation of the triple response in skin has been taught to medical students as indicating certain properties of cutaneous arterioles and capillaries, modern knowledge puts much of the theory in doubt and it deserves new experimental investigation.◄]

General Reflexes from Somatic Afferents

The whole picture of circulatory responses to stimulation of somatic afferents, from muscle and skin, has been studied by Johansson (13). At low frequencies of stimulation, the effects were mainly depressor, with fall of blood pressure, slowing of the heart and peripheral vasodilation. This is called the *somatic depressor reflex*. High-intensity, high-frequency stimulation, presumably imitating violent pain, however, produced pressor, rather than depressor, responses. This is the *somatic pressor reflex*. Both reflexes were diffuse in their effect, although the kidney vessels showed a response to the high-intensity stimulation only. The reflexes probably are through the depressor and pressor centers in the medulla.

There is no doubt that many more reflexes regulating the blood flow of the tissues in man await discovery, and chapters on this subject in future textbooks will have to be much longer.

REFERENCES

1. Jones, J. J.: The Bainbridge reflex, J. Physiol. 160:298, 1962.
2. Aviado, D. M., Jr.; Li, T. H.; Kalow, W.; Schmidt, C. F.; Turnbull, G. L.; Peskin, G. W.; Hess, M. E., and Weiss, A. J.: Respiratory and circulatory reflexes from the perfused heart and pulmonary circulation of the dog, Am. J. Physiol. 165:261, 1951.
3. Daly, I. de B.; Ludaney, G.; Todd, A., and Verney, E. B.: Sensory reception in the pulmonary vascular bed, Quart. J. Exper. Physiol. 27:123, 1937.
4. Dawes, G. S., and Comroe, J. H., Jr.: Chemoreflexes from the heart and lungs, Physiol. Rev. 34:167, 1954.
5. Aviado, D. M.: Some controversial cardiovascular reflexes, Circulation Res. 10:831, 1962.
6. Irving, L.: Respiration in diving mammals, Physiol. Rev. 19:112, 1939.
7. Scholander, P. F.: The master switch of life, Scient. Am., December, 1963, p. 92.
8. Scholander, P. F.; Hammel, H. T.; de Messurier, H.; Hemmingsen, E., and Garey, W.: Circulatory adjustments in pearl divers, J. Appl. Physiol. 17:184, 1962.
9. Gaskell, P., and Burton, A. C.: Local postural vasomotor reflexes arising from the limb veins, Circulation Res. 1:27, 1953.
10. Yamada, S.: Effects of positive tissue pressure on blood flow of the finger, J. Appl. Physiol. 6:495, 1954.
11. Yamada, S., and Burton, A. C.: Effect of reduced tissue pressure on blood flow of the fingers; the veni-vasomotor reflex, J. Appl. Physiol. 6:501, 1954.
12. Wallis, W.; Borenman, R., and Honig, C. R.: A veni-venomotor response to local congestion, J. Appl. Physiol. 18:593, 1963.
13. Johansson, B.: Circulatory responses to stimulation of somatic afferents, Acta physiol. scandinav. (supp. 198) 57:1, 1952.

23

Mechanism of Control of Peripheral Blood Vessels

The Three Possible Effector Mechanisms

THREE WAYS have been suggested by which the effector mechanism of the central cardiovascular reflexes might change the resistance of vascular beds:

1. *Local release of noradrenaline* (and possibly adrenaline) at the sympathetic nerve endings, in the immediate vicinity of vascular smooth muscle, causing its contraction.

2. *The release of adrenaline (and possibly noradrenaline) by the adrenal medulla.* The substance released upon arrival of the impulses in the sympathetic splanchnic nerves circulates and causes contraction of *distant* vascular smooth muscles. This action of adrenaline as a hormone is well established.

3. *The distant effects of noradrenaline* (and possibly adrenaline) that is released at sympathetic nerve endings, and then circulates to produce effects on distant vascular smooth muscle. This was suggested by W. B. Cannon, a pioneer in research on the action of sympathetic nerves. He called the humoral substance mediating the nervous action *sympathin* and distinguished an excitatory vasoconstrictor substance, *sympathin E,* now to be associated with noradrenaline, and an inhibitory (on some organs) substance, *sympathin I,* which would, to some extent, now be associated with adrenaline. This third mechanism, the distant action of noradrenaline released from nerve endings, is now largely discounted, and it seems that the action of a "sympathin" is confined to the immediate neighborhood of the endings themselves.

Celander (1) directly compared relative effec-tiveness in causing vasoconstriction in muscle, in skin and in kidney blood vessels of the cat (as well as dilation of the iris and contraction of the nictitating membrane), by the following methods:

a) The intrinsic sympathetic nerves to the organs or tissue were stimulated at different frequencies of maximal electrical stimuli.

b) The sympathetic splanchnic nerves to both adrenal glands were similarly stimulated, causing secretion of adrenaline (and some noradrenaline).

c) Different concentrations of adrenaline were infused intravenously.

d) Different concentrations of noradrenaline were infused intravenously.

The results are shown in Figures 23–1 and 23–2. The results on different target organs all show the following common features:

1. In every case the greatest effectiveness was shown by stimulation of the intrinsic sympathetic nerves, in that the maximal vasoconstrictor effect exceeded that produced by the other methods.

2. Infusions of adrenaline were slightly more effective than those of noradrenaline, for the same concentrations, in producing vasoconstriction in renal and skin vessels. [►Results in the literature and on other organs are controversial on this matter, noradrenaline being sometimes considered to be the more effective vasoconstrictor agent.◄]

3. On muscle vessels, the effects of stimulating the sympathetic nerves and of infusion of noradrenaline were purely vasoconstrictor; while stimulating the adrenal medulla to secretion, or infusion of adrenaline, has a dilator effect at low frequencies of stimulation, or with low concentrations of infusion, but a constrictor effect for higher frequencies or concentrations.

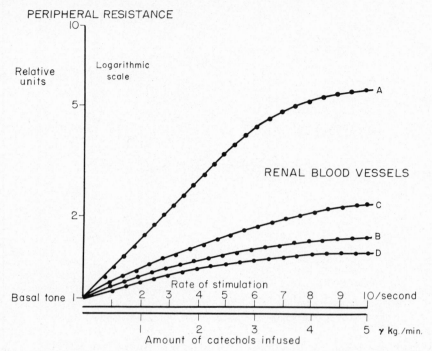

Fig. 23-1.—Relative effectiveness of *(A)* electrical stimulation of vasoconstrictor nerve fibers to the kidney or *(B)* to both adrenal medullae, *(C)* infusions of l-adrenaline and *(D)* infusions of l-noradrenaline. (From Celander [1].)

Fig. 23-2.—Blood vessels of muscle. *A,* electrical stimulation of sympathetic vasoconstrictor nerves to muscle. *B,* to both adrenal glands. *C,* l-adrenaline. *D,* l-noradrenaline. Note the dilation effect of adrenaline at low concentrations, absent for noradrenaline. (From Celander [1].)

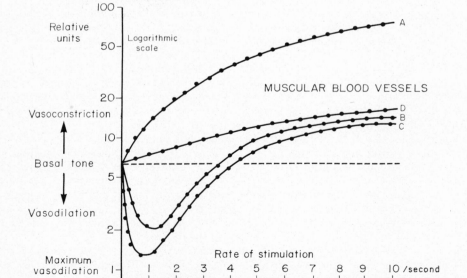

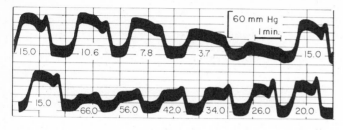

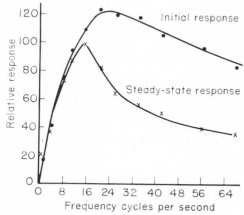

Fig. 23-3.—**Top,** the increase in resistance (from the rise in arterial pressure, using a constant flow pump) produced in the vascular bed of the isolated rabbit ear (electrical stimulation of the nerve plexus on the central artery). Time runs from right to left. There is a spike response, due to constriction of the arteriovenous anastomoses, followed by a steady-state response, due to constriction of metarterioles. **Bottom,** dependence of effect on frequency of stimuli. (From Stinson [3].)

4. The maximal effects of stimulation of the sympathetic nerves are at a frequency of between 10 and 15 stimuli per sec. There is much other evidence that the impulse frequency in the sympathetic vasoconstrictor system is very low (2) (i.e., 2–3 impulses per sec) and that the full range of physiological effect is obtained by frequencies up to 10 impulses per sec (3). Higher frequencies actually produce less response (Fig. 23–3).

As to the third possibility listed—that is, the action of noradrenaline from nerve endings as a circulating hormone (sympathin E) producing distant effects—this seems to have been eliminated as a possibility by Celander. He used the denervated nictitating membrane of the cat as a very sensitive indicator of circulating adrenaline or noradrenaline. In spite of massive stimulation of the sympathetic chains, plus the splenic and the renal nerves, no effect on the nictitating membrane of the same animal (cat) was observed in 18 experiments. Yet intravenous injection of as little as 0.1 μg of adrenaline or noradrenaline caused the membrane to contract. Evidently there is local destruction of the sympathetic neurohumor, at the place where it is released from the nerves, by an enzyme (monoaminoxidase or 0-methyltransferase). "Circulating sympathin" is, then, of little or no physiological importance. Indeed, it would be most inconvenient if it were.

Adrenaline and Noradrenaline

Modern knowledge of adrenaline and noradrenaline is largely based on the work of von Euler (4), for which he received the Nobel Prize.

Noradrenaline and adrenaline are chemically very closely related phenolic-alkyl amines (synonyms: norepinephrine or arterenol, and epinephrine). Noradrenaline differs from adrenaline only in having no methyl group on the phenol ring; hence the name "no-R(radical)-adrenaline."* Electron microscopy has shown that adrenaline and noradrenaline are stored in the adrenal gland, and in sympathetic nerve endings, as *chromaffin granules* of an average size of 0.3–0.4 μ. The active substance is enclosed within a membrane. The contents of the granules can be released by various procedures. After prolonged stimulation of the splanchnic nerves to the adrenals, the granules can be seen to be pale and empty, and often are fragmented, at the membrane of the cells. [▶How the nerve impulse causes release of noradrenaline and adrenaline is not known, although Ca^{++} ions probably play a mediating role, as they do in muscle.◀] From both cat adrenal glands, Celander found, by assay against injected noradrenaline, that about 5 μg per min per 1 kg of

*This is a convenient mnemonic, not a scholarly translation of the German "N (nitrogen) ohne Radikal."

TABLE 23–1.—VASCULAR EFFECTS ON CIRCULATION OF DIFFERENT VASCULAR
BEDS OF ADRENALINE (A) AND NORADRENALINE (NA)*†

| HORMONE | ORGAN | | | | | | |
	Coronaries	Muscle	Skin	Lung	Liver	Brain	Kidneys
NA	D?	C	C	C	0–C	C	C
A	0–D	D–C	C	C?	D	0	C

*According to von Euler.
†C = constrictor, reducing blood flow; D = dilator, increasing blood flow; 0 = no effect.

cat was released for a frequency of 10 impulses per sec.

Von Euler assayed the content of noradrenaline, as well as of adrenaline, in the adrenal glands of many species. In man, only about 15–20% is noradrenaline; but in cats (including one lion!), it was up to 50% of the total catecholamines. Tumors of the adrenal (pheochromocytomas) usually are very high in noradrenaline, rather than in adrenaline.

In nerves, the highest content of catechols is found in the endings, compared with the nerve trunks, and it is almost exclusively noradrenaline, with adrenaline and dopamine only in minute amounts.

The physiological actions of noradrenaline and adrenaline are very different. [►*Noradrenaline is a pure vasoconstrictor substance*, for it either causes vasoconstriction or has little or no effect on all types of blood vessels.◄] *In contrast, adrenaline is a constrictor on skin and kidney vessels but a dilator, in low concentrations, on muscle vessels, on the liver vessels and on the coronary circulation.* With high concentration of adrenaline, the effect may become constrictor. Indeed, certainly in man (from the work of Barcroft and Swan [5]), the intravenous infusion of adrenaline always lowers the *total* peripheral resistance. It is a mistake to think, then, of adrenaline as, over all, a vasoconstrictor substance. The dilator effect on muscle, which makes up 50% or more of the total body weight in most animals, overshadows the constrictor effects on skin, kidney, etc.

Adrenaline is a hormone with important metabolic effects as well as vascular effects, whereas noradrenaline appears to have no metabolic effects. The dilator effects of adrenaline are thought to be related to its metabolic effects. Whole systems and theories of action of the catecholamines have been built (as by Ahlquist, Burn, etc.) on the existence of more than one type of receptor in smooth muscle, vascular or visceral (α and β receptors, and "indifferent receptors" in all

tissues), but discussion of these is more suited to textbooks of pharmacology.

Table 23–1 gives a summary of some of the vascular effects of adrenaline and noradrenaline that have been measured.

On the isolated heart, noradrenaline produces acceleration, as does adrenaline more strongly; but in the intact animal, noradrenaline usually produces bradycardia, probably because of the vagal slowing by the carotid sinus reflex as the response to the rise of blood pressure. Injection of adrenaline produces cardiac acceleration in the intact animal, probably because the rise of blood pressure and the reflex elicited are much less.

Adrenaline and noradrenaline are very quickly taken up or destroyed in passing through peripheral vascular beds, for *intra-arterial injection*, in contrast to intravenous, usually produces very little cardiac effect, although marked effects are observed in the limb supplied by that artery. Evidently, there are very many receptor sites in the walls of the small blood vessels, some of which, when the catecholamines are "captured," produce contraction of smooth muscle, but others of which may produce no effects. [►This concept, due to Burn and Rand, helps explain the complicated interactions of adrenaline and noradrenaline with analogous drugs which, while not themselves active, can greatly modify the effects of adrenaline and noradrenaline. There is competition, with the active amines, between the "active" and "inactive" receptor sites. The field is so complicated that research pharmacologists will be kept happy arguing with each other for many years.◄]

Rhythmic Activity in the Sympathetic Vasoconstrictor System of Man

The best place to study the activity of the sympathetic vasoconstrictor system of man is in the digital circulation (fingers and toes), for the flow here is entirely through vessels of the skin (no muscle, no bone flow). Also, here the control by the nerves overshadows any direct chemical effect. For example, while a chemical dilator such

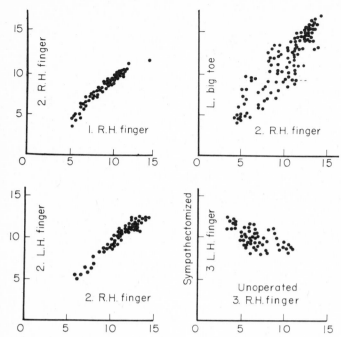

Fig. 23-4.—Proof that the sympathetic vasoconstrictor system acts en masse in its rhythmic activity. The amplitude of the volume pulsation in fingers and toes from moment to moment (in arbitary units on the graphs) is very highly positively correlated, except when a limb has been sympathectomized, in which case there is negative correlation (because the denervated vessels follow the changes of blood pressure produced by the rest of the vessels). (From Burton [6].)

as nitrite (sodium nitrite under the tongue or sniffing the vapor of amyl nitrite) produces a profound general vasodilation on many areas of the body (e.g., the blush area of the face, neck and upper thorax), the digital blood flow is drastically reduced. The fall of arterial pressure, produced by the vasodilation elsewhere, elicits the carotid sinus reflex, and the vasoconstrictor tone of the vessels is overwhelming.

The fluctuations in tone of the digital vessels is very easily recorded by the digital plethysmograph, which records the increased volume in the capillaries and venules due to the pulsation that persists even after passage through the resistance vessels, the arterioles. The amplitude of this finger-volume pulse greatly diminishes as the tone of the arterioles increases, and vice versa. Indeed, actual measurements of flow, by the venous-occlusion plethysmographic method, simultaneously with the finger-volume pulse, have established that the correlation with flow is very great (so long as venous pressure is not altered). The fluctuations in the magnitude of this volume pulse therefore can indicate the arrival of volleys of impulses in the sympathetic vasoconstrictor nerves (6).

Fig. 23-5.—Right, the rhythmic vasoconstrictions mediated by the sympathetic vasoconstrictor nerves of man, as recorded by the finger-volume pulse. *A–E,* the thermal state of the subject, from cold *(A)* to very warm *(E).* Dots over the records indicate transient cardiac accelerations accompanying the vasoconstrictions. **Left,** dependence of the rhythm on the environmental temperature. (From Burton and Taylor [7].)

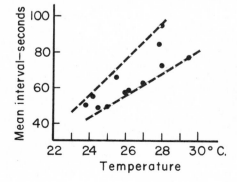

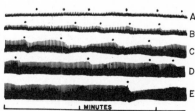

Such observations show that, physiologically, the system discharges en masse, for every one of the vasoconstrictions (decrease in volume pulse) of the fingers is accompanied by a correlated vasoconstriction in the toes, and also in many visceral vessels (Fig. 23–4). There is also a simultaneous, although often slight, increase in heart rate; so the cardiac sympathetics share in this *mass discharge*. By special methods, it can be shown that enough blood vessels constrict at the same time to cause a short-lasting rise of blood pressure. In a sympathectomized limb, the correlation is absent or negative; the vessels of that limb simply respond to the level of blood pressure.

The rhythm of vasoconstrictions, representing volleys in the nerves, varies from 5 or 10 per min. in vasoconstriction to as infrequently as 1 every 3–5 min in complete vasodilation. The chief determinant of this rhythm is the requirement for peripheral blood flow in the interests of temperature regulation; that is, in warm surroundings or with heavily insulated clothing, when heat loss threatens to fall below heat production, the vessels remain dilated for long periods with only an occasional vasoconstriction (Fig. 23–5). In the

cold, the volleys may occur at a rate up to 10 per min. In this case, the vessels have no time to dilate appreciably between volleys and remain in a state of vasoconstriction. (The rhythm can still be counted, however, by the rhythmic cardiac accelerations.)

We see, then, that at least in these digital vessels, the gradation of vasomotor tone is accomplished, not by a steady discharge in the sympathetic nerves, but by a rhythmic discharge, the frequency of which is modified to result in different degrees of average tone. Probably this rhythmic activity represents a characteristic of the vasomotor center, for a similar rhythm of afferent impulses (e.g., from fluctuations of skin temperature) does not produce such an effect (7). [►It is likely that the so-called *Traube-Hering waves*, which are rhythmical changes in arterial blood pressure (superimposed upon the respiratory fluctuations), reflect the same characteristic property of the centers.◄]

Active Vasodilation

There is no doubt that in the control of the caliber of the resistance vessels, modifications of

Fig. 23-6.—The relative ranges of vasoconstrictor and vasodilator tone in muscle and in skin vessels. The resistance for muscle vessels ranges from *A* under vasoconstrictor tone to *B* under active dilator tone. For skin vessels, it is from *C* under vasoconstrictor tone to the level of *D* when there is no vasoconstrictor tone. (From Celander and Folkow [8].)

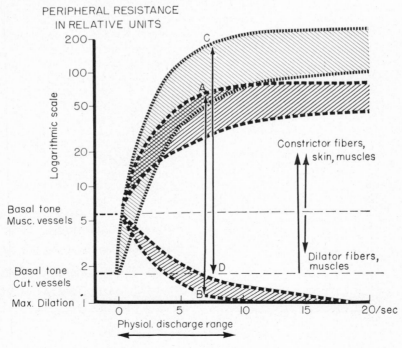

active vasoconstrictor tone dominate; that is, vasodilation may be considered as the result of inhibition of existing constrictor tone. However, after many years of research by Barcroft and Swan (5) and others, the existence of active neural vasodilator effects in man must be recognized. The proof depends largely on showing that interrupting the pathway of sympathic nerves (e.g., by sympathectomy or complete local anesthesia) results in a maximal blood flow in a limb that is not as great as was seen in maximal dilatation produced by reflex physiological means (as by exposure to heat). Interrupting the nerves removes the possibility of the effect of those nerves which cause active dilatation, as well as of those causing vasoconstriction.

In animals, such nerves have been found emerging from the dorsal roots, and electrical stimulation causes an extra dilatation even when vasoconstrictor tone is absent. In muscle, electrical stimulation of sympathetic nerves causes vasodilation. Figure 23–6 shows the relative importance of constrictor and active dilator nervous action in the vessels of muscle and skin of the cat (8). The *sympathetic dilator fibers* are cholinergic; so their action can be blocked by atropine. They seem to exist only to the muscle vessels, not to skin. *Parasympathetic dilator fibers* are well known to the tongue, salivary glands, external genital organs and possibly the bladder and rectum, that is, their distribution is cranial and sacral.

A new factor suggested in the mechanism of vasodilation is the polypeptide *bradykinin*, which is released during the activity of the thermal sweat glands (9) (it was discovered in connection with secretion of the salivary glands). [▶This is certainly a very potent vasodilator of peripheral vessels, and it may be physiologically important in thermal vasodilation (e.g., in hot environments). It apparently does not take part in the activity of carotid sinus buffer reflexes.◀]

Decline of Vascular Reactivity in Hemorrhagic Shock

The sequelae of hemorrhage, called *hemorrhagic shock*, have been a favorite topic and subject of research by physiologists for many years. [▶Success in understanding, particularly in understanding *irreversible shock*, has been astonishingly small; the elaborate theories centered on "vicious cycles" of a sequence of effects have very little basis in proved fact. For example, an increase in loss of blood proteins through the capillary wall is often included as a key step toward irreversibility; yet no convincing evidence that this actually occurs has been advanced.◀]

To study shock in animals, a major artery is connected to an external reservoir which may be set to a desired level above the heart of the animal which then bleeds into the reservoir until the mean blood pressure falls to the standard value represented by this level. Levels as low as 30–40 mm Hg for periods up to an hour are usually employed. The level of the reservoir is then raised, to reinfuse the blood back into the circulation, and the subsequent course of the blood pressure is then recorded. If the hypotensive level of blood pressure and the period of hypotension have not been too great, this reinfusion is followed by recovery of the animal and the normal blood pressure is maintained. If, however, they exceed critical values, the blood pressure is not maintained and progressively falls, even though all the original blood that was taken into the reservoir was returned eventually, together with added transfusions of blood. This condition is called "irreversible shock," and its counterpart is seen in patients who have suffered a considerable loss of blood.

There is no controversy as to the acute compensatory reactions that occur in response to hemorrhage. Because the capillary pressure falls below the standard 25 mm Hg that is in equilibrium with the colloidal osmotic pressure (see the volume on kidney and water balance,* especially regarding the Starling-Landis hypothesis), fluid will move from the tissues to the blood stream to make up the deficit of blood volume. This is proved by the hemodilution (fall of hematocrit) that follows hemorrhage. The compensatory effects of the carotid sinus reflex, in response to the hypotension, of intense peripheral vasoconstriction and of tachycardia, are also indisputable. The controversy centers on what factors eventually produce the irreversibility.

[▶It is reasonable to suppose that ischemia, and consequent anoxia, of certain tissues is responsible. But of what tissues—the peripheral blood vessel walls; some organ, such as the liver or kidney, which might produce a toxic circulating substance; the intestinal epithelium, invaded by anaerobic organisms producing an endotoxin; or possibly cells of the central nervous system? For many years the theory was that the liver put out a

---

*Pitts, R. F.: *Physiology of the Kidney and Body Fluids* (2d ed.; Chicago: Year Book Medical Publishers, Inc., 1968).

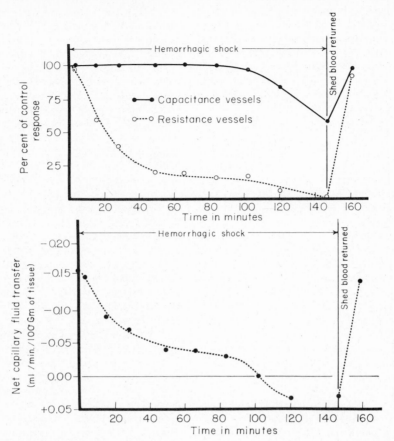

Fig. 23-7.—Top, the decline in reactivity (response to sympathetic stimulation) of the blood vessels of the hind limb of a cat produced by a period of hypotension. That of the capacitance vessels (venous vessels) was deduced from the decrease in volume of the limb on stimulation. **Bottom,** the net filtration from tissues to blood stream (in millimeters per minute per 100 Gm of tissue), which was deduced from the steady rate of change of limb volume. (From Mellander and Lewis [10].)

vasodilator material (VDM) that was to blame, but this theory is now no longer held, since VDM is identified with ferritin, and large amounts of ferritin can be injected into the circulation without any deleterious physiological effect. Invasion of the intestines and blood stream by anaerobic bacteria (clostridia) (theory of Jacob Fine) undoubtedly may be a factor, because intestinal blood flow here ceases (critical closure) in hypotension.◄]

It has recently been shown (10) that hypotensive shock results in a progressive loss of the reactivity of peripheral vessels to sympathetic stimulation of the precapillary "resistance vessels" and the postcapillary "volume vessels," both of which assist, by vasoconstriction, in the compensatory process (Fig. 23–7). The results applied to the blood flow in the hind parts of the cat (i.e., mostly muscle vessels), and stimulation of the lumbar sympathetic trunks was used to measure the reactivity of the vessels in terms of decrease in flow (increase in peripheral resistance). The movement of fluid into the blood from the tissues was also measured. As the period of hypotension progressed, this movement decreased until it actually reversed, that is, the blood was losing water to the tissues. On raising the blood pressure, reactivity and fluid shifts returned to normal; so the stage of irreversibility had evidently not been reached. It was noted that the decline in constrictor reactivity was much more rapid for the precapillary "resistance vessels" than for the postcapillary "volume vessels," and this could explain the change in fluid shift (net filtration transfer). If the precapillary resistance fell while the postcapillary resistance was maintained, the capillary pressure would rise and reverse the direction of filtration.

Research on the factors responsible for irreversible shock must continue, and probably a completely new approach is required. Certainly, a differential decrease in reactivity of the peripheral vessels, probably due to local anoxia, is an important factor.

Protective Agents against Shock

A great deal of research has been done by the standard method of lowering blood pressure to a standard level for a standard length of time, then determining how the subsequent course of recovery and irreversibility could be modified. The results are most confusing and very easily misinterpreted.

To physiologists brought up on the idea that the sympathetic nervous system has the function of equipping the animal for *fight or flight,* it is shocking to be told that sympathectomized animals, or those where the action of the sympathetic nerves have been blocked by drugs, withstand the shocking procedure remarkably better if the nerve blockade precedes the hemorrhage. Confusion is made worse by learning of the enthusiasm of many for treatment of *hypotensive shock* by infusion of noradrenaline or adrenaline, for this would seem to be based on an opposite idea to the use of blocking agents.

It is important to realize that the way in which hypotensive shock is usually studied in experimental laboratories makes the results, although valuable as basic information, very difficult to apply to the practical problem of treating patients who have suffered serious loss of blood, either by external hemorrhage or into their own traumatized tissues. Considering this, the experimental finding that blocking the sympathetic effects may give protection in experimental shock may be reconciled with the important physiological protection by the sympathetic system for animals in natural conditions.

An older method of studying hypertensive shock was to bleed the animal, withdrawing a standard percentage of his blood volume (say 20%), and then to follow the recovery. If the tests are done in this way, exactly the opposite result, as to the effect of blocking agents, is found; that is, the mortality is very greatly increased after sympathetic blockade! The explanation is simple. Removal of a standard percentage of the blood volume (or a standard volume of blood) produces a much more profound hypotension if the compensatory sympathetic reflexes are not operating than if they are. Thus it may be concluded that the apparent protection by sympathetic blockade from shock, given in the standard way of producing a given level of hypotension, is obtained simply because this level is reached after a very small blood volume has been lost, compared with animals without blockade. The animals with sympathetic blockade have suffered far less loss of blood volume.

The question is: What are the conditions that apply to patients in the hospital? To the animals in natural conditions, having to fight or flee, the maintenance of arterial blood pressure is vital. If the blood pressure falls enough to impair the function of the brain (and brain circulation is closely proportional to arterial blood pressure), the animal will lose the fight or be overtaken in flight. On the other hand, if the victim of hemorrhage is brought into the protected environment of a hospital ward, the level of arterial blood pressure may not be of such urgent vital importance. (In fact, arterial hypotension for short periods is used deliberately by surgeons to give them "bloodless fields.") Again, it would seem that, on the average, those brought to the hospital would have suffered a similar loss of blood volume, rather than had hypotension to a standard level. For these reasons, few would suggest that sympathetic blocking agents had any place in the treatment of shock. Of course, the *replacement of blood volume by transfusion with blood or blood substitutes* remains the keystone of treatment.

One change in the older teaching, found particularly in textbooks of nursing, must be made, that is, regarding the *dangers of heating the patient in hemorrhagic shock.* During World War I, it was advocated that soldiers found on the battlefield should at once be kept very warm, by heaters and blankets, and rushed into especially hot casualty wards. H. C. Bazett,* a medical officer in France at that time, concluded, on the basis of physiological knowledge and from personal observation, that this advice was completely wrong. He noted that the men who were bypassed and left in the cold of the battlefield made remarkably good recoveries, compared with those picked up immediately and kept very warm.

This is not to advocate the *use of cold in shock,* although hypothermia was used by the French authorities in transporting shock casualties to

---

*Personal communication.

hospitals in the war in Indochina, apparently with advantage. The paramount treatment remains the *replacement of blood volume* as soon as possible, after which it may matter little whether the patient is warm or cold. The emphasis should be on the dangers of heat for the patient *before* this replacement of blood volume has been made. The dangers of heating are much greater than of allowing the patient to be cold, even to the point of hypothermia. Overheating, especially the application of heat to the extremities, where the afferents from temperature receptors have most effect in temperature regulation, can inhibit the intense protective vasoconstriction which is produced by the buffer reflexes as a compensation for the fall of arterial pressure. This is a case of one homeostatic mechanism (that of temperature regulation) disastrously interfering with another homeostatic mechanism (that of arterial blood pressure). In normal physiology, such interferences between systems are remarkably few; but in abnormal physiological states, they may be fatal.

Sensitization after Denervation

W. B. Cannon enunciated a general law that, after the nervous connections to an effector organ are cut, the organ becomes more sensitive to its peculiar physiological stimulus (e.g., skeletal muscle becomes sensitized to circulating acetylcholine after its motor nerve is cut). The law has been shown to be very general. Sensitization occurs not only to the peculiar stimulus but to other types of stimulus also; for example, denervated cells in the central nervous system become sensitive not only to convulsant agents but to depressants also (Stavraky [11]).

[►The application of this law to denervation of vascular smooth muscle has not been so clear-cut. After sympathectomy, patients show a very great dilatation of the vessels in the denervated limb, but there is a partial restoration of the vascular tone in 6–12 weeks. The nature of this restoration is not understood. Reflex vasoconstriction or vasodilation is completely absent, or very slight if the sympathectomy has been adequate, and the patients suffer from postural hypotension (Chapter 21, Fig. 21–9). Astonishingly, Barcroft and Swan (5) have found that, in patients with complete lumbar sympathectomy, the reflex activity returns almost to normal some 9 months after the operation. It seems hardly possible that rein-

nervation by regeneration of neurons can have occurred. The facts must be accepted even though the mechanism is mysterious. A gradual return of the stores of catecholamines in heart, spleen, kidney, liver and salivary gland 2–4 months after sympathectomy has been shown in animals, but this store may not be directly involved in nervous control.◄]

A very complete review (citing 390 references) of the nervous control of the blood vessels has been written by Folkow (12).

REFERENCES

1. Celander, O.: The range of control exercised by the sympatho-adrenal system, Acta physiol. scandinav. (supp. 116) 32:1, 1954.

2. Folkow, B.: Impulse frequency in sympathetic vasomotor fibres correlated to the release and elimination of the transmitter, Acta physiol. scandinav. 25:49, 1952.

3. Stinson, R. H.: Electrical stimulation of the sympathetic nerves of the isolated rabbit ear and the fate of the neurohormone released, Canad. J. Biochem. & Physiol. 39:309, 1961.

4. von Euler, U. S.: *Noradrenaline: Chemistry, Physiology, Pharmacology and Clinical Aspects* (Springfield, Ill.: Charles C Thomas, Publisher, 1956).

5. Barcroft, H., and Swan, H. J. C.: *Sympathetic Control of Human Blood Vessels* (Physiological Society Monograph No. 1) (London: Edward Arnold, 1953).

6. Burton, A. C.: The range and variability of the blood flow in the human fingers and the vasomotor regulation of body temperature, Am. J. Physiol. 127:437, 1939.

7. Burton, A. C., and Taylor, R. M.: A study of the adjustment of peripheral vascular tone to the requirements of the regulation of body temperature, Am. J. Physiol. 129:565, 1940.

8. Celander, O., and Folkow, B.: A comparison of sympathetic vasomotor fibre control of the vessels within the skin and the muscles, Acta physiol, scandinav. 29:241, 1954.

9. Fox, R. H.; Goldsmith, R.; Kidd, D. J., and Lewis, G. P.: Bradykinin as a vasodilator in man, J. Physiol. 157:589, 1961.

10. Mellander, S., and Lewis, D. H.: Effect of hemorrhagic shock on the reactivity of resistance and capacitance vessels and on capillary filtration transfer in cat skeletal muscle, Circulation Res. 13:105, 1963.

11. Stavraky, G. W.: *Supersensitivity Following Lesions of the Nervous System* (Toronto: University of Toronto Press, 1961).

12. Folkow, B.: Nervous control of the blood vessels, Physiol. Rev. 35:629, 1955.

24

Local Autonomous Circulatory Control: Autoregulation, Reactive Hyperemia

Autoregulation

SOME CASES of what is called *autoregulation* of the blood flow of organs have already been discussed. That of the *coronary vessels* is a very good example (Chapter 17). Here the control is overwhelmingly by the level of oxygen tension reaching the tissues. If the demand for oxygen exceeds the supply, the oxygen tension of the tissues (as of the coronary vascular muscle) falls, and this automatically decreases vascular tone, so that the resistance to flow falls.

The case of *regulation of brain blood flow* is less dramatic. The vasomotor tone of intracranial arterial vessels seems to be far less, and far less variable, than that of peripheral vessels. Indeed, very little evidence of nervous vasomotor control has been found. Even perfusion with adrenaline and noradrenaline seems to have relatively little effect. [►It is thought that *serotonin*, known to be released in damage to blood platelets and probably from other cells, may have more effect.◄] As pointed out in Chapter 1, the requirements for energy, and thus for blood flow, of the brain are much less variable than for other organs. The carotid sinus reflex keeps the arterial pressure, which is the driving pressure for blood flow of the brain, at a constant value. This being so, a relatively constant resistance to flow of the cerebral vascular bed will insure the required constant flow.

The cerebral arterial vessels do, however, show a dilatation if the carbon dioxide partial pressure of the blood is increased, as has been demonstrated in man by arteriography. A reduction of oxygen tension is not markedly dilating; but increase of oxygen tension above that of air, as when pure oxygen is breathed, does tend to cerebral vasoconstriction ("oxygen poisoning").

Autoregulation of blood flow of the kidney is a puzzling case. The graph of flow versus driving pressure for the kidney is approximately linear, indicating a relatively constant resistance to flow except for a small passive decrease of resistance, due to distensibility as the transmural pressure rises with the arterial pressure. However, after the arterial pressure exceeds about 100 mm Hg, flow increases very little, even if the pressure is as high as 200 mm Hg. This indicates a progressive increase in resistance to flow as the pressure rises above 100 mm Hg, which could not possibly be a passive effect.

If the perfusing fluid of a kidney is changed from blood of normal hematocrit, when autoregulation is seen, to blood with lower hematocrit and finally to plasma or Ringer's solution alone, the feature of autoregulation described above becomes less and less marked. With zero hematocrit in the perfusate (i.e., plasma or Ringer's solution), there is no evidence of autoregulation at all, and the flow-pressure relation is approximately linear even up to very high arterial pressures. This was at first interpreted as evidence that the presence of red cells was necessary for autoregulation in the kidney and that these cells produced the effect by the anomalous character of the viscosity of blood (axial accumulation, etc.). However, this ingenious and plausible theory stimulated a great deal more research. When it was shown that, even with Ringer's solution as perfusate, autoregulation still occurred if the perfusate carried sufficient oxygen, the theory was discredited. This was accomplished by doing the experiment under several atmospheres of pressure of pure oxygen, so that the oxygen dissolved in the solution substituted for that carried by the red cells in blood. It is, therefore, not the physical, hemodynamic effects of the presence of red cells in the perfusate of the kidney that is necessary for autoregulation, but the oxygen-carrying capacity of the blood that the cells provide. (Curves of flow versus pressure for the kidney are given in the volume on kidney and water balance* in this series.) [▶The autonomous regulation of the kidney circulation thus appears to represent another case of regulation by the oxygen tension of the tissue cells. The puzzling feature is that it appears to operate only in a high range of blood pressure and of high blood flow, that is, above that of normal physiology. Reduction of blood flow of the kidney does not appear to cause vasodilation, but rather to elicit the production of pressor agents (e.g., angiotonin in the renal theory of hypertension) which increase the level of systemic blood pressure. This may result in increases in the blood flow in the particular kidney where ischemia was produced (e.g., by a Goldblatt clamp on the renal artery) and so achieve some local homeostasis of blood flow. However, this local homeostasis is achieved at the cost of eventual damage from hypertension to the rest of the vascular bed, including that of the other kidney. Perhaps the very great blood flow of the kidneys required for the excretion of urine, rather than for the metabolic needs of the kidney tissue (these would require much less than the actual flow), is so essential to the organism that this inconvenient noncooperative kind of autonomy is necessary.◀]

Reactive Hyperemia in Muscle Vessels

The classic example of local control of peripheral resistance to ensure a constant level of supply of oxygen is that of skeletal muscle, where measurements of flow are easily made, in man, by the use of the *venous-occlusion plethysmograph*. The history of this most useful method is to be found in a monograph by Barcroft and Swan (Chapter 23, ref. 5). A plethysmograph (fullness recorder) is simply a container in which a limb can be sealed by the use of a rubber sleeve at the entrance or,

more conveniently but not so accurately in practice, by a continuous rubber or plastic "skin" over the whole appendage. The increase of volume of that appendage (finger or toe, foot or hand, leg or arm) is recorded by the forcing of the air, or water, that fills the space in the plethysmograph outside the tissue into a volume recorder. It has been the custom to use water kept at a "physiological temperature" (e.g., 33° C) rather than to use air, although air transmission is much more convenient and the fears that it would introduce serious error due to changes of volume of air with temperature are, in practice, not justified. Instead of recording the changes of volume, the volume is sometimes kept constant and the small changes in pressure in the plethysmograph are recorded by sensitive electromanometers. This is convenient, but not so sound theoretically as recording the change of volume, keeping the pressure constant.

As long as there is a steady state of the circulation in the appendage, its volume will not change. If, however, there is a change in the tone of the blood vessels, the content of blood in the whole vascular bed (most of it is on the venous side) will alter, and this will be reflected as a change of volume recorded by the plethysmograph; that is, a vasoconstriction will be shown as a decrease in volume, a vasodilation as an increase. This use of the plethysmograph is informative, but only as to the changes in vascular volume; caution must be exercised in interpreting this in terms of changes of flow or of resistance to flow. For example, if the limb is lowered below the heart, the volume will increase, owing to extra filling of the veins under the hydrostatic factor, but the flow may, and usually does, decrease.

The addition by Brodie in 1905 of a cuff, just outside the plethysmograph, which, when inflated to pressures from, say, 10 mm Hg to 60 mm Hg, occluded the veins, makes it possible to measure the rate of arterial inflow unequivocally in milliliters per minute.

This venous-occlusion cuff must be inflated suddenly. Then, at that moment, outflow is prevented, and consequently the blood that flows in via the arteries must stay there, to increase the volume of the appendage. The volume record therefore shows a progressive rise, and the slope of this rise is a measure of arterial inflow (Fig. 24–1). Later, the rate of rise decreases, for two reasons: first, as the venous pressure dammed back behind the occlusion rises, the pressure gradient from the artery to this point decreases and the arterial inflow decreases accordingly;

---

*Pitts, R. F.: *Physiology of the Kidney and Body Fluids* (2d ed.; Chicago: Year Book Medical Publishers, Inc., 1968).

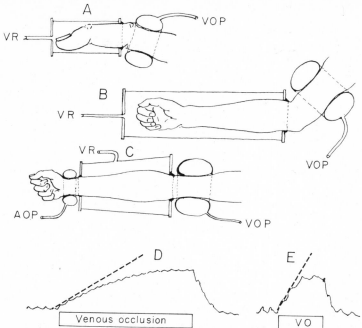

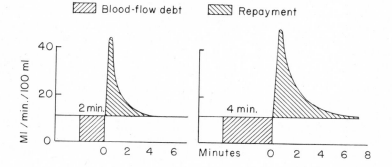

Fig. 24-1.—Illustrating types of plethysmographs for measuring blood flow by venous occlusion. **A,** for finger (skin flow). **B,** for lower arm plus hand. **C,** for forearm alone (mostly muscle flow). **D,** typical record of the changes of volume when the veins are occluded in hand or forearm. **E,** typical record for the finger, where the venous reservoir is much smaller and a new steady state is reached in a few heartbeats. The broken line is the initial tangent from which the rate of arterial inflow is estimated. *VR,* connection to volume recorder. *VOP,* connection to supply of venous-occlusion pressure (e.g., 60 mm Hg). *AOP,* to arterial-occlusion pressure (e.g., 160 mm Hg). *VO,* venous occlusion.

second, when the pressure in the veins behind the occlusion reaches that in the occluding cuff, or a fraction of a millimeter of mercury higher, the veins under the cuff begin to open, so that outflow is resumed. Soon the outflow increases to equal the arterial inflow (which will now be less than normal), at which time the volume of the appendage will no longer change; that is, a new steady state has been reached. It is the *initial rate of increase of volume* at the moment of venous occlusion that is a true measure of arterial inflow.

It was thought that it could be assumed that muscle flow made up about 70% of the total flow in the forearm (the remainder being to skin and some to bone); so, to study the reactions of muscle vessels, plethysmographs that included just the forearm were used, with a cuff blown up to well above the arterial pressure at the wrist. For the hand, the proportion was thought to be about 50% muscle, 50% skin flow. In the finger,

Fig. 24-2.—Schematic diagram illustrating how reactive hyperemia in muscle (human forearm or calf) pays back the blood-flow debt incurred during a period of ischemia. The corresponding areas above and below the horizontal lines on the graphs are approximately equal.

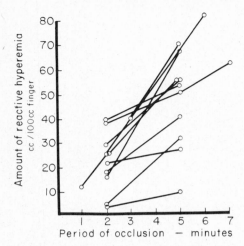

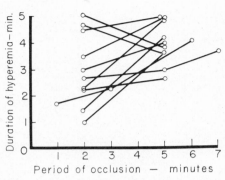

Fig. 24-3.—Reactive hyperemia in the fingers (skin flow). **Left,** showing that the extra blood flow after occlusion increases with the duration of the occlusion but is variable in different subjects. **Right,** showing that the duration of the hyperemia is not well correlated with the duration of the occlusion. Only about 50% of the blood-flow debt, on the average, is repaid. (From Patel and Burton [1].)

the flow is exclusively to skin. By comparison of results on forearm, hand and skin, the very different reactions of the different vessels were deduced. It is now known that the assumption of fixed proportions of the total flow to these different categories of vessel is not justified and that the proportions in the forearm can differ greatly in different conditions of vasomotor tone.

The results for the forearm, after the arterial flow is stopped for several minutes (by a cuff on the upper arm inflated to above arterial pressure) are shown schematically in Figure 24–2. Immediately upon release, the flow increases to a much higher value than before period of complete ischemia and thereafter slowly declines to the original value. The vessels have evidently greatly dilated during the ischemia.

There is a quite remarkable correspondence of the extra volume that flows after the ischemia to the *blood-flow debt* incurred during the occlusion (i.e., the total volume that would have flowed during that period). Increasing the duration of occlusion results in a greater hyperemia, that is, a greater "repayment" of the debt. The increase is mainly in the duration of the increased flow, rather than in the magnitude of the increase. Reactive hyperemia also occurs in the finger, but here the flow debt is seldom repaid in full (only about 50% on the average [1]) and the duration of the hyperemia is not closely correlated with duration of the occlusion (Fig. 24–3).

The explanation of the phenomena lies, most likely, in the accumulation of the products of anaerobic metabolism in the blood vessel wall during the occlusion, these products being vasodilator. Carbon dioxide is the most likely agent, although lactic acid and increased hydrogen ion concentration (lowered pH) could also be important. Alternatively, one might postulate that low oxygen tension was the dilating agent. This, however, seems to be excluded as the agent that maintains the dilatation during the postocclusion hyperemia, for McNeill (2) has shown that the venous oxygen saturation actually rises above the preocclusion level in this period. This is because the oxygen consumption (increased at first in making up the oxygen debt) decreases faster in the hyperemia period than does the blood flow.

[►The theory based on the accumulation of dilator substances has encountered one difficulty. The course of the reactive hyperemia is not influenced as one would expect, if, during the period of occlusion, flow of low P_{O_2} perfusate is maintained, which might be expected to prevent the accumulation of the metabolites by flushing them out. The theory can be retained by supposing that the limiting factor in diffusion of the metabolites is not the rate of blood flow, as long as there is a trace of this, but, rather, some barrier to diffusion between cells and the blood stream.◄]

Reactive Hyperemia as a General Principle

Physiologists are tempted to teach reactive hyperemia, based on vasodilation by accumulation of anaerobic metabolites, as a general principle applying to the circulation of all tissues and organs. However, reactive hyperemia is well established only for the vessels of muscle and, in a much less dramatic way, for skin vessels. [►In the mesenteric circulation and for the liver, there is no clear evidence that flow is increased above normal after a period of partial or complete ischemia. Indeed, in the case of the kidney, there may well be an accumulation of constrictor, rather than dilator, agents during ischemia, making it very difficult to re-establish the normal blood flow after it has been interrupted.◄]

Exercise Hyperemia in Muscle

During a muscular contraction, the blood flow of the forearm may either decrease or increase, according to the strength of the contraction. A weak contraction increases the flow; a strong contraction is ischemic. Immediately upon the muscle's becoming relaxed after a contraction, the flow rises to high values (Fig. 24–4). During rhythmic exercise, the average flow rises to an intermediate value. The reduction during the contraction is undoubtedly due to mechanical squeezing of the blood vessels by the muscle tension (compare the same phenomenon in coronary blood flow). In exercise, the muscle blood flow spurts through the vessels in the brief periods of relaxation but is almost stopped during the contractions. During the contraction of the calf muscles, the volume of the muscles shrinks, owing to the action of the muscle pump upon the veins.

Fig. 24-4.—Exercise hyperemia in the human calf muscle. *Closed-circle line,* mean flow. *Crossed line,* flow during relaxation. *Open-circle line,* flow during a few seconds of sustained contraction. (From Barcroft, H., and Swan, H. J. C.: *Sympathetic Control of Human Blood Vessels* [London: Edward Arnold, 1953].)

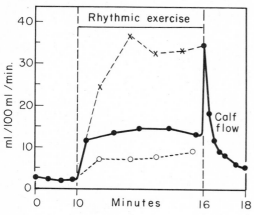

During relaxation periods between contractions, the volume increases, owing to refilling of the veins (3, 4).

The Hunting Reaction of Lewis, an Autonomous Local Control in Vessels of Digits

A most interesting phenomenon in the circulation of the fingers and toes was discovered by Sir Thomas Lewis (5). It has been shown also in the ear of the rabbit and in the legs of other animals. When a digit is immersed in ice-cold water, the blood flow (e.g., as indicated by the excess temperature of the skin over that of the water, or by calorimetry [Greenfield]) initially falls to a low value, but after 5 or 10 min. there is a sudden vasodilation (Fig. 24–5). The skin temperature and the blood flow rise to a comparatively high value, which is not, however, sustained but is followed by another period of vasoconstriction, and so on, rhythmically. This "hunting" between vasoconstriction and vasodilation continues for as long as the local cold is applied. The vasodilation is certainly protective of the tissues against their freezing.

Many attempts have been made, particularly by Greenfield (6), to elucidate the mechanism of this reaction. The dilatation is certainly due to the opening-up of the arteriovenous anastomoses (Chapter 6), which play so great a role in the extreme variability of blood flow of the digits. Grant, by direct observation, verified this for the same phenomenon in the rabbit ear. Sir Thomas Lewis thought that an axon reflex was involved; but, since the phenomena persist after complete degeneration of the sympathetic nerves (although with modifications), this is ruled out. Periodic cold block of the sensory nerves was suggested, but the timing of the periods of pain and relief that are experienced does not support this. [►It is possible that a biophysical explanation applies, depending

Fig. 24-5.—Periodic cold vasodilation in fingers immersed in ice water (the hunting reaction of Lewis), as indicated by the skin temperature of the finger. RT = room temperature. (Redrawn from Lewis [5].)

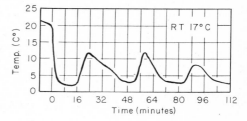

on the change in resistance to flow in the capillary bed according to the blood temperature (viscosity increases very greatly with fall of temperature). With the increased resistance in the cold, the pressure at the junction of the arteriovenous shunt with the terminal artery would rise and might open the sphincter-like glomus of the shunt. The increased flow of warm blood through the shunt would, by conduction, warm the capillary vessels, reducing the viscosity of blood there. However, this would eventually reduce the pressure at the shunt, which would once more close under its prevailing constrictor tone (critical closure). Definitive confirmatory evidence is hard to obtain, but what exists does support this theory. For example, precooling the blood in the arm and hand postpones the occurrence of the next vasodilation, whereas on almost any other theory this might be expected to increase the cold stimulus and so accelerate the hunting.◀]

Whatever the mechanism, this local autonomous control does provide a local protection against frostbite. Skiers must have noticed the periodic painfully cold sensation interrupted by periods of warmth (vasodilation) in fingers, toes, cheeks and ears. The local protection is at the expense of the thermal economy of the whole animal, for the heat loss increases significantly during these periods of cold vasodilation.

Change in Circulation at Birth— Control of the Ductus Arteriosus

Few subjects are of such importance to the medical student as knowledge of the anatomy of the fetal circulation and the most remarkable change in the first few hours or days after birth. Such knowledge gives insight regarding many congenital cardiac defects. The student is referred to the excellent article by Dawes on the changes in circulation at birth (7) or to his more recent textbook (8).

The initiation of the many changes that occur is, of course, the first expansion of the lungs with air. This expansion lowers the pulmonary vascular resistance by a factor of as much as 30 times, according to Dawes, and immediately the flow of blood in the pulmonary circuit, which in the fetus is very slight, becomes an important hemodynamic factor, resulting in a redistribution of the pressures in the left and right heart and in the major arteries. Attempts to explain the closure of the ductus arteriosus (the anastomosis between pulmonary artery and aorta) on hemodynamic

grounds alone have not been very successful, since there seems little evidence that there is a valvelike action of the ductus walls. In contrast, the closure of the foramen ovale (the opening between the two atria) can be explained as the result of a rise in the pressure in the left atrium relative to that in the right atrium, for the septum forms a flaplike valve.

Various theories have been advanced as to the stimulus that is effective in closing the ductus arteriosus, which is endowed with contractile cells in its walls. Attempts to obtain evidence of a neurogenic mechanism have failed. Studies by Dawes and his colleagues on the circulation of the lamb at birth have probably supplied the answer (9). Earlier work had shown that asphyxia and anoxia could result in narrowing the lumen of the ductus arteriosus, but *the true physiological stimulus seems to be a rise of oxygen tension.* Before the change, the saturation in the pulmonary artery side of the ductus arteriosus is about 50%; in the aorta it is about 60%. In the completely changed adult circulation, it rises to 60 or 70% on the pulmonary side and to 98% on the aortic side. A most convincing demonstration of the local effect of a rise in oxygen tension in the ductus arteriosus has been provided by Assali and his co-workers (10). Figure 24–6 is reproduced from their work on perfusion of an isolated ductus arteriosus with different oxygen pressures in the perfusing blood. Measurements in vivo on the unanesthetized fetal lamb when the lungs were ventilated with different mixtures of gases have shown the same effects.

It is to be noted that the constrictor effect on the ductus arteriosus of increasing the oxygen tension of the blood is not merely in the physio-

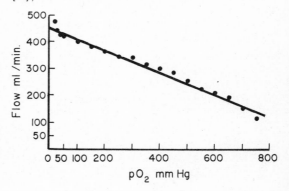

Fig. 24-6.—Relation between blood flow (average of five consecutive experiments) and P_{O_2} in perfusion of the isolated ductus arteriosus of the fetal lamb. (From Assali *et al.* [10].)

logical range but continues to be graded up to the oxygen tension of pure oxygen, and to hyperbaric oxygen.

In human beings the rise of oxygen tension in the blood when the lungs expand at birth is the trigger that leads to closure of the ductus. The most convincing evidence is from surveys of population at sea level and at high altitudes by Penazola *et al.* in Colombia, South America. These surveys have indicated that above 10,000 feet the incidence of "patent ductus arteriosus" is 30 times as great as at sea level. The rise of oxygen tension in the blood at such altitudes, when the lungs expand, is evidently not sufficient to reach the threshold for contraction of the smooth muscle of the ductus in some infants. Figure 24–6, while it shows the gradual response of the ductus up to very high oxygen pressure, gives a false impression as to the remarkable sensitivity, in vivo, of the ductal wall to slight increases in oxygen tension.

Gillman and Burton (11) perfused the isolated ductus, or alternatively the "preductal" region of the aorta of neonatal pigs, guinea pigs, rabbits and cats, and used the resistance to flow as a measure of closure of the ductus, or of narrowing of the nearby aorta. When the oxygen tension in the perfusing solution and water bath was changed from equilibration with 95% nitrogen, 5% carbon dioxide to equilibration with air, the ductus closed so promptly that graduated resistance measurements were impossible, except for a few seconds. However, the less violent degree of narrowing of the preductal aorta gave an index of the "oxygen-contraction sensitivity" of this nearby tissue (Fig. 24–7). Gillman noted large differences in oxygen sensitivity in different species; the pig vessels responded most violently and with a low threshold of Po_2; next came the guinea pig; then the rabbit; the cat; and finally the dog, where no oxygen contraction was ever seen, even to pure oxygen. [►There must be some other mechanism, perhaps by sympathetic nerves, that initiates the closure of the ductus in puppies, unless the conditions of these experiments on isolated vessels somehow inhibited the response in dog vessels, yet not in the vessels of other species.◄]

Even more noteworthy than the species differences in sensitivity were the changes in the few days after birth in each species, shown in Figure 24–6. Three or four days after birth, the oxygen contraction of the preductal aorta has fallen to the level of a negligible response, as in the same vessels for the rest of the animal's life.

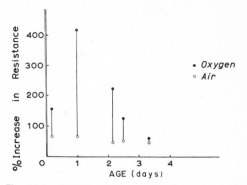

Fig. 24-7.—Relative contraction to O_2 of the aorta of guinea pigs as affected by neonatal age of the animal. The isolated vessels were perfused with solutions equilibrated with 5% carbon dioxide, 95% N_2 (base line), air, or 5% carbon dioxide and 95% oxygen. The points are the mean of five vessels at each age. (Redrawn from Gillman and Burton [11].)

By listening for the distinctive murmur of blood rushing through an open ductus, investigators have found that in the normal human infant in the first few days of life, the degree of closure may fluctuate. The breathing of low-oxygen mixtures can cause the ductus to reopen. After about three weeks, the normal closure becomes anatomical and irreversible. [►The knowledge that the oxygen tension is the stimulus should open the possibility of administering high-oxygen mixtures as a therapeutic measure when the ductus does not close normally (although this may be difficult to diagnose early enough). Certainly, infants born at high altitude might benefit by a brief period of oxygen administration at birth in order to reduce the incidence of patent ductus.◄]

Incidentally, Gillman found that the oxygen-contraction sensitivity of the preductal region of the aorta, although far less than that of the ductus, might explain *"infantile aortic coarctation,"* which is high on the list of congenital cardiac defects. (This condition caused death in one out of 12,000 cases of children under 15 in Toronto). The coarctation (narrowing) almost invariably occurs in the region of the aorta that is close to the ductus. [►It could be due to a "spilling-over," in the course of development, of these specialized oxygen-sensitive-contractile cells of the ductus itself, or a translocation of these cells from ductus to aortic wall.◄] Another example of pathology due to a response to raised Po_2 is "retrolental hyperplasia." The use of pure oxygen in incubators for premature infants caused infantile blindness in unknown, but certainly large, numbers of babies before this was discovered. The mechanism may well be by vasoconstriction of blood vessels of the retina which are especially oxygen sensitive at birth, but not later. An atmosphere of no more than 40% oxygen in incubators has proved safe for premature babies.

Here, then, we have a quite remarkable example of highly specialized "adaption." Cells that possess a unique sensitivity to rise of the oxygen tension of the blood stream, responding by violent contraction, are situated in this special region of the circulation (i.e., the walls of the ductus arteriosus) to fulfill their function (closure of the ductus) at this special time (at birth and a few days thereafter). The C.C.D.M.C. must have done a remarkable job on this particular mechanism, which is, of course, absolutely essential to the survival of mammalian species.

REFERENCES

1. Patel, D. J., and Burton, A. C.: Reactive hyperemia in the human finger, Circulation Res. 4:710, 1956.
2. McNeill, T. A.: Venous oxygen saturation and blood flow during reactive hyperemia in the human forearm, J. Physiol. 134:195, 1956.
3. Barcroft, H., and Dornhorst, A. C.: Blood flow through the human calf during rhythmic exercise, J. Physiol. 109:402, 1949.
4. Barcroft, H.; Greenwood, B., and Whelan, R. F.: Blood flow and venous oxygen saturation during sustained contraction of the forearm muscles, J. Physiol. 168:848, 1963.
5. Lewis, T.: Observations upon the reactions of the vessels of the human skin to cold, Heart 15:177, 1930.
6. Greenfield, A. D. M.: The Circulation through the Skin, in Handbook of Physiology, Sec. 2, Vol. II: Circulation (Washington, D.C.: American Physiological Society, 1963), Chap. 39, pp. 1325–1351.
7. Dawes, G. S.: Changes in circulation at birth, Brit. M. Bull. 172:148, 1961.
8. Dawes, G. S.: Foetal and Neonatal Physiology (Chicago: Year Book Medical Publishers, Inc., 1968).
9. Born, G. V. R.; Dawes, G. S.; Mott, J. C., and Remick, B. R.: The constriction of the ductus arteriosus caused by oxygen and by asphyxia in newborn lambs, J. Physiol. 132:304, 1956.
10. Assali, N. S.; Morris, J. A.; Smith, R. W., and Manson, W. A.: Studies on ductus arteriosus circulation, Circulation Res. 13:478, 1963.
11. Gillman, R. G., and Burton, A. C.: Constriction of the neonatal aorta by raised oxygen tension, Circulation Res. 19:755, 1966.

Finale

If there is still a reader, it is suggested that he reread Chapter 1 and decide what he now thinks of the work of the C.C.D.M.C.

William Harvey, in *Exercitatio Anatomica de Motu Cordis et Sanguinis in Animalibus* (1628), in which he developed his great discovery of the circulation, gave his own assessment of the importance of what he had written in its application to medicine:

"Finally, reflecting on every part of medicine, physiology, pathology, semeiotics (symptomatology), therapeutics, when I see how many questions can be answered, how many doubts resolved, how much obscurity illustrated, by the truth we have declared, the light we have made to shine, I see a field of such vast extent in which I might proceed so far, and expatiate so widely, that this my tractate would not only swell out into a volume, which was beyond my purpose, but my whole life, perchance, would not suffice for its completion."*

I know much more than Harvey,
Could argue with Poiseuille,
But yet with deference;
For I have built on libraried stores
Of reference on reference.

*Cited from Mallock, A.: *William Harvey* (New York: Paul B. Hoeber, Inc., 1929).

Index